Quick Look Nursing:

Pathophysiology

Second Edition

Bernadette Madara, EdD, BC, APRN
Associate Professor
Southern Connecticut State University
New Haven, Connecticut

Vanessa Pomarico-Denino, MSN, APRN
Family Nurse Practitioner, Specializing in Women's Health
Medical Associates of North Haven, LLC
North Haven, Connecticut

JONES AND BARTLETT PUBLISHERS
Sudbury, Massachusetts
BOSTON   TORONTO   LONDON   SINGAPORE

10/07

World Headquarters
Jones and Bartlett Publishers
40 Tall Pine Drive
Sudbury, MA 01776
978-443-5000
info@jbpub.com
www.jbpub.com

Jones and Bartlett Publishers Canada
6339 Ormindale Way
Mississauga, Ontario L5V 1J2
Canada

Jones and Bartlett Publishers International
Barb House, Barb Mews
London W6 7PA
United Kingdom

Jones and Bartlett's books and products are available through most bookstores and online booksellers. To contact Jones and Bartlett Publishers directly, call 800-832-0034, fax 978-443-8000, or visit our website www.jbpub.com.

Substantial discounts on bulk quantities of Jones and Bartlett's publications are available to corporations, professional associations, and other qualified organizations. For details and specific discount information, contact the special sales department at Jones and Bartlett via the above contact information or send an email to specialsales@jbpub.com.

The authors, editor, and publisher have made every effort to provide accurate information. However, they are not responsible for errors, omissions, or for any outcomes related to the use of the contents of this book and take no responsibility for the use of the products and procedures described. Treatments and side effects described in this book may not be applicable to all people; likewise, some people may require a dose or experience a side effect that is not described herein. Drugs and medical devices are discussed that may have limited availability controlled by the Food and Drug Administration (FDA) for use only in a research study or clinical trial. Research, clinical practice, and government regulations often change the accepted standard in this field. When consideration is being given to use of any drug in the clinical setting, the health care provider or reader is responsible for determining FDA status of the drug, reading the package insert, and reviewing prescribing information for the most up-to-date recommendations on dose, precautions, and contraindications, and determining the appropriate usage for the product. This is especially important in the case of drugs that are new or seldom used.

Production Credits

Executive Editor: Kevin Sullivan
Acquisitions Editor: Emily Ekle
Associate Editor: Amy Sibley
Editorial Assistant: Patricia Donnelly
Production Editor: Karen Ferreira
Senior Marketing Manager: Katrina Gosek

Associate Marketing Manager: Rebecca Wasley
Cover Design: Tim Dziewit
Composition: Shepherd, Inc.
Manufacturing and Inventory Coordinator: Amy Bacus
Printing and Binding: Malloy, Inc.
Cover Printing: Malloy, Inc.

Library of Congress Cataloging-in-Publication Data
Madara, Bernadette.
    Pathophysiology / Bernadette Madara, Vanessa Pomarico-Denino.—2nd ed.
        p. ; cm.—(Quick look nursing)
    Rev. ed. of: Pathophysiology / Eileen M. Crutchlow . . . [et al.]. c2002.
    Includes bibliographical references and index.
    ISBN-13: 978-0-7637-4932-3
1. Physiology, Pathological—Textbooks. 2. Nursing. I. Pomarico-Denino, Vanessa.
II. Title. III. Series.
    [DNLM: 1. Pathology—Nurses' Instruction. 2. Diagnostic Techniques and Procedures—
    Nurses' Instruction. QZ 4 M178p 2008]
    RB113.M25 2008
    616.07—dc22
                                                            2007015729
6048

Printed in the United States of America
11 10 09 08 07   10 9 8 7 6 5 4 3 2 1

Dedication

We dedicate this book to our students,
who have challenged and inspired us.

CONTENTS

PREFACE

This book is intended for undergraduate nursing students and registered nurses re-entering the practice area or beginning a new area of practice. It is useful as a reference book because of its format and design. Each section includes an overview of the body system's anatomy and physiology along with common laboratory and diagnostic tests pertinent to that system. Chapters address commonly occurring adult health deviations and are organized to include an overview, pathophysiology, and goals of treatment. References for each section are included at the end of the book. We trust that you will find this book useful.

ABOUT THE AUTHORS

Bernadette Madara, EdD, BC, APRN
Dr. Bernadette Madara is a professor of nursing at Southern Connecticut State University in New Haven, Connecticut. She is an APRN with Board Certification in medical-surgical nursing. Dr. Madara has taught on both the undergraduate and graduate levels.

Vanessa Pomarico-Denino, MSN, APRN
Vanessa Pomarico-Denino is a Family Nurse Practitioner specializing in Women's Health at Medical Associates of North Haven, LLC. She received an Associate's Degree in Nursing at the University of Bridgeport and went on to earn her Bachelor's Degree as well as her Master's Degree in Nursing at Southern Connecticut State University (SCSU). Vanessa taught both undergraduate and graduate nursing at SCSU and provided women's health services at their student health center for several years. She remains an active guest lecturer in their Family Nurse Practitioner program. She is a Clinical Instructor and preceptor for SCSU family nurse practitioner students as well as the Yale School of Nursing.

ACKNOWLEDGMENTS

Sincere thanks to Vanessa, the coauthor of this book who made this journey a pleasure. Her dedication to teaching and life-long learning is valued! A special thank you to my mother and husband who supported me during this project.

And finally thank you to the staff at Jones and Bartlett especially Karen Ferreira, production editor, who believed in this project and helped it to become a reality.

Bernadette

Learning patho is not always easy, and my involvement with this book has brought back many memories of when I was a nursing student. I would like to thank Beth Delucia, LPN, who saw the nurse in me when I did not. I also want to thank Donna Sandillo, RN, and Carole Ruggiero, RN—two of my "study buddies"—and in memory of Nancy Quinn Fredericks, RN. Our study sessions were a source of laughter, education, and therapy that strengthened the bond of our friendships.

And to my husband, David, whose unwavering love, patience, and support has helped me get to where I am today.

vpd

Part I

Fluid and Electrolyte Balance

Vanessa Pomarico-Denino, MSN, APRN

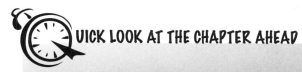

QUICK LOOK AT THE CHAPTER AHEAD

Fluids are distributed in various compartments in the body, with movement back and forth to maintain homeostasis. This movement is a result of variations in hydrostatic pressure and osmotic forces, especially in interstitial and intravascular compartments. The fluid environment serves as the medium for exchange and distribution of electrolytes and nutrients and elimination of waste products from cellular metabolism.

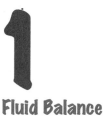

Fluid Balance

TERMS
- [ ] active transport
- [ ] edema
- [ ] hydrostatic pressure
- [ ] insensible losses
- [ ] osmolality
- [ ] osmosis
- [ ] osmotic (oncotic) pressure
- [ ] third spacing

Figure 1-1   Movement of water across cell membranes.

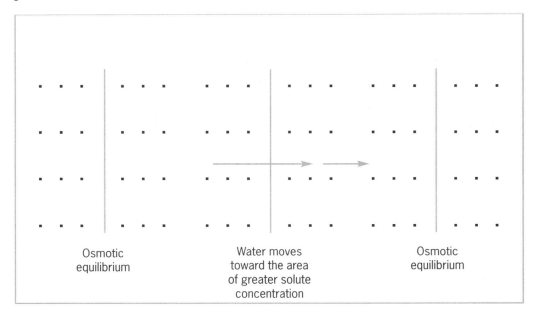

Osmotic equilibrium

Water moves toward the area of greater solute concentration

Osmotic equilibrium

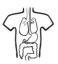

DISTRIBUTION

Water makes up the largest component in the body and comprises approximately 60% of body weight. The three main fluid compartments are *intracellular, extracellular,* and *intravascular.* The intracellular compartment comprises fluids within cells, whereas the extracellular compartment comprises all the fluid outside the cells. This compartment is further divided into two smaller compartments: the interstitial (between cells) and the intravascular (blood plasma). Other extracellular compartments include those areas of the body containing smaller amounts of fluid such as lymphatic, synovial, cerebrospinal, pericardial, and others. These smaller compartments are important in particular diseases or conditions but are less so in terms of overall fluid and electrolyte balance and maintenance of homeostasis.

The percentage of total body water varies with age and amount of body fat. The greater the percentage of body fat, the lesser the amount of water present. Infants have a proportionally larger percent of total body water, which makes them particularly vulnerable to shifts in fluid levels and dehydration. Their rapid metabolic rate, greater body surface area, and immature renal function also contribute to their susceptibility to fluid imbalances. This percentage decreases after 12 months of age and continues to decrease until adolescence. The elderly have proportionally smaller percentages of body water due to higher amounts of body fat, less lean tissue, and reduced ability of organ systems to compensate to maintain homeostasis. These variations are particularly important during periods of illness or stress, making the elderly especially vulnerable to dehydration, electrolyte imbalance, and system dysfunction.

> ☑ The percentage of total body water varies with age and amount of body fat. The greater the percentage of body fat, the lesser the amount of water present.

> ❗ Infants have a proportionally larger percent of total body water, which makes them particularly vulnerable to shifts in fluid levels and dehydration. Their rapid metabolic rate, greater body surface area, and immature renal function also contribute to their susceptibility to fluid imbalances.

Daily fluid intake varies from person to person within a range of 2,400 to 3,200 mL, with roughly two-thirds obtained by oral intake of fluids and one-third obtained through food and water of oxidation (300 to 400 mL). Daily output balances intake in approximately the same proportions—two-thirds through urine and one-third through **insensible losses.** It is important to take insensible losses into account during periods of illness, such as diarrhea, ventilator-assisted breathing, diaphoresis, and fever, because these losses may be significantly increased.

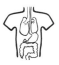

FLUID MOVEMENT

Movement of water between the intracellular and extracellular fluid compartments is primarily affected by osmotic forces. Because water moves freely across cell membranes (i.e., toward the side with the greatest solute or particle concentration), an equilibrium

> ☑ Movement of water between the intracellular and extracellular fluid compartments is primarily affected by osmotic forces.

ordinarily exists between compartments. Sodium (Na$^+$) is the most abundant extracellular ion and is responsible for maintaining osmotic balance in that compartment. Potassium (K$^+$) performs the same role in the intracellular compartment. The osmotic force of intracellular proteins and **active transport** of ions out of the cell are additional forces contributing to this process.

Plasma proteins play an important role in maintaining **osmolality** through plasma oncotic pressure in the intravascular compartment. These osmotic forces are balanced by **hydrostatic pressure** in the vascular compartment. Forces that favor movement of water out of the capillary and into the interstitial compartment are vascular hydrostatic pressure and interstitial fluid **osmotic (oncotic) pressure.** Forces that favor movement of water into the capillary from the interstitial compartment are interstitial hydrostatic pressure and vascular (plasma) osmotic pressure. The major forces for this filtration process are within the capillary membrane because plasma proteins do not readily cross it. Under normal circumstances, hydrostatic pressure exceeds capillary oncotic pressure at the arterial end of the capillary, causing water to move into the interstitial space. Consequently, hydrostatic pressure is lower than capillary oncotic pressure at the venous end of the capillary. This causes fluid to be reabsorbed back into the vascular system. Changes in capillary membrane permeability may alter this process by allowing plasma proteins to enter the interstitial space. Water follows, and edema results.

Fluid volume imbalances (i.e., deficits or excesses) that occur may involve either changes in volume only or changes in volume and concentration. The causes of these differ, as will laboratory values, and affect the treatment prescribed. The nurse's role in assessing and educating the patient and monitoring the effectiveness of management is crucial. See p. 9, Figure 1-2, for manifestations of fluid volume deficit (dehydration) and fluid volume overload (circulatory overload).

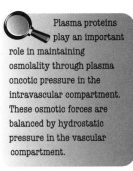

Plasma proteins play an important role in maintaining osmolality through plasma oncotic pressure in the intravascular compartment. These osmotic forces are balanced by hydrostatic pressure in the vascular compartment.

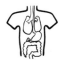

EDEMA

Edema is a problem of fluid distribution, not necessarily one of fluid overload. It results when forces favoring movement of fluid from the vascular (or lymphatic) compartment exceed those retaining fluid within that compartment. The most common mechanisms causing edema are increased hydrostatic pressure, decreased plasma oncotic pressure, increased capillary membrane permeability, and lymphatic obstruction. Any condition that increases blood volume or that causes venous or lymphatic obstruction can cause edema, including tumors, advanced pregnancy, tight clothing, and Na^+ and H_2O retention. Conditions such as tissue injury, infection, and allergies cause inflammation and increase capillary permeability, causing edema. Any condition that either prevents the formation of plasma proteins, particularly albumin as found in cirrhosis, or leads to their loss, such as chronic renal failure, causes edema. In all these situations, the balance between hydrostatic and oncotic pressures in capillaries and interstitial fluid has been altered. It is not uncommon for more than one condition to coexist. It is important to understand the basic path ... ses involved so that nursing assessment is ... measures can be instituted to alleviate

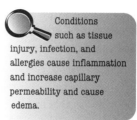

Conditions such as tissue injury, infection, and allergies cause inflammation and increase capillary permeability and cause edema.

... s favoring movement of fluid from the
... mpartment exceed those retaining fluid

... ses to current in a particular ody because tissue perfu- ased trans- s. One way ... understand the ... structures and characteristics of involved tissues/organs and then to recall the physiological processes/functions of the organ system or area of the body. Visualizing the consequences of the presence of fluid (and resultant pressure) on that organ system, tissue, or area of the body is helpful in proper assessment of a

It is not uncommon for more than one condition to coexist. It is important to understand the basic pathophysiological processes involved so that nursing assessment is thorough and various measures can be instituted to alleviate the edema.

patient. For example, fluid accumulation in the brain is life threatening because the bony skull is hard and cannot expand, except in infants. Therefore, any intracranial pressure buildup from even small amounts of fluid causes compression of the softer tissue, the brain. On the other hand, fluid accumulation in the abdomen, such as ascites, may not create observable abdominal distention until 2 or more liters are present. This is because there is room in the abdominal cavity for greater amounts of fluid to collect before tissue/organ compression causes physiological disturbances.

 It is also important for nurses to understand the consequences of edema in a particular organ system or part of the body because pressure from edema can impair tissue perfusion, leading to hypoxia and decreased transport of nutrients and waste products.

 Fluid accumulation in the abdomen, such as ascites, may not create observable abdominal distention until 2 or more liters are present.

A term often used in clinical situations is **third spacing,** which means that fluid is leaving one compartment and moving elsewhere. Ordinarily, it has not left the body but has become sequestered and is unavailable for use in maintaining fluid balance. When this occurs, signs of dehydration may be present. Third spacing is used in describing large fluid shifts. Common examples are postoperative patients and persons with significant burns. When large amounts of fluid move from the vascular space into the interstitial space, it is then followed by a reverse fluid shift; therefore, care must be taken to avoid circulatory overload while attempting to compensate for the initial reduced circulating volume.

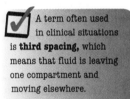

A term often used in clinical situations is **third spacing,** which means that fluid is leaving one compartment and moving elsewhere.

Edema is often referred to as either *pitting* or *brawny*. Pitting edema can be compressed by finger pressure, resulting in a "dent" or pit in the subcutaneous tissue. Brawny edema is firm and noncompressible. It accompanies tissue injury, and the fluid includes clotting factors, hence its character.

Management

The goal of management is to reduce or eliminate the edema, thereby preventing (further) tissue injury. Determining the cause or causes is

Figure 1-2   Percent of body weight due to water.

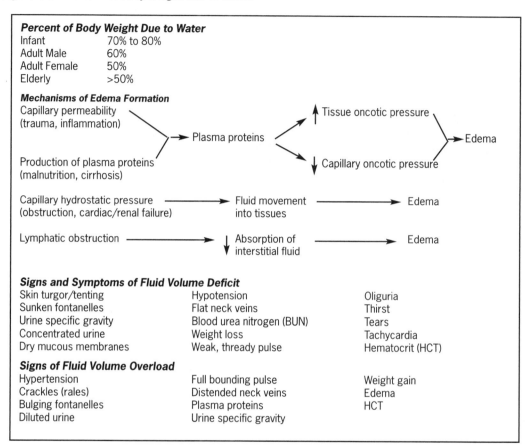

Percent of Body Weight Due to Water
Infant   70% to 80%
Adult Male   60%
Adult Female   50%
Elderly   >50%

Mechanisms of Edema Formation
Capillary permeability
(trauma, inflammation)
                     ↘
                       → Plasma proteins ↗ ↑ Tissue oncotic pressure ↘
                                                                        → Edema
Production of plasma proteins ↗   ↘ ↓ Capillary oncotic pressure ↗
(malnutrition, cirrhosis)

Capillary hydrostatic pressure ———→ Fluid movement ———————→ Edema
(obstruction, cardiac/renal failure)   into tissues

Lymphatic obstruction ———————————→ ↓ Absorption of ———————→ Edema
                                      interstitial fluid

Signs and Symptoms of Fluid Volume Deficit
Skin turgor/tenting   Hypotension   Oliguria
Sunken fontanelles   Flat neck veins   Thirst
Urine specific gravity   Blood urea nitrogen (BUN)   Tears
Concentrated urine   Weight loss   Tachycardia
Dry mucous membranes   Weak, thready pulse   Hematocrit (HCT)

Signs of Fluid Volume Overload
Hypertension   Full bounding pulse   Weight gain
Crackles (rales)   Distended neck veins   Edema
Bulging fontanelles   Plasma proteins   HCT
Diluted urine   Urine specific gravity

essential. Treatment may be supportive though proper positioning or use of compression stockings. Treatment also includes therapeutic use of diuretics and restricted sodium intake.

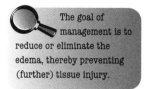

The goal of management is to reduce or eliminate the edema, thereby preventing (further) tissue injury.

Electrolytes play a key role in maintaining homeostasis. Any alteration or imbalance of fluids or electrolytes can lead to severe health consequences and altered disease states. Approximately 60% of the total body weight is comprised of fluids found in the body. Any change, however slight, in the concentrations of electrolytes can adversely affect muscle and nerve cells as well as cellular functions.

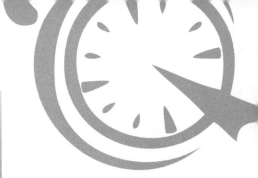

2

Electrolyte Balance: Part 1

TERMS
- [ ] **Chvostek's sign**
- [ ] **diffusion**
- [ ] **filtration**
- [ ] **hyponatremia**
- [ ] **hypertonic**
- [ ] **hypotonic**
- [ ] **isotonic**
- [ ] **natriuretic hormone**
- [ ] **osmosis**
- [ ] **Trousseau's sign**

Figure 2-1 Normal serum values of major electrolytes.

Normal Serum Values of Major Electrolytes*

Na+	135 to 145 mEq/L	Mg	1.8 to 2.4 mEq/L
Cl−	104 to 110 mEq/L	PO4	2.5 to 4.5 mg/dL
K+	3.5 to 5 mEq/L	Albumin	3.5 to 5.5 mg/dL
Ca++	4.5 to 5.5 mEq/L	Urine specific gravity	1.010 to 1.030

*There are slight variations in published normal values; use those of the lab with which you are affiliated.

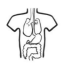

SODIUM, CHLORIDE, AND WATER BALANCE

The balance of sodium (Na+) and water is closely related because of the osmotic relationship between the two. Water balance is regulated by the antidiuretic hormone (ADH) from the posterior pituitary, and Na+ is regulated by aldosterone produced by the adrenal cortex.

Thirst is experienced when water loss equals 2% or more of body weight or when there is an increase in osmolality. Osmolality can be increased by either a reduction in water or an increase in Na+. Osmoreceptors are located in the hypothalamus and are stimulated by increases in osmolality and decreases in blood volume. Oral fluids increase blood volume and decrease osmolality. Osmoreceptor stimulation also causes an increased release of ADH, which then increases renal tubular permeability to water and increases its reabsorption. This causes an increased concentration of urine. If fluid (blood) volume is decreased, centrally located volume and pressure-sensitive receptors (baroreceptors) are stimulated, which also stimulates the release of ADH.

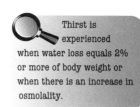
Water balance is regulated by the antidiuretic hormone (ADH) from the posterior pituitary, and Na+ is regulated by aldosterone produced from the adrenal cortex.

Thirst is experienced when water loss equals 2% or more of body weight or when there is an increase in osmolality.

Oral fluids increase blood volume and decrease osmolality.

Na$^+$ is the most powerful cation in extracellular fluid (ECF), and chloride is the most powerful ECF anion. In addition to its primary role in maintenance of osmolality, Na$^+$ also helps to maintain neuromuscular irritability, acid–base balance, various cellular chemical reactions, and membrane transport. Chloride (Cl$^-$) neutralizes the positive charge of Na$^+$ and is passively transported along with the active transport of Na$^+$. Bicarbonate is the other major ECF anion, and its concentration varies inversely with that of Cl$^-$.

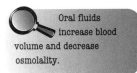

Oral fluids increase blood volume and decrease osmolality.

Na$^+$ concentrations are regulated by the kidneys via aldosterone, a mineralocorticoid synthesized and secreted by the adrenal cortex, and atrial natriuretic factor, a **natriuretic hormone** from the atrial muscle of the heart. These affect tubular reabsorption of Na$^+$. (Note: The former increases it and the latter decreases it.) When Na$^+$ is conserved, potassium is lost. Atrial natriuretic factor is released when there is an increase in atrial pressure. A similar hormone in the left ventricle of the brain, called *brain natriuretic peptide,* is released in response to increases in blood volume and causes natriuresis, vasodilation, and inhibition of aldosterone.

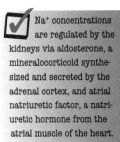

Na$^+$ concentrations are regulated by the kidneys via aldosterone, a mineralocorticoid synthesized and secreted by the adrenal cortex, and atrial natriuretic factor, a natriuretic hormone from the atrial muscle of the heart.

Aldosterone secretion is also influenced by blood volume (increased with decreased renal perfusion). In addition, the renin–angiotensin system is stimulated by reductions in blood volume and renal perfusion. Activation of this system causes an increase in aldosterone release (increased Na$^+$ and H$_2$O reabsorption) and vasoconstriction, both of which serve to increase circulating blood volume and improve renal perfusion.

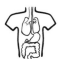

ALTERATIONS IN SODIUM, CHLORIDE, AND WATER BALANCE

Alterations in Na$^+$ and water balance are closely linked because Na$^+$ imbalances can develop as a result of water imbalances and vice versa. Usually, these changes are discussed in terms of tonicity. (Some authors use the terms *tonicity* and *osmolality* interchangeably.)

Isotonic alterations occur when changes in both solutes and water are proportionally the same as body fluids such as blood loss, severe wound drainage, or excessive administration of intravenous normal saline. Isotonic losses produce the classic signs of dehydration or fluid volume deficit. Isotonic excesses are usually iatrogenic (excessive intravenous fluid administration, glucocorticoid administration), and signs of fluid volume excess or circulatory overload become evident.

> Isotonic alterations occur when changes in both solutes and water are proportionally the same as body fluids such as blood loss, severe wound drainage, or excessive administration of intravenous normal saline.

Hypertonic alterations develop when there is excess solute concentration (increased osmolality). Hypernatremia is usually caused by an excess of Na^+ or a deficit of H_2O. When this occurs, water is drawn out of the cells, causing cellular dehydration. This hypertonicity can lead to symptoms of hypervolemia if the causative agent is increased Na^+ or ingestion of $NaHCO_3$, or hypovolemia if the causative agent is decreased H_2O from a fever or diabetes insipidus. Hyperchloremia (too much sodium and too little bicarbonate) accompanies hypernatremia or a deficit in bicarbonate (metabolic acidosis). These conditions have no specific symptoms.

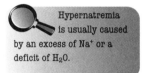
Hypernatremia is usually caused by an excess of Na^+ or a deficit of H_2O.

Hypotonic alterations occur with a deficiency of Na^+ (**hyponatremia**) or an excess of water. The loss of osmotic pressure in the ECF causes movement of water into the cell, or intracellular edema. This hypotonicity can lead to signs of hypovolemia if the causative agent is a decrease in Na^+, or signs of hypervolemia if the causative agent is excess water. Hyponatremia is usually caused by extrarenal losses through vomiting and nasogastric drainage or by iatrogenic causes such as diuretics or excessive enemas. Hyponatremia interferes with cellular depolarization and repolarization, resulting in nonspecific clinical manifestations of headache, malaise, lethargy, confusion, and apprehension. Hypochloremia, loss of Cl^-, occurs as a result of hyponatremia or elevated bicarbonate levels. This is seen in metabolic alkalosis, vomiting, and loss of hydrochloric acid. Use of diuretics or restricted sodium intake can be accompanied by hypochloremia. Hyponatremia is not uncommon in high-risk groups (elderly and infants/children) and should be suspected if there is an unexplained change in mental status or lethargy.

> Use of diuretics or restricted sodium intake can be accompanied by hypochloremia.

MANAGEMENT

The goal of management is to normalize fluid and electrolyte levels, prevent complications of imbalances, and treat the underlying cause.

Table 2-1 Sodium Imbalances

Normal	Cause	Clinical Manifestations
Sodium 135–145 mEq/L	*Hyponatremia:*	*Hyponatremia:*
	Diuretic therapy	Serum level < 135 mEq/L
	Sodium-restricted diet	Muscle cramps
	Renal failure	Weakness
	Excessive GI losses (vomiting, NG tube, diarrhea)	Lethargy or coma
		Hypernatremia:
	Exercise or diaphoresis	Serum level > 145 mEq/L
	Hypernatremia:	Polydipsia
	Burns	Oliguria or anuria
	Watery diarrhea	High specific gravity
	NPO or poor PO intake	
	Diabetes	
	Hypertonic tube feedings	

GI, gastrointestinal; NG, nasogastric; NPO, nothing by mouth; PO, oral.

Electrolytes are essential for normal cellular functioning and help to maintain normal fluid balance in tissues and cells. Certain electrolytes are needed for conduction of nerve impulses and muscle contraction. Any increase or decrease in the concentration of electrolytes can lead to acidosis or alkalosis. Imbalances can occur as a result of poor diet or fluid intake, vomiting, diarrhea, or certain drugs.

3

Electrolyte Balance: Part II

TERMS
- ☐ hypercalcemia
- ☐ hyperkalemia
- ☐ hypermagnesemia
- ☐ hypocalcemia
- ☐ hypokalemia
- ☐ hypomagnesemia

Figure 3-1   Isotonic intravenous solutions.

Isotonic IV Solutions

D_5NS
Normal saline (NS) (0.9%)
Ringer's lactate
Lipids

Hypotonic IV Solutions

D_5W
0.45% saline (half strength)

Hypertonic IV Solutions

3% saline
Total parenteral nutrition

Common Chemical Symbols

Na^+	Sodium	Fe	Iron
K^+	Potassium	Mg	Magnesium
P	Phosphorus	SO_4	Sulfate
PO_4	Phosphate	NH_3	Ammonia
Cl^-	Chloride	NH_4	Ammonium
HCl	Hydrochloric acid	OH	Hydroxide
H^+	Hydrogen	Ca^{++}	Calcium
O_2	Oxygen	CO_2	Carbon dioxide
HCO_3	Bicarbonate	H_2CO_3	Carbonic acid

Dietary Intake of Electrolytes

	Average Daily	Minimal Requirement
Na^+	5 to 6 g	500 mg
K^+	40 to 150 mEq	40 mEq

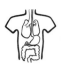

ALTERATIONS IN POTASSIUM, CALCIUM, AND PHOSPHATE

Potassium

Potassium (K^+) is the major intracellular electrolyte (cation). The balance between intracellular and extracellular K^+ levels is maintained by an active transport system. The primary role of K^+ is maintaining the resting potential of cell membranes, which allows for transmission and conduction of nerve impulses, maintenance of cardiac rhythm, and skeletal and smooth muscle contraction. It also plays a role in glycogenesis. Most K^+ is located in the small intestine, with a moderate amount found in gastric secretions and lesser amounts in other body fluids. Diet provides the source of potassium.

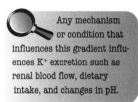

The primary role of K^+ is maintaining the resting potential of cell membranes, which allows for transmission and conduction of nerve impulses, maintenance of cardiac rhythm, and skeletal and smooth muscle contraction.

The kidneys regulate the balance of potassium in the body, and K^+ is excreted via passive transport. This occurs as Na^+ is reabsorbed and is related to the concentration gradient between the plasma and the distal tubular cells. Therefore any mechanism or condition that influences this gradient influences K^+ excretion such as renal blood flow, dietary intake, and changes in pH. Mechanisms for tubular conservation of K^+ are weak.

Any mechanism or condition that influences this gradient influences K^+ excretion such as renal blood flow, dietary intake, and changes in pH.

During states of acid–base imbalance, K^+ and hydrogen (H^+) shift back and forth, in an inverse relationship, across the cell membrane to maintain a healthy balance of these cations. In other words, when there is excess H^+ in the extracellular fluid during states of acidosis, H^+ crosses into the cell, causing K^+ to leave, which results in hyperkalemia. Conversely, when there is a deficit of H^+ in the extracellular fluid during states of alkalosis, H^+ leaves the cell, causing K^+ to enter the cell, which results in hypokalemia. Renal excretion is affected in these conditions to either conserve or eliminate K^+ as necessary.

Aldosterone also plays a role in K^+ balance because it is released when K^+ levels are high. This causes renal conservation of Na^+ and excretion of K^+. Insulin facilitates the passage of K^+ into liver and muscle cells. This fact should be recalled when patients are receiving insulin for management of diabetes, particularly if they have other disorders that might be influenced by this mechanism.

 Insulin facilitates the passage of K^+ into liver and muscle cells.

Hypokalemia

Serum **hypokalemia,** a potassium deficiency that develops when serum potassium falls below 3.5 mEq/L, can result from either loss of K^+ from the body or shifts of K^+ into the cell from alkalosis or insulin administration. This can occur due to inadequate oral intake of at least 10–30 mEq/day, transcellular shifts that redistribute K^+ from extracellular to intracellular compartments, or through diuresis. The loss of K^+ through the gastrointestinal tract is usually minimal but can become excessive in the presence of vomiting and diarrhea. Diarrhea can cause the loss of 100 to 200 mEq K^+/day. Vomiting or nasogastric tube drainage can result in hypokalemia primarily due to the kidneys' response to blood volume depletion and metabolic alkalosis.

> Vomiting or nasogastric tube drainage can result in hypokalemia primarily due to the kidneys' response to blood volume depletion and metabolic alkalosis.

It is difficult to measure the amount of total body K^+ because only serum K^+ is available for such determinations. Total body losses may be present yet not reflected in the serum level due to the body's maintenance of the balance between extracellular fluid and intracellular fluid levels and its passive excretion by the kidneys. Therefore, extreme care must be taken by all health care providers to monitor patient status in regard to this electrolyte. Dietary deficiencies are rare under normal circumstances but may become important if intake is severely restricted or occurs in the presence of certain comorbidities or medication use (most diuretics). Because K^+ is not stored in the body, daily intake is essential. This becomes important if patients are to take nothing by mouth for longer than a few days. Other causes of hypokalemia include renal disease and certain antibiotics.

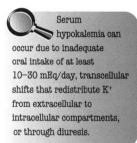

Serum hypokalemia can occur due to inadequate oral intake of at least 10–30 mEq/day, transcellular shifts that redistribute K^+ from extracellular to intracellular compartments, or through diuresis.

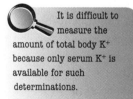

It is difficult to measure the amount of total body K^+ because only serum K^+ is available for such determinations.

Hypokalemia affects carbohydrate metabolism and renal function as well as neuromuscular and cardiac function. The latter two are most obvious with a decrease in neuromuscular excitability (due to hyperpolarization of the cell membrane), which manifests as skeletal and smooth muscle atony such as ileus, abdominal distention, nausea and vomiting, and weakness as well as cardiac dysrhythmias due to delayed ventricular repolarization (bradyrhythmias, reflecting delayed repolarization). Other causes of hypokalemia include diuretic therapy (not K⁺-sparing), nasogastric tube suction, vomiting and diarrhea, and primary hyperaldosteronism. Alcoholism also contributes to this state. Hypokalemia increases the risk of digitalis toxicity. Acute losses create more symptoms than gradual losses.

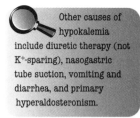

Other causes of hypokalemia include diuretic therapy (not K⁺-sparing), nasogastric tube suction, vomiting and diarrhea, and primary hyperaldosteronism.

Management   The goal of management is to prevent and/or replace losses and treat underlying conditions. Dietary supplementation may be indicated. Because intravenous (IV) K⁺ is so irritating to the veins, concentrations greater than 40 mEq should not be used. The usual dilution is 20 to 40 mEq/L. It is imperative to avoid rapid IV administration. The maximum K⁺ replacement is 40 to 80 mEq with 20 mEq daily commonly prescribed for maintenance.

Hyperkalemia

Hyperkalemia is relatively uncommon and occurs when the serum concentration of K⁺ exceeds 5.5 mEq/L. It is most likely to be caused by accidental ingestion, excessively rapid administration, extensive cellular destruction, or changes in cell membrane permeability, acidosis, or renal failure. Early manifestations would be those related to increased neuromuscular irritability (due to hypopolarization of the cell membrane) such as restlessness, intestinal cramping, diarrhea, and electrocardiogram changes. Other early symptoms include muscle weakness in the lower extremities and paresthesias. Severe hyperkalemia can cause some of the same manifestations as deficiency states, such as bradycardia and progressive conduction disturbances, with more rapid repolarization leading to ventricular fibrillation. Because of the overlap between the roles of calcium and K⁺ on membrane potentials, manifestations of hyperkalemia may also be influenced by calcium levels.

Early manifestations would be those related to increased neuromuscular irritability (due to hypopolarization of the cell membrane) such as restlessness, intestinal cramping, diarrhea, and electrocardiogram changes.

Management   The goal of management is to normalize K⁺ levels by treating the causative disease or condition, preventing its accumulation, or enhancing its excretion through the use of exchange resins such as IV

Table 3-1   Potassium Imbalances

	Cause	Clinical Manifestations
Normal, 3.5–5.5 mEq/L	*Hypokalemia:* Diuretic therapy Poor diet Primary hyperaldosteronism Excessive GI losses (vomiting, NG tube, diarrhea) Healing stage of severe burns Alcoholism *Hyperkalemia:* Rapid infusion of IV K^+ Excessive oral intake Tissue trauma or burns Renal failure K^+-sparing diuretics ACE inhibitors	*Hypokalemia:* <3.5 mEq/L *Hyperkalemia:* <5.5 mEq/L Paresthesias or lower extremity weakness Progressive conduction changes in ECG Bradycardia

ACE, angiotensin-converting enzyme; ECG, electrocardiogram; GI, gastrointestinal; NG, nasogastric.

sodium bicarbonate, 10% IV calcium gluconate, 500 mL of 10% glucose, or dialysis.

Calcium

The amount of calcium (Ca^{++}) circulating in the blood is small (1%); approximately 99% of calcium is found in teeth and bones. Of the 1%, approximately two-fifths is in ionized form and available for physiological functions. It plays an important role in blood clotting, hormone secretion, receptor function, nerve transmission, and muscular contraction. Phosphorus (P) is also found in the bones, with small amounts in circulation in the form of phospholipids and others. It also helps in cellular metabolism and acts as a buffer in acid–base balance. These two ions have an inverse relationship to each other.

Ca^{++} is introduced to the body through the gastrointestinal tract and is absorbed from the small intestine. Vitamin D helps with absorption of calcium that is stored in bone. It is also regulated by parathyroid hormone (PTH) and calcitonin (a thyroid hormone). Excess calcium is excreted in urine and stool.

The balance between Ca^{++} and P is mediated by PTH, vitamin D, and calcitonin, which regulate their absorption (from gastrointestinal tract, bone, and renal), deposition, and excretion. PTH is released in

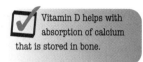
Vitamin D helps with absorption of calcium that is stored in bone.

response to low serum Ca^{++} levels and causes renal reabsorption of Ca^{++} and excretion of P. It also stimulates renal activation of vitamin D, which increases gastrointestinal absorption, renal reabsorption, and bone absorption of Ca^{++}. These hormones also regulate the exchange of Ca^{++} with P between the bones and the serum. Low levels of Ca^{++} and P cause bone resorption osteoclasts, thereby releasing more Ca^{++} and P into the circulation. Calcitonin is secreted to prevent Ca^{++} levels from becoming too high by stimulating osteoblasts, which causes formation of new bone and decreases serum Ca^{++} levels. The amount of ionized versus bound serum Ca^{++} is influenced by pH. Acidosis causes increases in serum Ca^{++}, whereas alkalosis causes decreased levels.

Hypocalcemia

Hypocalcemia occurs when ionized Ca^{++} drops below 4 mg/dL. This can occur from decreased gastrointestinal absorption, decreased dietary intake, multiple blood transfusions (citrate, used to prevent clotting in the bag, binds with Ca^{++}), pancreatitis (an increase in free fatty acids binds Ca^{++}), vitamin D deficiency, removal of the parathyroid glands, alkalosis, and hypoalbuminemia (decreases bound Ca^{++} levels). Other causes include inability to mobilize stored calcium and renal failure.

Manifestations, either acute or chronic, are primarily related to neuromuscular excitability due to a decrease in membrane threshold potential. They present as confusion, paresthesias, muscle spasms, or hyperreflexia. Two clinical signs often assessed are Chvostek's and Trousseau's signs (see p. 24, Table 3-2). Severe signs are convulsions, tetany, electrocardiographic changes (prolonged QT), increased bowel sounds, and cramps.

Hypercalcemia

Hypercalcemia exists when levels rise above 12 mg/dL and is most commonly caused by hyperparathyroidism; bone metastasis with breast, prostate, and cervical cancer (many tumors produce PTH); sarcoidosis (increases vitamin D levels); and excess vitamin D. Symptoms are related to loss of cell membrane excitability and often are nonspecific, including weakness, fatigue, anorexia, nausea, constipation, renal stones, and electrocardiographic changes (short-ened QT, bradyrhythmia). The two most common causes are neoplasm of the bone and hyperparathyroidism.

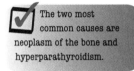

The two most common causes are neoplasm of the bone and hyperparathyroidism.

Management

The goal of management in both hypo- and hypercalcemia is to identify and treat the underlying pathology. With hypocalcemia, oral Ca^{++} supplements or IV Ca^{++} gluconate may be used. Phosphate intake may be reduced if indicated. Oral PO_4 preparations or other medications may be used with hypercalcemia.

Phosphorus

Phosphate (PO_4) is an intracellular anion that is essential to muscle and red blood cell function. It is an important component of adenosine triphosphate, which is the major source of energy for many cellular processes. Ca^{++} functions with PO_4 to support formation of bone. PO_4 is found in dietary sources and is eliminated through urine. Absorption of PO_4 is decreased with food sources containing calcium, magnesium, and aluminum, which bind phosphate.

Hypophosphatemia

Hypophosphatemia occurs when levels drop below 2.5 mg/dL and is usually caused by PO_4 deficiency due to renal excretion (hyperparathyroidism) or intestinal malabsorption. PO_4 is easily found in many food sources, so hypophosphatemia is rare. Vitamin D deficiency, Mg^{++} or aluminum antacids, or alcohol abuse are also attributable causes of this condition. Severe depletion causes abnormal function of bone, cardiac, and respiratory systems. Manifestations of hypophosphatemia include paresthesia, malaise, diminished reflexes, muscle weakness, and confusion.

 Manifestations of hypophosphatemia include paresthesia, malaise, diminished reflexes, muscle weakness, and confusion.

Hyperphosphatemia

Hyperphosphatemia occurs with blood levels greater than 4.5 mg/dL and is usually associated with endogenous or exogenous phosphorus intake, renal failure, cellular destruction (PO_4 is an intracellular ion), or hyperparathyroidism (from increased P reabsorption). There may be deposition of Ca^{++} and P in soft tissue. Acute or chronic renal failure is the leading cause of hyperphosphatemia, but it can also be caused by hypoparathyroidism, adrenal insufficiency and hyperthyroidism. Other contributing factors include chemotherapy, respiratory or metabolic acidosis, and excessive laxative use. Clinical manifestations are similar to those of hypocalcemia and are rarely seen alone.

Management

The goal of management in both of these conditions is to identify and treat the underlying pathology. Aluminum hydroxide or aluminum carbonate binds to PO_4 and causes intestinal excretion; therefore, they are not used as frequently due to the risk of aluminum toxicity. Dialysis is used for renal failure.

Magnesium

Magnesium (Mg^{++}) is an intracellular ion stored in muscle and bone, with 30% stored in the cells. A very small amount is found in serum. It is regulated by the kidneys and plays an important role in the release of acetylcholine at neuromuscular junctions, affecting neuromuscular excitability. **Hypomagnesemia** occurs at values of less than 1.5 mEq/L and results in increased excitability and tetany (similar to signs of Ca^{++} deficits). Chronic alcoholism is a major risk factor for hypomagnesemia, which may also be accompanied by hypokalemia. **Hypermagnesemia** (>2.5 mEq/L) is rare and is caused by renal failure or excess intake through cathartics and antacids, especially in the elderly. Signs are those related to decreased neuromuscular excitability.

Management

The goal of management is to treat the cause and normalize values. IV administration of $MgSO_4$ may be required with hypomagnesemia. Treatment of hypermagnesemia is achieved by the IV administration of Ca^{++}, which is a direct antagonist of Mg^{++}. Dialysis may also be used.

Table 3-2   Calcium Level (normal, 9.0–10.0)

	Cause	Clinical Manifestations
Hypocalcemia	Hypoparathyroidism	Serum level <8.5 mg/dL
	Acute pancreatitis	Paresthesias
	Hypomagnesia	Abdominal cramps
	Malabsorption	Hyperreflexia
	Vitamin D deficiency	Positive Chvostek's and
	Renal failure	Trousseau's signs
	Rapid transfusion of	Tetany
	citrated blood	Laryngospasms
		ECG changes
Hypercalcemia	Hyperparathyroidism	Serum level >10.5 mg/dL
	Neoplasm of bone	Polyuria, polydipsia
	Renal insufficiency	Flank pain/signs of kidney
	Excessive vitamin D	stones
		Decreased neuromuscular
	Excessive dietary calcium	excitability
	Thiazide diuretics	CNS depression, stupor,
		or coma
		ECG changes

CNS, central nervous system; ECG, electrocardiographic.

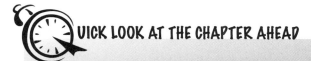

QUICK LOOK AT THE CHAPTER AHEAD

Maintenance of acid-base balance is critical for life and health and is achieved through various buffer systems and compensatory mechanisms of the lungs and kidneys. These imbalances can range from mild to severe and life threatening, and there is a narrow therapeutic window. Regulation of the pH is due to the concentration of hydrogen in the blood. When there are changes in the concentration of this ion, imbalances occur.

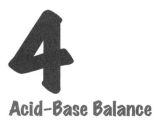

Acid-Base Balance

TERMS
- [ ] acid
- [ ] acidosis
- [ ] alkalosis
- [ ] base
- [ ] Kussmaul's respiration
- [ ] metabolic acidosis
- [ ] metabolic alkalosis
- [ ] respiratory acidosis
- [ ] respiratory alkalosis

Figure 4-1 Common causes of respiratory acidosis.

Common Causes of Respiratory Acidosis

- Chronic obstructive pulmonary disease
- Pneumonia
- Severe asthma
- Hypoventilation (thoracic surgery and others)
- Central nervous system depression (drugs, injury)

Common Causes of Respiratory Alkalosis

- Early salicylate poisoning
- Congestive heart failure
- Central nervous system disorders
- Head trauma

Common Causes of Metabolic Acidosis

- Ketoacidosis (diabetes mellitus, starvation)
- Renal failure
- Diarrhea
- Tissue anoxia (cardiac arrest and others)
- Intestinal decompression
- Salicylate poisoning

Common Causes of Metabolic Alkalosis

- Vomiting
- Bulimia
- Renal impairment
- Excess use of bicarbonate antacids

Signs and Symptoms of Acidosis

Metabolic
  Headache
  Lethargy
  Kussmaul's respiration
  Anorexia
  Nausea/vomiting
  Diarrhea
  Abdominal discomfort

Respiratory
  Restlessness
  Apprehension
  Headache
  Lethargy
  Muscle twitching
  Tremors
  Convulsions/coma

Signs and Symptoms of Alkalosis

Metabolic
  Weakness
  Muscle cramps
  Hyperreflexia
  Confusion
  Slow/shallow respiration
  Tingling of the fingers/toes
  Dysrhythmias
  Coma/death

Respiratory
  Dizziness
  Confusion
  Paresthesias
  Convulsions
  Coma

pH of Selected Body Fluids

Gastric	1.0 to 3.0		Cerebrospinal fluid	7.32
Urine	5.0 to 6.0		Blood	7.35 to 7.45
Bile	7.6 to 8.6		Pancreatic	7.1 to 8.2

Laboratory Values*

$Paco_2$	35 to 45 mm Hg		O_2 saturation	>95%
Pao_2	80 to 100 mm Hg		HCO_3	23 to 27 mEq/L
pH	7.35 to 7.45			

*There are slight variations in published normal values; use those of the laboratory with which you are affiliated.

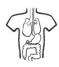

HYDROGEN IONS AND pH

Hydrogen ions maintain membrane integrity and speed of enzymatic reactions. Their concentration is expressed as pH. When there is a higher number of hydrogen ions, the solution is more acidic, which lowers pH. Conversely, when there is a lower number of hydrogen ions, the solution is more basic, which raises the pH. Acids are produced as a byproduct when protein, carbohydrate, and fat metabolize.

 Regulation of the pH is due to the concentration of hydrogen in the blood. When there are changes in the concentration of this ion, imbalances occur.

 The respiratory and renal systems have primary responsibility for maintaining pH within a normal range.

The respiratory and renal systems have primary responsibility for maintaining pH within a normal range. The lungs excrete volatile acids (carbonic acid) by eliminating carbon dioxide (CO_2), whereas the kidneys excrete nonvolatile acids such as sulfuric, phosphoric, and organic by regulating bicarbonate. Buffer systems assist in this process.

 The respiratory and renal systems have primary responsibility for maintaining pH within a normal range.

Buffer Systems

Buffers absorb excess **acid** (H^+) or excess **base** (OH^-) without a significant change in pH. They work as pairs, each containing a weak acid and a weak base. The carbonic acid–bicarbonate buffer system is the most important extracellular buffer system. Hemoglobin is an important buffer in erythrocytes. Phosphorus and protein are the primary intracellular buffers. Most buffer systems disassociate rapidly in response to changes in pH. The carbonic acid–bicarbonate buffer system acts in both the lungs and the kidneys. As the Pa_{CO_2} increases in the blood, more carbonic acid is formed. The lungs compensate for this by blowing off CO_2, and the kidneys compensate by either reabsorbing bicarbonate or producing more. The respiratory response

 The lungs compensate for this increase in carbonic acid by blowing off CO_2, and the kidneys compensate by either reabsorbing bicarbonate or producing more.

begins within minutes or hours. The renal response occurs within hours or days. Conversely, if the ratio between bicarbonate (HCO_3) and carbonic acid (H_2CO_3) shifts toward the basic side, H^+ is conserved or produced by the kidneys and the lungs retain CO_2 (allowing more carbonic acid to be formed). The lungs respond similarly to changes in nonvolatile acid levels, which compensates for it. This response takes a little longer. When the body is adequately compensating for changes in pH, the pH of the blood is normal but there are variations in the levels of HCO_3 or $Paco_2$ and other blood chemistry values. This compensation may also be reflected in changes in respiratory rate and depth and pH of the urine. The elderly respond less quickly to changes in pH.

> When the body is adequately compensating for changes in pH, the pH of the blood is normal but there are variations in the levels of HCO_3 or $Paco_2$ and other blood chemistry values.

Proteins carry negative charges and are buffers for H^+. Hemoglobin is an excellent intracellular buffer because it binds readily with H^+ and CO_2. In addition, the kidney regulates amounts of PO_4 and ammonia in response to changes in the pH of the blood, which allows H^+ to be excreted in the urine. These systems work in conjunction with the

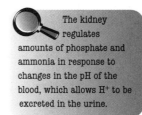

The kidney regulates amounts of phosphate and ammonia in response to changes in the pH of the blood, which allows H^+ to be excreted in the urine.

H^+ ion and bicarbonate renal mechanisms previously described to effect a normal pH and maintain homeostasis. Shifts in K^+ and H^+ ions in acidosis or alkalosis also assist in buffering. In acidosis, H^+ cannot be excreted without another cation being retained. Because K^+ is the ion retained, hyperkalemia develops in acidosis. Additionally, when excess H^+ moves into the cell, K^+ leaves, further contributing to hyperkalemia. The reverse happens with alkalosis, resulting in hypokalemia. Ca^{++} is also affected by serum pH. More Ca^{++} is bound with serum proteins in an alkalotic state; therefore hypocalcemia accompanies alkalosis, and hypercalcemia accompanies acidosis.

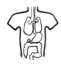

ACID BASE IMBALANCES

Imbalances can be manifested as either acidosis or alkalosis and may be of respiratory, metabolic, or mixed origin. **Acidosis** is the result of either a loss of base or excess acid; **alkalosis** is the result of either excess base or loss of acid. Imbalances of respiratory origin are compensated for by the kidneys; imbalances of metabolic origin are compensated for by the lungs and/or the kidneys (if they are not the cause of the problem).

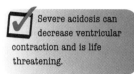

The body compensates for metabolic acidosis by increasing the respiratory rate, thereby releasing CO_2 and lowering the amount of carbonic acid.

In **metabolic acidosis** either noncarbonic acids increase or bicarbonates decrease. The body compensates by increasing the respiratory rate, thereby releasing CO_2 and lowering the amount of carbonic acid. In addition, the kidneys excrete H^+ by binding it with

Severe acidosis can decrease ventricular contraction and is life threatening.

ammonia or phosphate. If acidosis is severe, the buffers may not be able to compensate effectively. Severe acidosis can decrease ventricular contraction and is life threatening. Uncompensated metabolic acidosis exists with pH < 7.35 and HCO_3 < 23 mEq/L. Causes of metabolic acidosis include diarrhea, lactic acidosis, diabetic and alcoholic ketoacidosis, salicylate poisoning, and starvation.

 Metabolic alkalosis may occur with hypokalemia, bulimia, Cushing's syndrome, or renal impairment.

Metabolic alkalosis is usually the result of excess loss of acid that can occur with vomiting or gastric suctioning or ingestion of excessive bicarbonate. It may also occur with hypokalemia, bulimia, Cushing's syndrome, or renal impairment. When the acid loss is accompanied by loss of fluids and electrolytes, renal compensatory mechanisms are not effective because the kidneys are also trying to compensate for the lost fluids and electrolytes. These two mechanisms work at cross-purposes, the result of which is excretion of H^+ (to balance the loss of K^+), reabsorption of HCO_3 (to balance the loss of Cl^-), and a worsening of the alkalosis. Correction can be achieved if extracellular volume is expanded with intravenous sodium chloride (NaCl) and K^+, thereby allowing the kidney to use its buffers to correct the alkalosis. Metabolic alkalosis also inhibits the respiratory center and decreases the rate and depth of respirations, causing CO_2 retention and consequent formation of carbonic acid. Clinical manifestations vary depending on the cause. Metabolic alkalosis exists when pH > 7.45 and HCO_3 > 26 mEq/L. If compensated, the Pa_{CO_2} may be greater than 40 mm Hg and the K^+ and Cl^- may be below normal.

Respiratory acidosis occurs when ventilation is depressed, causing CO_2 retention and consequent increases in carbonic acid, resulting in acidosis. Causes of respiratory acidosis include drug overdoses, head injuries, disorders of the respiratory muscles, chronic obstructive pulmonary disease, pulmonary edema, and respiratory distress syndrome. If it is acute, renal compensatory mechanisms are inadequate because they take time to become effective. Hemoglobin buffers help, and depending on the cause there may be an initial increase in respiratory rate. Laboratory values in acute, uncompensated respiratory acidosis show slightly lowered pH, increased Pa_{CO_2}, and normal or slightly increased HCO_3 due to delayed renal response. Chronic respiratory acidosis is adequately compensated for by the kidneys, and the laboratory values indicate normal pH, elevated Pa_{CO_2}, and elevated HCO_3. Clinical manifestations depend on acuity of onset and severity. The respiratory center gradually adapts to prolonged elevations of CO_2 so the respiratory rate, although initially increased, may be normal or depressed. Cyanosis does not occur unless there is also hypoxemia.

> Causes of respiratory acidosis include drug overdoses, head injuries, disorders of the respiratory muscles, chronic obstructive pulmonary disease, pulmonary edema, and respiratory distress syndrome.

> If it is acute, renal compensatory mechanisms are inadequate because they take time to become effective.

> Laboratory values in acute uncompensated respiratory acidosis show slightly lowered pH, increased Pa_{CO_2}, and normal or slightly increased HCO_3 due to delayed renal response.

Respiratory alkalosis is the most common acid–base imbalance and occurs with alveolar hyperventilation and excessive loss of CO_2. Common causes include high altitude, hysteria, early salicylate poisoning, hypermetabolic states, congestive heart failure, central nervous system disorders, head trauma, fever, and thyrotoxicosis. Improper use of ventilators can cause iatrogenic respiratory alkalosis. Cellular buffers provide immediate response, although these are not very effective. Renal buffers, however, are effective. Laboratory values show pH > 7.45, Pa_{CO_2} < 38 mm Hg, and a normal HCO_3; if compensated, the pH is normal and the HCO_3 decreased.

MANAGEMENT

The goal of management in all four conditions is to return the pH to normal as rapidly and as safely as possible and to treat the underlying cause so recurrences are prevented. Each condition has additional treatment options. Severe metabolic acidosis may be treated with $NaHCO_3$ administration. Metabolic alkalosis is treated with intravenous administration of Na^+, Cl^-, and K^+ to replace volume and electrolytes. Respiratory acidosis is treated by trying to restore normal ventilation; mechanical ventilation may be required. Oxygen must be administered with care so the respiratory center is not further depressed. Treatment in respiratory alkalosis varies depending on the cause. With hysteria, breathing into and exhaling from a paper bag helps to restore CO_2 levels.

PART I · QUESTIONS

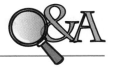

1. Which of the following groups is most at risk for fluid volume deficits?
   a. School-aged children
   b. Infants
   c. Middle-aged women
   d. Athletes

2. Which of the following is the best example of third spacing?
   a. Edema following a sprain
   b. Rales
   c. Pedal edema
   d. Ascites

3. Which of the following conditions increases fluid needs?
   a. Anorexia
   b. Hypertension
   c. Renal failure
   d. Fever

4. Which of the following is *most* likely to result in edema?
   a. Low albumin levels
   b. Low hemoglobin levels
   c. Decreased blood volume
   d. Decreased hydrostatic pressure

5. What is a common consequence of hypokalemia?
   a. Tetany
   b. Ileus
   c. Thirst
   d. Paresthesias

6. You just received the lab reports on your patients and you notice that Mrs. T. has a K^+ level of 5.2. What would you do?
   a. Nothing; it's within the normal range.
   b. Suggest use of a K^+ supplement to her health care provider.
   c. It's at the bottom of the normal range; suggest dietary modifications.
   d. It's elevated; report it to her health care provider.

7. Which of the following is the major intracellular ion?
   a. Na^+
   b. K^+
   c. Cl^-
   d. HCO_3

8. What is a common sign of hyponatremia?
   a. Confusion
   b. Diarrhea
   c. Muscle spasms
   d. Insomnia

9. What often accompanies acidosis?
   a. Hypokalemia
   b. Hyperkalemia
   c. Hypocalcemia
   d. Hypercalcemia

10. Someone with emphysema is at risk for what?
    a. Respiratory acidosis
    b. Respiratory alkalosis
    c. Metabolic acidosis
    d. Metabolic alkalosis

11. What is the kidneys' role in maintaining acid–base balance?
    a. Excrete or conserve bicarbonate
    b. Regulate carbon dioxide levels
    c. Influence respiratory rate
    d. Increase or decrease renal output

12. Someone with vomiting is at risk for what?
    a. Respiratory acidosis
    b. Respiratory alkalosis
    c. Metabolic acidosis
    d. Metabolic alkalosis

13. What causes an increase in blood volume and a decrease in osmolality?
    a. Oral fluids
    b. Decreased secretion of ADH
    c. Vasoconstriction
    d. Decreased renal perfusion

14. A patient who is taking hydrochlorothiazide is at increased risk for which of the following?
  a. Hypernatremia
  b. Hypokalemia
  c. Hyperchloremia
  d. Hypochloremia

15. Hyperparathyroidism can cause
  a. Hyperphosphatemia
  b. Hypophosphatemia
  c. Hypercalcemia
  d. Hypocalcemia

16. A patient is receiving a blood transfusion. The nurse knows to monitor labs for
  a. Hypomagnesemia
  b. Hypocalcemia
  c. Hyperkalemia
  d. Hypokalemia

17. The most common acid–base imbalance is
  a. Respiratory acidosis
  b. Respiratory alkalosis
  c. Metabolic acidosis
  d. Metabolic alkalosis

PART I · ANSWERS

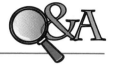

1. **The correct answer is b.** The greater the proportion of body water, the greater the risk. Choices a, c, and d are at no particular risk. Athletes may be more so if doing strenuous exercise in high temperature environments and if not replacing their fluids periodically.

2. **The correct answer is d.** When large amounts of fluid become sequestered in a body compartment and therefore are unavailable for body processes, it is referred to as third spacing. Choices a, b, and c are not examples of third spacing, which ordinarily refers to large fluid shifts.

3. **The correct answer is d.** Fever increases metabolism and therefore increases fluid needs. Choices a, b, and c do not increase fluid needs.

4. **The correct answer is a.** An important function of albumin is to maintain osmotic pressure. Choices b, c, and d do not cause edema.

5. **The correct answer is b.** Ileus results from the decreased peristalsis that is a consequence of reduced neuromuscular function and is one of the earlier clinical signs of hypokalemia. Tetany results from hypocalcemia, thirst is associated with hypernatremia, and paresthesias sometimes occur with respiratory alkalosis.

6. **The correct answer is d.** It is important to report even small variations in potassium outside the normal values for your institution due to the importance of this electrolyte in cardiac function. The other choices are incorrect because although normal values vary from lab to lab, the commonly accepted normal range is from 3.5 to 5.

7. **The correct answer is b.** Potassium is the major intracellular ion. Sodium is the major extracellular ion. Although important, neither choice c nor d is considered to be a major ion.

8. **The correct answer is a.** Confusion often occurs early and is especially important to watch for in the elderly. The other choices are incorrect because diarrhea occurs with hyperkalemia, muscle spasms occur with hypocalcemia, and insomnia is not relevant.

9. **The correct answer is b.** In acidosis, as hydrogen enters the cell, it causes potassium to leave, resulting in hyperkalemia. The other choices are incorrect because hypokalemia results in muscle weakness, atony, and electrocardiographic changes; hypocalcemia causes tetany, and hypercalcemia causes muscle weakness and renal stones.

10. **The correct answer is a.** Decreased ventilation causes CO_2 retention, resulting in an increase in carbonic acid and respiratory acidosis. The other choices are incorrect because respiratory alkalosis occurs with increased exhalation of CO_2 and metabolic acidosis and metabolic alkalosis both have metabolic etiologies.

11. **The correct answer is a.** Bicarbonate–carbonic acid is the major buffer system. The other choices are incorrect because the lungs regulate carbon dioxide levels, the central nervous system influences respiratory rate, and an increase or decrease in renal output is a function of the glomerular filtration rate and overall kidney function.

12. **The correct answer is d.** Metabolic alkalosis occurs because there is loss of gastric acid. The other choices are incorrect because respiratory acidosis is due to CO_2 retention, respiratory alkalosis is due to loss of CO_2, and metabolic acidosis is due to excess acid or loss of base.

13. **The correct answer is a.** Drinking fluids increases blood volume and decreases osmolality due to release of ADH by osmoreceptor stimulation

14. **The correct answer is b.** Hydrochlorothiazide is a diuretic that causes hypokalemia

15. **The correct answer is c.** PTH regulates the balance between calcium and phosphate. Overstimulation of the thyroid causes an increase in serum calcium

16. **The correct answer is b.** Citrate is a common preservative found in blood transfusions that is used to prevent clotting in the bag, and it binds with calcium

17. **The correct answer is b.**

Part II

Immune Disorders

Bernadette Madara, BC, APRN

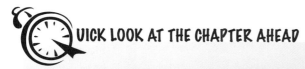

Immune system functions include protecting the body against invasion by foreign substances, such as microorganisms like bacteria; maintaining homeostasis by removing damaged cells; and destroying tumor cells. Inflammation is not synonymous with infection, although the two terms are often erroneously used interchangeably. **Colonization** (i.e., the presence of microorganisms without cellular injury) alone does not produce inflammation—cell injury initiates the inflammatory process.

Any cellular injury produces a nonspecific inflammatory response that is generally local but can also be systemic. Infection is only one activity that causes cell injury and inflammation. Other ways a cell can be injured include surgery, hypoxia, trauma, exposure to toxins, or temperature extremes. Regardless of the mechanism of injury, the result is the same: inflammation. When the immune system is overactive, damage to the body from the inflammatory response can occur, such as in autoimmune diseases and hypersensitivity reactions or allergies. By contrast, a weak immune system leads to opportunistic infections and possibly sepsis and malignant disease.

5

Immune Response

TERMS
- [ ] **chemical mediators**
- [ ] **colonization**
- [ ] **complement system**
- [ ] **cyclooxygenase**
- [ ] **extrinsic pathway**
- [ ] **fibrinous exudate**
- [ ] **granuloma**
- [ ] **inflammatory response**
- [ ] **interleukin-1**
- [ ] **intrinsic pathway**
- [ ] **leukocytosis**
- [ ] **leukotrienes**
- [ ] **mast cells**
- [ ] **phagocytosis**
- [ ] **prostaglandins**
- [ ] **purulent exudate**
- [ ] **serous exudate**

Figure 5-1 Inflammatory response.

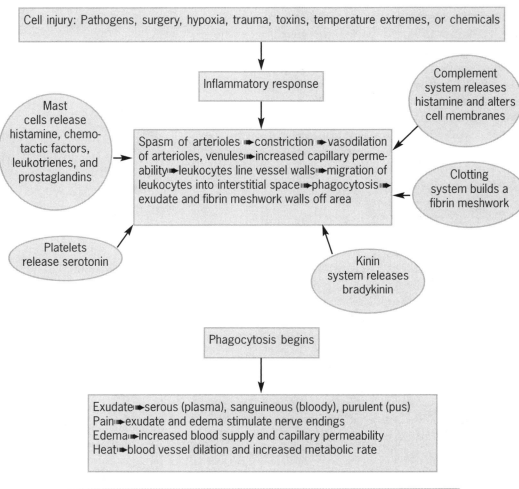

Cell injury: Pathogens, surgery, hypoxia, trauma, toxins, temperature extremes, or chemicals

Inflammatory response

Mast cells release histamine, chemotactic factors, leukotrienes, and prostaglandins

Complement system releases histamine and alters cell membranes

Spasm of arterioles ➡ constriction ➡ vasodilation of arterioles, venules ➡ increased capillary permeability ➡ leukocytes line vessel walls ➡ migration of leukocytes into interstitial space ➡ phagocytosis ➡ exudate and fibrin meshwork walls off area

Clotting system builds a fibrin meshwork

Platelets release serotonin

Kinin system releases bradykinin

Phagocytosis begins

Exudate ➡ serous (plasma), sanguineous (bloody), purulent (pus)
Pain ➡ exudate and edema stimulate nerve endings
Edema ➡ increased blood supply and capillary permeability
Heat ➡ blood vessel dilation and increased metabolic rate

 Inflammation is not synonymous with infection, although the two terms are often erroneously used interchangeably.

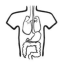

INFLAMMATORY RESPONSE

The **inflammatory response**, indicated by the suffix "-itis," begins immediately after cell injury when arterioles in the region briefly go into

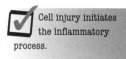

spasm and constrict to limit bleeding and the extent of the injury. This vasoconstriction is immediately followed by arteriolar and venular vasodilation, which bring increased blood flow to the injured area in an attempt to dilute toxins and provide the area with neutrophils, monocytes, nutrients, and oxygen. As capillary permeability increases, leukocytes line the vessel walls in preparation for emigration into the surrounding tissue. At the same time leukocytes are lining the vessel walls, endothelial cells lining the capillaries and venules react to biochemical mediators that cause these tiny vessels to retract. This retraction makes space for the leukocytes to emigrate, a process by which leukocytes migrate into the interstitial space to begin the process of **phagocytosis,** or the engulfing and digesting of bacteria in order to clean up cellular debris. Also during this time, fibrinogen transforms into fibrin, which is used to wall off the injured area so that bacteria/toxins are contained, a meshwork for new cells to use in the healing process is formed, and blood clotting begins if blood vessels have been damaged.

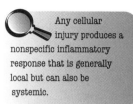

Cell injury initiates the inflammatory process.

Any cellular injury produces a nonspecific inflammatory response that is generally local but can also be systemic.

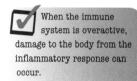

When the immune system is overactive, damage to the body from the inflammatory response can occur.

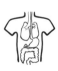

MAST CELLS AND CHEMICAL MEDIATORS

The cells mainly responsible for the inflammatory response are called **mast cells.** In response to cell injury caused by mechanical factors such as surgery, chemical irritants such as toxins, or IgE hypersensitivity reactions, mast cells activate the inflammatory response by immediately releasing their granular content into the injured area along with **chemical mediators,** including histamine, neutrophil chemotactic factor, and eosinophil chemotactic factor of anaphylaxis. As part of this initial response, platelets release serotonin. Temporary blood vessel dilation and increased permeability are caused by histamine and serotonin, whereas neutrophils and eosinophils, which are phagocytes, are attracted to the area by the release of neutrophil and eosinophil chemotactic factors.

Other chemical mediators synthesized by mast cells are leukotrienes (slow-reacting substances of anaphylaxis) and prostaglandins. **Leukotrienes** are acidic, sulfur-containing lipids released from the mast cell membrane that produce a slower and more prolonged inflammatory response by creating reactions that mirror the action of histamine.

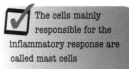

The cells mainly responsible for the inflammatory response are called mast cells

Prostaglandins have many functions. They can cause actions similar to histamine, inhibit the inflammatory response, produce fever and pain, or promote platelet aggregation. The enzyme **cyclooxygenase** is necessary for the production of prostaglandins. If this enzyme is blocked, as occurs with nonsteroidal antiinflammatory drugs (NSAIDs) and aspirin (ASA) use, the inflammatory response is blunted.

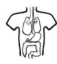

PLASMA PROTEIN SYSTEM

The complement system, the clotting system, and the kinin system are also important mediators of the inflammatory response. Each system contains proenzymes that produce a cascade of events when activated, much like a row of dominoes falling after the first domino is pushed. Plasma enzymes rapidly inactivate many of the mediators of the inflammatory response to prevent widespread, uncontrolled tissue damage.

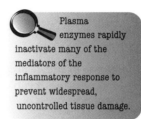

Plasma enzymes rapidly inactivate many of the mediators of the inflammatory response to prevent widespread, uncontrolled tissue damage.

The **complement system** is made up of about 20 different plasma proteins that remain inactive until stimulated by cell injury, byproducts from invading bacteria, or an antigen–antibody reaction. Once activated, these proteins aid in the inflammatory process by causing the release of histamine from mast cells and basophils, altering cell membranes so lysis can occur, and coating the surface of cells so that phagocytosis can occur.

The clotting system (cascade), through a chain reaction, is responsible for building a fibrin meshwork that traps exudates, microorganisms, and foreign material at the site of cellular injury. The clotting cascade can be activated by the **intrinsic pathway**, which reacts to vascular injury, or the **extrinsic pathway**, which reacts to chemical mediators released from damaged endothelial cells. Regardless of the mechanism of activation, the result is a fibrin clot. The infection is contained, phagocytosis is more easily accomplished, and bleeding is controlled because of this fibrin meshwork.

Bradykinin, which is part of the final plasma protein system—the kinin system—is responsible for many actions that are similar to the actions produced by histamine and prostaglandin. Some of these actions include increasing vascular permeability and induction of pain.

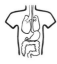

ACUTE INFLAMMATORY RESPONSE

Acute inflammation produces fever, leukocytosis, and an increase in plasma proteins. **Interleukin-1,** a substance produced by neutrophils and macrophages that acts on the hypothalamus, is primarily responsible for fever production. Fever has both beneficial and harmful effects. Although fever can create an environment that kills some microorganisms, it can also make the host more sensitive to endotoxins produced by some bacteria. The process by which the number of circulating white blood cells is increased is called **leukocytosis.**

> Although fever can create an environment that kills some microorganisms, it can also make the host more sensitive to endotoxins produced by some bacteria.

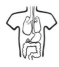

CHRONIC INFLAMMATORY RESPONSE

If the inflammatory response lasts weeks or longer, it is termed *chronic.* Chronic inflammation can occur because the acute inflammatory process was unsuccessful at repairing cellular damage, chemical irritants persisted, or the invading microorganism was difficult to kill. The inflammatory response will continue as long as the invading bacteria are present.

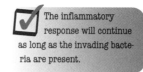
The inflammatory response will continue as long as the invading bacteria are present.

Granuloma formation is a classic sign of chronic inflammation. A **granuloma** is formed when giant cells (fused macrophages) engulf large foreign particles. The granuloma is encased by a collagen network and may eventually calcify. Inside the granuloma, the debris decays and forms a liquid that eventually diffuses out of the granuloma, leaving just the thick-walled casing.

 Granuloma formation is a classic sign of chronic inflammation.

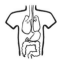

SIGNS AND SYMPTOMS OF THE INFLAMMATORY RESPONSE

Regardless of the cause, the signs and symptoms of the inflammatory response are similar: An exudate is formed; pain, heat, and swelling are present; and ideally healing will begin. The exudate is composed of plasma, blood cells, and products of phagocytosis.

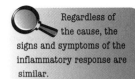 Regardless of the cause, the signs and symptoms of the inflammatory response are similar.

The exudate dilutes toxins produced by dying cells and bacteria, transports plasma (proteins and white blood cells) to the injured area, and carries away cellular debris.

Serous exudate is a watery fluid made of plasma. If the inflammation continues, then the exudate becomes thick and clotted and is called **fibrinous exudate.** Bacterial infections commonly lead to **purulent** (suppurative) **exudate,** which is composed of leukocytes, pus, and dead cells. The accumulation of exudate causes swelling and pain as nerve fibers are stimulated by chemical mediators such as prostaglandins and bradykinin. Warmth of the inflamed area is caused by an increased blood supply to the area.

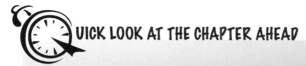
Many microorganisms live on the internal and external exposed surfaces of the human body without causing harm. When the normal balance of microorganisms is disrupted or the body is subjected to noncolonized virulent microorganisms that cause injury or pathological changes, an infection results. Viruses, bacteria, mycoplasmata, fungi, parasites, rickettsiae, and chlamydiae are some of the common organisms associated with the infectious process.

6

Infectious Microorganisms

TERMS
- ☐ aerobes
- ☐ anaerobes
- ☐ bacteria
- ☐ chain of infection
- ☐ fungi
- ☐ helminths
- ☐ mycoplasmata
- ☐ protozoa
- ☐ spirochetes
- ☐ viruses

Figure 6-1 Microorganisms.

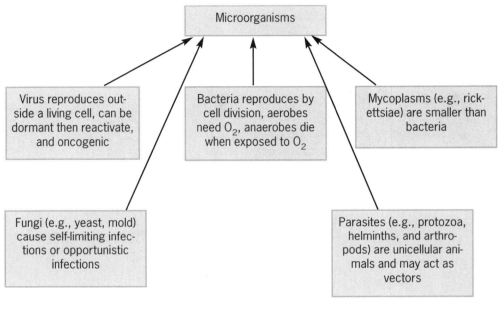

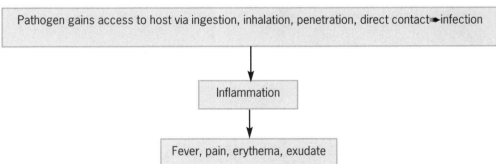

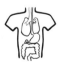

PATHOLOGY

Viruses are the smallest pathogens; they can reproduce outside of a living cell and are composed of a protein coat that surrounds a nucleic acid core of either ribonucleic acid (RNA) or deoxyribonucleic acid (DNA). Some viruses (e.g., herpes virus) are continually shed from the infected cell's surface, whereas others cause the host cell's death during replication. A virus may remain dormant after host cell invasion only to replicate and produce symptoms of the disease months or years after the initial infection. Some retroviruses that belong to the oncogenic group are capable of transforming normal cells into malignant cells during their replication process.

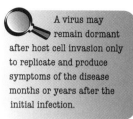
A virus may remain dormant after host cell invasion only to replicate and produce symptoms of the disease months or years after the initial infection.

Bacteria contain both RNA and DNA, have a rigid cell wall, and reproduce by cell division. Spore production allows survival in a latent state until growing conditions are favorable. **Aerobes** require oxygen for growth and metabolism, whereas **anaerobes** die when exposed to oxygen. The shape of the cell wall identifies the bacteria as coccus (i.e., spherical), spirillum (i.e., helical), or bacillus (i.e., elongated). Some bacteria have flagella, which are whip-like appendages that allow them to move

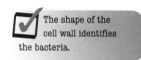
The shape of the cell wall identifies the bacteria.

through blood and lymph fluid. Gram-positive bacteria acquire a purple stain when exposed to a basic dye, whereas gram-negative bacteria do not accept the stain.

A special class of bacteria, called **spirochetes,** is an anaerobic gram-negative rod capable of movement by filaments that cover the entire cell wall. Spirochetes can cause human infection through contact with infected animals or contaminated surroundings (*Leptospira*, causing Weil's syndrome), through the bite of an arthropod vector (*Borrelia*, causing Lyme disease), or person-to-person contact (*Treponema pallidum*, causing syphilis).

Mycoplasmata, one-third smaller in size than bacteria, are also capable of reproducing independently. Unlike bacteria, they do not have a rigid cell wall. Some are capable of causing pneumonia. Typhus and Rocky Mountain spotted fever are caused by rickettsiae, which are microorganisms that depend on the host cell for nutrients, multiply by cell division, and have a rigid cell wall. Human infection is caused through the bite of an infected arthropod.

Most **fungi,** which include yeast and molds, cause infections that are self-limiting and involve the skin and subcutaneous membranes, but they can also cause opportunistic infections. Some of the illnesses associated with fungi are athlete's foot and *Candida* infections.

Parasites include protozoa, helminths, and arthropods. **Protozoa** are minute unicellular animals responsible for diseases such as malaria and amebic dysentery. Transmission of protozoa may be from human to human, by arthropod vector, or through contaminated water or food. **Helminths** are worm-like parasites that are transmitted through the ingestion of fertilized eggs or larval penetration of the skin. The infection can involve many organ systems. Helminth infections are most common in developing countries.

Parasitic arthropod vectors include ticks, mosquitoes, and biting flies as well as localized tissue inflammation from burrowing ectoparasites such as mites, lice, and chiggers. Ectoparasites are transmitted as immature or mature arthropods or eggs through contact with infected clothing, bedding, or grooming articles such as hair brushes.

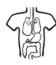

PATHOLOGY OF INFECTION

The **chain of infection** includes virulence of the pathogen, transmission to the host, and entry into the host. Once these conditions are met, the pathogens can cause an infection. Virulence of a pathogen refers to its disease-causing potential. Transmission from the reservoir (i.e., where the pathogen lives) to the host can occur through direct or indirect contact, airborne droplets (e.g., tuberculosis), or a vector (e.g., Lyme disease).

Pathogens gain access to the body through inhalation, ingestion, direct contact, and penetration. A healthy respiratory tract contains functional cilia that sweep invading microorganisms and dust away from the lungs, whereas coughing removes invaders from the lower respiratory tract. Enzymes, naturally occurring antibiotics in respiratory

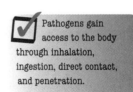

Pathogens gain access to the body through inhalation, ingestion, direct contact, and penetration.

secretions, and alveolar macrophages mitigate most respiratory tract pathogens. Influenza, pneumonia, and the common cold result when these natural defenses are rendered ineffective by smoking, respiratory diseases, or an ineffective immune system.

Ingestion of contaminated food or water is responsible for introducing a wide variety of pathogens into the body, including those responsible for hepatitis A, food poisoning, and cholera. Normally, low gastric pH, enzymes, peristalsis, and intestinal flora protect the body from ingested pathogens. Medications that reduce gastric acid increase the chance of an infection caused by ingested pathogens.

Some pathogens can live for hours or weeks on hard surfaces such as bed rails and tables and are transmitted easily. Direct contact is also responsible for sexually transmitted diseases and for infections passed from mother to child during childbirth, which may cause severe congenital defects involving the neurological system in newborns.

Any break in the skin or mucosal surface leaves the body open to infection. These breaks may result from dry, chapped skin, scratches, burns, bites, intravenous drug use, surgery, trauma, or medical procedures. Antibiotic therapy may result in the development of a superimposed infection as the balance of the body's normal flora is disrupted. For example, a fungal infection is likely to develop if a patient is taking three antibiotics.

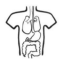

SIGNS AND SYMPTOMS OF INFECTION

The clinical signs and symptoms of an infection can be specific to the site, such as nausea, vomiting, and diarrhea for a gastrointestinal infection, or reflective of the general inflammatory process, such as fever, malaise, and myalgia. The signs and symptoms presented provide a picture of the struggle between the pathogen and immune system.

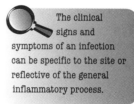

The clinical signs and symptoms of an infection can be specific to the site or reflective of the general inflammatory process.

Fever, pain, erythema (i.e., redness), swelling, and exudate formation are classic signs of an infection in otherwise healthy adults. Infection in elderly and immunocompromised patients may be represented by a normal or low-grade temperature, malaise, changes in mental status, weakness, fatigue, and weight loss.

Infection in elderly and immunocompromised patients may be represented by a normal or low-grade temperature, malaise, changes in mental status, weakness, fatigue, and weight loss.

Fever is generally considered harmless and in fact may be beneficial, producing enhanced movement of macrophages, stimulation of interferon production, T-cell activation, and destruction of some pathogens, if the body temperature does not rise above 104°F in otherwise healthy adults. Rectal temperatures above 100.4°F generally indicate serious illness in children 1 to 36 months of age, and elevations of 2°F above baseline (around 97.6°F) in the elderly require immediate medical attention, as does a mild fever in immunocompromised patients, such as those on oral prednisone or with bone marrow suppression.

> Rectal temperatures above 100.4°F generally indicate serious illness in children 1 to 36 months of age, and elevations of 2°F above baseline (around 97.6°F) in the elderly require immediate medical attention, as does a mild fever in immunocompromised patients.

The four stages of a fever are a prodromal period, a chill, a flush, and finally defervescence. The patient may complain of headache, fatigue, malaise, and aches and pains during the prodromal stage. These vague symptoms are followed by vasoconstriction, which results in pallor and a feeling of being cold. The chill stage produces shaking, which increases the metabolic rate and body temperature. The third stage produces cutaneous vasodilation, resulting in a feeling of warmth and flushing. The final stage, defervescence, produces diaphoresis. During a fever the patient's respiratory and heart rates also increase, and dehydration may develop because of diaphoresis and tachypnea. Delirium and confusion may result during a fever, especially in the elderly, because of a reduced supply of oxygen to the brain. An explanation of the inflammatory process is presented in Chapter 5.

Leukocytes, or white blood cells (WBCs), have specific functions involving the inflammatory process, namely, to defend the body against infection and to clean up the byproducts of inflammation and infection. They travel via the circulatory system to the site of inflammation or infection by responding to chemical signals released by damaged cells. The total leukocyte count in a healthy adult is between 5,000 and 10,000/mm³ of blood. Leukocytes are divided into phagocytic granulocytes (i.e., neutrophils, eosinophils, and basophils) and agranulocytes (i.e., phagocytic monocytes, phagocytic macrophages, and immunocytic lymphocytes). Colony-stimulating factors produced by endothelial cells, fibroblasts, and lymphocytes are responsible for the production, maturation, and function of leukocytes.

All leukocytes come from stem cells in the bone marrow. Granulocytes are released from the bone marrow as mature cells, whereas agranulocytes are released as immature cells. Leukocyte production is increased in response to biological triggers, such as infection, strenuous exercise, fever, stress, and tachycardia, and psychological triggers, such as pain and anxiety.

7

Leukocytes

TERMS
- [ ] agranulocytes
- [ ] alveolar macrophages
- [ ] B cells
- [ ] bands
- [ ] basophils
- [ ] dendritic cells
- [ ] eosinophils
- [ ] granulocytes
- [ ] histiocytes
- [ ] Kupffer's cells
- [ ] Langerhans' cells
- [ ] leukocytes
- [ ] lymphocytes
- [ ] macrophages
- [ ] mesangial cells
- [ ] microglia
- [ ] monocytes
- [ ] mononuclear phagocyte system
- [ ] natural killer cells
- [ ] neutrophils
- [ ] osteoclasts
- [ ] phagocytosis
- [ ] primary lymphoid organs
- [ ] reticuloendothelial system
- [ ] secondary lymphoid organs
- [ ] segs
- [ ] splenic pulp
- [ ] stabs
- [ ] T cells

Figure 7-1 Leukocytes.

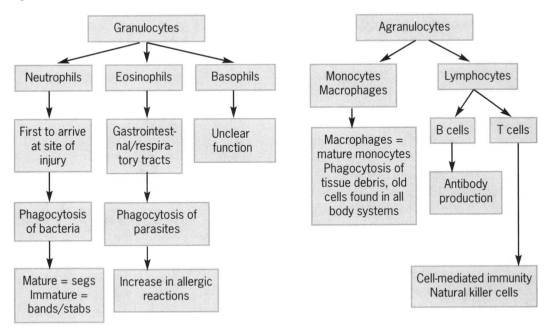

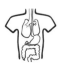

PATHOPHYSIOLOGY

Granulocytes are leukocytes that contain cytoplasmic granules, which contain enzymes and multilobar nuclei. The enzymes in granulocytes have several functions, including killing invading microorganisms, cleaning up the resulting debris, and releasing chemical mediators involved in the inflammatory process. The three types of granulocytes are neutrophils, eosinophils, and basophils.

Neutrophils, also called *polymorphonuclear leukocytes,* make up approximately 55% of the total WBC count and are the first to arrive at the site of cell injury, generally within 90 minutes. They remain the primary leukocytes at the

> All leukocytes come from stem cells in the bone marrow.

> The three types of granulocytes are neutrophils, eosinophils, and basophils.

inflammatory site until the monocytes/macrophages arrive and take over 6 to 12 hours after the initial injury. Neutrophils have a short lifespan of approximately 48 hours and are charged with the phagocytosis of bacteria and small particles of debris. Hydrogen peroxide and hypochloric acid, which are highly toxic and damaging to cells, are produced during the phagocytic process. Each neutrophil is capable of ingesting up to 20 bacteria before it becomes inactive and dies. As dead neutrophils are phagocytized by monocytes, they release enzymes that help prepare the site for healing. Mature neutrophils are called **segs,** whereas immature neutrophils are called **bands** or **stabs** and are released from the bone marrow when the inflammatory response is activated.

Eosinophils, which make up 1% to 3% of the total WBC count, are found mainly in the gastrointestinal and respiratory tracts where they protect the body from parasitic infections by secreting toxic enzymes that destroy the invader. Eosinophils live approximately 30 minutes (when circulating) to 12 days (in tissue). Eosinophils also increase in response to an allergic reaction.

Basophils are not phagocytic and account for between 0.3% and 0.5% of the WBC count. Basophils contain substances also found in mast cells, such as bradykinin, serotonin, histamine, heparin, and leukotrienes, and are involved in an allergic response or stress, although their function is unclear.

Agranulocytes, which are WBCs that do not contain lysosomal granules, include monocytes, macrophages, and lymphocytes. Monocytes and macrophages are called the **mononuclear phagocyte system,** formerly known as the **reticuloendothelial system. Monocytes, macrophages** that have matured, are the largest WBC and account for 3% to 8% of the WBC count. Their function is phagocytosis of tissue debris and large particles such as some parasites, whole red blood cells, and dead neutrophils. If the foreign matter cannot be phagocytized, the macrophages simply encapsulate it. Monocytes circulate for approximately 48 hours after being released by the bone marrow; they then migrate into tissue, where they mature into macrophages and live for months to years. Macrophages in the liver sinusoids are called **Kupffer's cells** and are a main defense against blood-borne pathogens. Macrophages are termed **histiocytes** in connective tissue, **alveolar macrophages** in the lung, and **microglia** in the nervous system. **Mesangial cells** are

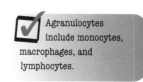

Agranulocytes include monocytes, macrophages, and lymphocytes.

macrophages in the kidney, **osteoclasts** in the bone, **Langerhans' cells** in the skin, and **dendritic cells** in lymphoid tissue.

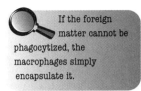

If the foreign matter cannot be phagocytized, the macrophages simply encapsulate it.

Lymphocytes comprise 20% to 30% of the WBC count and include **B cells,** which are involved with antibody production; **T cells,** which are involved with cell-mediated immunity; and natural killer cells. **Natural killer cells** act as surveillance agents. They are cytotoxic cells that do not need prior sensitization to attack foreign cells or cancer cells and are found in the spleen, lymph nodes, bone marrow, and blood. B cells and T cells are discussed further in Chapter 8.

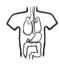

LYMPHOID ORGANS

The thymus gland and the bone marrow are called **primary lymphoid organs,** whereas the spleen, lymph nodes, tonsils, and Peyer's patches in the small intestine are called **secondary lymphoid organs.** Lymphoid tissue in the spleen, which contains macrophages and lymphocytes that filter and clean the blood, is called **splenic pulp.** White splenic pulp initially filters blood entering the spleen and is constructed of masses of lymphoid tissue that form clumps around arterioles in the spleen. Red splenic pulp is the residence of macrophages that digest old cells, pathogens, and debris. Red pulp macrophages are responsible for the breakdown of old red blood cells and the liberation/recycling of heme (from hemoglobin). From the red pulp, blood enters the venous sinuses and then the portal circulation.

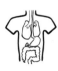

LYMPH NODES AND FLUID

Lymph nodes, which are clustered in the inguinal, axillary, and cervical areas of the body, group around lymphatic veins that collect lymph (i.e., interstitial fluid). Lymphocytes, monocytes, and macrophages develop and function in the lymph nodes. The function of these cells is to clean the lymph of pathogens and foreign matter. During the infectious process, the lymph nodes enlarge and become tender as they increase the production of macrophages.

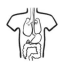

PHAGOCYTOSIS

The process of **phagocytosis** (i.e., ingestion of foreign particles by leukocytes) is initiated by chemical mediators that guide leukocytes to the area of pathogen invasion. The pathogens are first coated with complement or antibody so that they can be identified as foreign. Receptors on leukocytes bind to the coated pathogen, and then the leukocyte extends pseudopodia around the pathogen, totally engulfing it. The engulfed pathogen is called a *phagosome*. Intracellular cytoplasmic lysosomes then bind to the phagosome to create a phagolysosome. Once this process is complete, granulocytes release their contents, including oxygen radicals and lysosomal enzymes that digest the invading organism.

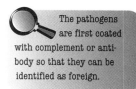

The pathogens are first coated with complement or antibody so that they can be identified as foreign.

QUICK LOOK AT THE CHAPTER AHEAD

An **antigen** is any substance recognized as foreign by the immune system and therefore capable of producing an immune response. Antigens may be proteins, polysaccharides, polypeptides, nucleic acids, or substances such as pollen or bee and snake venom. Cells and tissues, including red blood cells, also contain antigens that the body recognizes as "self" or "nonself." The **major histocompatibility complex** is a large cluster of genes located on chromosome 6, and it is the process by which the body codes its own antigens. **Human leukocyte antigens** are part of our individual genetic makeup, and the closer the human leukocyte antigen types are matched, the less chance of organ or tissue transplant rejection. If the immune system mistakes its own antigens as foreign, an autoimmune response results.

8

Antigens, Antibodies, and Immunity

TERMS
- [ ] acquired active immunity
- [ ] antibody
- [ ] antigen
- [ ] CD antigen
- [ ] cell-mediated immunity
- [ ] cytotoxic T cells
- [ ] effector cells
- [ ] helper T cells
- [ ] human leukocyte antigens
- [ ] humoral immunity
- [ ] hypersensitivity reaction
- [ ] IgA
- [ ] IgD
- [ ] IgE
- [ ] IgG
- [ ] IgM
- [ ] killer T cells
- [ ] major histocompatibility complex
- [ ] passive immunity
- [ ] regulator cells
- [ ] suppressor T cells

Figure 8-1 Immunity.

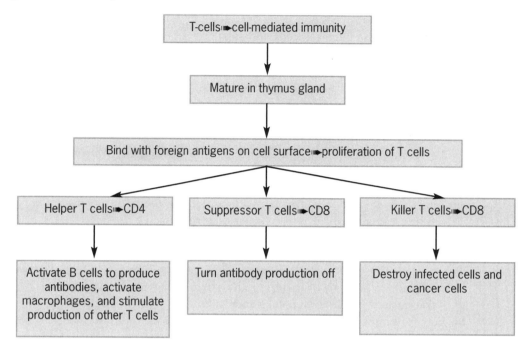

T-cells➠cell-mediated immunity

↓

Mature in thymus gland

↓

Bind with foreign antigens on cell surface➠proliferation of T cells

| Helper T cells➠CD4 | Suppressor T cells➠CD8 | Killer T cells➠CD8 |

↓ | ↓ | ↓

| Activate B cells to produce antibodies, activate macrophages, and stimulate production of other T cells | Turn antibody production off | Destroy infected cells and cancer cells |

If the immune system mistakes its own antigens as foreign, an autoimmune response results.

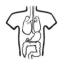

PATHOPHYSIOLOGY

T cells and B cells are produced in the bone marrow and thymus gland. These cells interact with antigens as they circulate between body fluid and peripheral lymphoid tissue (e.g., tonsils, lymph nodes, spleen, intestinal lymphoid tissue) to either destroy the invading substance (T-cell function) or produce antibodies (B-cell function).

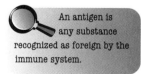

An antigen is any substance recognized as foreign by the immune system.

T-Cell Function

There are two major types of T cells: **regulator cells,** including helper T cells and suppressor T cells, and **effector cells,** or killer T
cells. The function of helper T cells is to
activate B cells to produce antibodies,

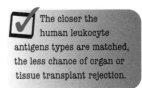

The closer the human leukocyte antigens types are matched, the less chance of organ or tissue transplant rejection.

whereas the suppressor T cells turn the antibody production off. **Cytotoxic T cells** are capable of destroying cells infected with viruses by
releasing lymphokines that destroy cell walls.

   T cells mature in the thymus gland and are the largest group of
lymphocytes, making up approximately 60% to 70% of the total lymphocyte count. **Cell-mediated immunity** is the responsibility of the T cells
and macrophages and is concerned with protecting the body against
viruses and cancer cells. These cells are also responsible for delayed
hypersensitivity and transplant rejections.

   T cells are activated when they bind with foreign antigens on the surface of a cell. These cell-surface antigens may occur naturally (e.g., when
a virus invades a host cell or on transplant tissue). Cell-surface antigens
may also occur when a foreign substance enters the body, is engulfed
by macrophages that then move the antigen fragments to the
macrophage's receptor sites, and then presents the antigen to the T cell.
Once activated by a specific antigen, the T cell divides and multiplies to
form **killer T cells** and helper T cells. Killer T cells destroy foreign antigen cells. Some killer T cells become memory killer T cells. These memory killer T cells "remember" a specific antigen so that upon subsequent
exposure, activation of cell-mediated immunity is rapid.

   Helper T cells have several functions, including stimulating the production of other T cells, activating macrophages, helping killer T cells,
and activating B cells to produce antibodies against the offending antigen. **Suppressor T cells** turn off the immune response by stopping the
activity of B cells and T cells.

   Proteins on the surface of the T cells, called *the cluster of differentia-
tion antigen* or **CD antigen,** enable the cells to be identified. Killer
T cells and suppressor T cells both have the CD8 marker (CD8 cells),
whereas helper T cells have the CD4 marker (CD4 cells).

B-Cell Function

Humoral immunity (antibody-mediated immunity) is controlled by
B lymphocytes, which eliminate bacteria, neutralize toxins produced by

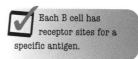

bacteria, prevent viral reinfection, and produce an immediate allergic response. B cells,
which mature in the bone marrow, differentiate into memory cells or immunoglobulin-
secreting (**antibody**) cells. Each B cell has
receptor sites for a specific antigen or antigens, and when it encounters the antigen(s),
the B cell activates and multiplies into either
an antibody-producing cell or a memory
cell. Although antibody-producing B cells
live only 24 hours, they produce millions of
antibody molecules before they die.

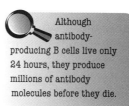

Each B cell has receptor sites for a specific antigen.

Although antibody-producing B cells live only 24 hours, they produce millions of antibody molecules before they die.

When an antigen is first introduced into the body, it takes between
48 and 72 hours for the antigen to be recognized as foreign and antibody
production by B cells to begin. Subsequent exposures to the antigen
produce a quick response because B memory cells "remember" the antigen as foreign, and antibody production is rapid. This response is
termed humoral immunity.

When the body makes its own antibodies, the person is said to have
acquired active immunity. Active immunity generally provides long, in
some cases lifelong, immunity. Antibody production may be the result
of exposure to a specific bacteria or virus or the result of immunization
with a small amount of killed or weakened (attenuated) organism or
toxin. Examples of active immunity acquired by vaccine include hepatitis B, poliomyelitis, and *Haemophilus influenzae.*

Passive immunity is obtained when a person receives antibodies
made outside the body by another person, animal, or recombinant
DNA. Examples of passive immunity include the transfer of antibodies
from mother to fetus across the placenta or through breast-feeding and
gamma globulin vaccinations. Passive immunity is short-lived but effective in preventing illness after exposure to snake or rat toxins and diseases such as hepatitis A and varicella.

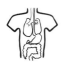

ANTIBODY CLASSIFICATIONS

There are five classes of immunoglobulins (antibodies): IgG, IgA, IgM,
IgE, and IgD. **IgG,** gamma globulin, is the most common of the
immunoglobulins and the only one to cross the placenta. It prevents
systemic infections from bacteria, viruses, and damage from toxins and

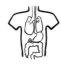

is used to provide passive immunity. **IgA** is found in saliva, tears, and gastrointestinal, bronchial, prostatic, and vaginal secretions and is responsible for protecting these areas against local viral and bacterial infections. **IgM** activates complement and is the first antibody formed when B cells initially encounter an antigen. **IgE** binds to mast cells and causes the release of histamine and other mediators of an allergic reaction, including anaphylaxis. The role of **IgD** is unclear, but it may be responsible for binding the antigen to the surface of the B cell, allowing for B-cell activation.

HYPERSENSITIVITY REACTION

Hypersensitivity reaction is an excessive immune response. This reaction may be immediate (within 30 minutes of exposure) or delayed, taking several days to develop. Hypersensitivity reactions occur because of activation of IgE and the release of inflammatory chemicals, including histamine and prostaglandins by mast cells and basophils. IgE-secreting B cells are numerous in the skin, lungs, and gastrointestinal tract. Activation of these B cells accounts for the signs and symptoms of allergic reactions, which include edema, increased mucous production, coughing, wheezing, laryngeal edema, vomiting, hives, redness, itching of the skin, and vascular collapse and shock in severe reactions.

 This reaction may be immediate (within 30 minutes of exposure) or delayed, taking several days to develop.

Anaphylaxis is a severe, life-threatening, systemic response to an antigen. Anaphylactoid reactions, which produce anaphylaxis-like reactions, do not involve IgE antibodies. The exact cause of these reactions is unknown. Substances that can produce an anaphylactoid reaction include diagnostic radiographs (contrast medium) used for some x-rays, drugs, and foods.

 Anaphylaxis is a severe, life-threatening, systemic response to an antigen.

Figure 8-2 Immunity.

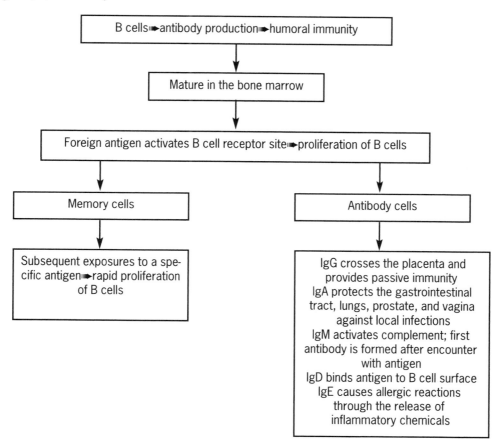

Delayed hypersensitivity is a local T-cell–mediated response to an offending allergen that occurs within 3 days of exposure and may involve a skin irritant such as poison ivy, lotions, tape, jewelry, or clothing. Memory T cells account for the increased severity of reactions on subsequent exposure. Purified protein derivative testing relies on a delayed hypersensitivity reaction.

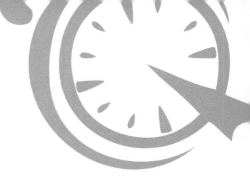

Lyme disease was first identified in 1975 in Old Lyme, Connecticut. Some deer and small mammals such as mice carry Ixodidae ticks, which act as a reservoir for the spirochete *Borrelia burgdorferi* and cause Lyme disease in humans. Lyme disease is the most common tick-borne illness in the United States. If a person is bitten by an infected tick that remains attached to the skin for at least 24 hours, the spirochete is transmitted and produces endotoxins that cause an inflammatory process involving the skin, musculoskeletal system, and central nervous system. This spirochete may remain localized at the site of the tick bite or may invade any tissue, accounting for the variety and severity of symptoms presented.

Systemic lupus erythematosus (SLE) is a chronic, multisystem, inflammatory disease of unknown cause affecting approximately 500,000 people in the United States. This is a disease that mainly affects young adult women, with African Americans, Hispanics, and Asians affected more than whites.

9

Lyme Disease and Systemic Lupus Erythematosus

TERMS
- [ ] **antinuclear antibody (ANA)**
- [ ] **erythema chronicum migrans**
- [ ] **Lyme disease**
- [ ] **systemic lupus erythematosus (SLE)**

Figure 9-1 Lyme disease and systemic lupus erythematosus.

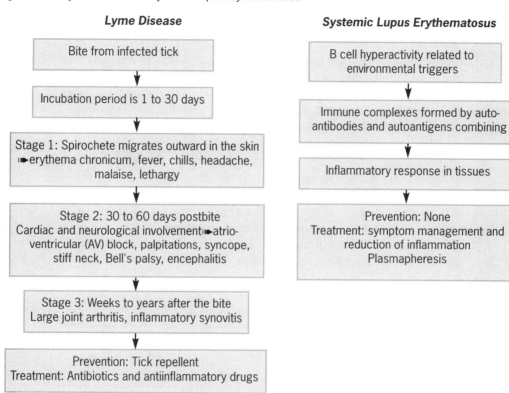

LYME DISEASE

Pathophysiology

There are three stages of infection with Lyme disease. After an incubation period of 1 to 30 days, stage one occurs when the spirochete migrates outward in the skin, resulting in the appearance of **erythema chronicum migrans,** the characteristic "bull's eye" rash some infected people develop. This expanding rash has a clear center at the site of the bite surrounded by a red ring and may reach

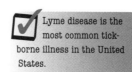

Lyme disease is the most common tick-borne illness in the United States.

a diameter of 50 cm. During this stage the spirochete may also spread to other sites by way of the lymph or blood. Other symptoms of the initial infection include fever and chills, headache, malaise, and lethargy. If the infection is undetected or untreated the disease becomes chronic, and cardiac and neurological involvement occur 2 to 3 months after the bite as part of the second stage of the disease. Symptoms of this stage of the infection include severe atrioventricular block, palpitations, syncope, stiff neck, photophobia, Bell's palsy, fatigue, encephalitis, and radiculoneuritis (i.e., inflammation of spinal nerves, producing pain and increased sensation) that can last 6 months or longer. If untreated, approximately 70% of people infected with Lyme disease develop arthritis, primarily of large joints as part of the third stage of the disease within weeks to years after the initial infection. Arthritis associated with Lyme disease may be in the form of arthralgia or, in 10% of people, a chronic inflammatory synovitis. The third stage of the disease is thought to be the result of treatment failure, relapses caused by persistent infection, or possibly an autoimmune reaction to the spirochete.

If the infection is undetected or untreated the disease becomes chronic, and cardiac and neurological involvement occur.

If untreated, approximately 70% of people infected with Lyme disease develop arthritis.

Cultures of the organism from tissue and blood confirm the diagnosis. The enzyme-linked immunosorbent assay (ELISA) can detect antibodies within 2 to 4 weeks after the appearance of the rash. The presence of the characteristic rash is also used to make the diagnosis.

Management

Prevention of Lyme disease involves avoiding tick-infested areas, using tick repellent, covering exposed skin, and checking for and removing ticks as soon as possible. Deer ticks are very small and hard to detect.

Treatment includes the use of antibiotics such as tetracycline, doxycycline, amoxicillin, cefuroxime, and erythromycin for 2 weeks for a stage one infection, 3 to 4 weeks for stages two and three infections. Antiinflammatory drugs may also be used.

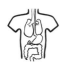

SYSTEMIC LUPUS ERYTHEMATOSUS

Pathophysiology

The pathology of SLE includes hyperactivity of B cells, which is thought to be triggered by environmental (e.g., hair dyes, hydralazine), hormonal (e.g., estrogen), genetic (e.g., familial tendency), and/or viral factors. In response to triggers, B cells produce a multitude of autoantibodies and autoantigens. These autoantibodies and autoantigens combine to form immune complexes against the body's own tissues, such as nucleic acids, red blood cells, platelets, coagulation proteins, and lymphocytes. It is postulated that hyperactivity of helper T cells and a diminished response of suppressor T-cell function set the stage for the B cells to overproduce, leading to hypergammaglobulinemia. The depositing of immune complexes in body tissues, such as the kidneys, brain, heart, lung, spleen, gastrointestinal tract, skin, peritoneum, and musculoskeletal system, sets up an inflammatory response leading to tissue destruction in these areas.

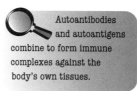

Autoantibodies and autoantigens combine to form immune complexes against the body's own tissues.

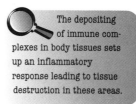

The depositing of immune complexes in body tissues sets up an inflammatory response leading to tissue destruction in these areas.

People with SLE have periods of remission and exacerbations of the disease, and the signs and symptoms depend on which body system(s) is involved. SLE can affect the body in many ways. Polyarthritis, for example, affects approximately 90% of people with SLE. Hand deformity and loss of function and femoral head avascular necrosis may also occur. Skin manifestations include the characteristic "butterfly" (malar) rash on the cheeks and bridge of the nose and sensitivity to ultraviolet light. Discoid SLE, which may be the only symptom, manifests itself as chronic cutaneous lesions on the head, scalp, and neck.

If SLE involves the renal system, glomerulonephritis and nephrotic syndrome may develop, leading to leg, abdominal, and eye edema and hypertension because the damaged kidneys are unable to effectively regulate fluid balance. Pleural effusion and/or pleuritis signals pulmonary involvement. Pericarditis occurs in approximately 40% of people with SLE. Up to 75% of people with SLE have neurological involvement,

ranging from seizures and psychosis to
depression. Anemia and thrombocytopenia
are indicative of hematological involvement.
Gastrointestinal involvement leads to
anorexia, nausea and vomiting, intestinal
ischemia, and pancreatitis. Buccal and
esophageal ulcerations are also possible.

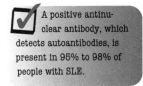 A positive antinuclear antibody, which detects autoantibodies, is present in 95% to 98% of people with SLE.

A positive **antinuclear antibody (ANA),** which detects autoantibodies, is present in 95% to 98% of people with SLE. When the cell is stained and examined under an ultraviolet microscope, a distinctive nuclear pattern is revealed. Other test results that may be abnormal during active SLE include an elevated sedimentation rate, decreased serum complement level, decreased red blood cell count, decreased white blood cell count, decreased platelet count, hematuria, and proteinuria.

Management

There is no way to prevent SLE; however, close medical surveillance is recommended for people in high-risk groups such as those of Hispanic, Asian, and African-American descent and those with family members who have SLE. Treatment is directed at symptom management and reduction of inflammation. Nonsteroidal antiinflammatory drugs are used to control inflammation, whereas antimalarial drugs control musculoskeletal and cutaneous symptoms. Corticosteroids are used to treat severe and/or acute symptoms. The use of sunscreen lotions is also advised. Recently, low-dose Cytoxan (Bristol-Myers Squibb, New York, NY) and prednisone therapy have been used to control symptoms and to avoid the necessity of high-dose corticosteroid use. Some patients may also benefit from plasmapheresis, a process similar to dialysis that removes antibodies from plasma, but this process is no more effective than conventional medication. Because exposure to the sun and ingestion of alfalfa sprouts have been implicated in exacerbations of SLE, avoidance of these factors is recommended for people with the disease.

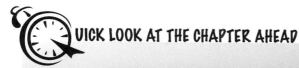

Acquired immunodeficiency syndrome (AIDS) is a result of cell-mediated (T cell) immune system failure caused by the proliferation of the **human immunodeficiency virus (HIV),** which replicates by invading T cells, thus weakening the immune system. Since it was first identified in 1981, HIV has reached pandemic proportions, currently infecting approximately 40 million people worldwide. HIV infection remains fatal, although both the quantity and quality of life have been vastly improved for people with the disease because of advances in pharmacotherapy.

10

Acquired Immunodeficiency Syndrome

TERMS
- ☐ acquired immunodeficiency syndrome (AIDS)
- ☐ human immunodeficiency virus (HIV)
- ☐ immune complex– dissociated *p24* assay
- ☐ OraSure HIV-1
- ☐ plasma viral load
- ☐ reverse transcriptase
- ☐ seroconversion

Figure 10-1 Acquired immunodeficiency syndrome.

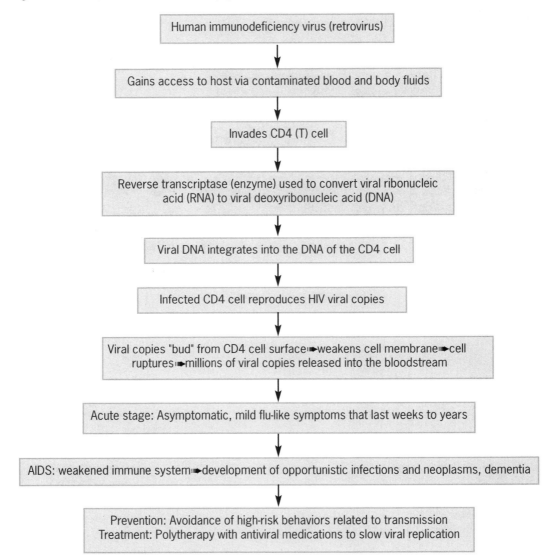

HIV is the second leading cause of death in the 24- to 44-year age group in the United States. Approximately 950,000 people in the United States are HIV positive and approximately 415,000 have AIDS. Women account for approximately 27% of new AIDS cases, up from 7% in 1985. African-Americans have the highest rate of new AIDS cases compared with other ethnic groups.

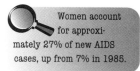
Since it was first identified in 1981, HIV has reached pandemic proportions, currently infecting approximately 40 million people worldwide.

HIV is transmitted through direct contact with infected blood, blood products, and body fluids, including breast milk, vaginal/cervical secretions, and semen. It is

Women account for approximately 27% of new AIDS cases, up from 7% in 1985.

also found in the cerebrospinal fluid and saliva of infected individuals. Two major types of the virus account for the majority of HIV infection: HIV-1 is found in most areas of the world and HIV-2 is found primarily in West African nations.

> HIV is transmitted through direct contact with infected blood, blood products, and body fluids, including breast milk, vaginal/cervical secretions, and semen.

The risk of acquiring HIV from a needlestick injury is approximately 1:300. The risk of HIV transmission increases if the needlestick injury is deep, occurs with a hollow-bore needle, if there was visible blood on the needle before the injury, and if the infected person was in an advanced stage of the disease. By contrast, estimated HIV infection rates from sharing needles with an HIV-infected individual are 1:150.

If an HIV-infected woman does not receive perinatal antiretroviral therapy, there is a 13% to 40% chance that her child will be HIV positive. Cesarean delivery decreases the risk of transmission, whereas a high maternal viral load and breast-feeding increases the risk of transmission.

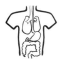

PATHOPHYSIOLOGY

As a retrovirus, HIV carries its genetic code for reproduction in its ribonucleic acid (RNA). Once inside the CD4 cell, it uses an enzyme called **reverse transcriptase** to convert this viral RNA to deoxyribonucleic acid

(DNA). The viral DNA is then integrated into the CD4 cell's DNA. As the infected CD4 cell reproduces, it inadvertently produces viral copies. As the virus replicates inside the CD4 cell, it buds from the CD4 cell surface, destroying the cell membrane and releasing millions of viral copies into the bloodstream.

Chemokine receptors (CCR5 and CXCR4) have yielded new insight into the HIV infectious process. Chemokines are peptides that are present on leukocytes. Research has shown that the virus which causes human immunodeficiency uses these chemokine receptors (CCR5 and CXCR4) to gain entry into CD4 cells. There is an inactivating mutation in the *CCR5* gene that provides resistance to HIV infection. If a person with this mutation does become infected, the disease progresses slowly.

The **plasma viral load,** or number of viral particles per milliliter of blood, is an indicator of clinical progression of the disease. A viral load below 10,000 copies per milliliter signals control of the disease and a low probability of disease progression. In contrast, a viral load above 100,000 copies per milliliter signals a poor prognosis and a high likelihood that the disease will progress rapidly. The aim of antiviral therapy is to reduce the viral load to a level at which the body's immune system can keep the virus in check. Treatment failure is indicated by a rising viral load even in the absence of symptoms.

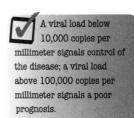

A viral load below 10,000 copies per millimeter signals control of the disease; a viral load above 100,000 copies per millimeter signals a poor prognosis.

In the acute stage of the disease process, the infected person is asymptomatic except for short-lived (2 weeks or less), mild, flu-like symptoms. During the asymptomatic phase of the infection, which may last a few weeks or 8 to 10 years depending on the strength of the person's immune system and the amount of virus transmitted during infection, the body's T cells are numerous enough to keep the virus in control and the person remains symptom free, although he or she is still able to transmit the virus to others. During the persistent generalized lymphadenopathy stage, the person presents with several enlarged extra inguinal lymph nodes.

 During the asymptomatic phase of the infection, an individual is still able to transmit the virus to others.

Eventually, the number of viral cells will greatly outnumber healthy T cells, resulting in a weakened immune system and the development of opportunistic infections, neurological disease, and neoplasms characteristic of AIDS. The term *AIDS* is applied when a person is infected with HIV and has a CD4 cell count of less than 200/mm³. Illnesses associated with AIDS include Kaposi's sarcoma, wasting syndrome, and opportunistic infections such as candidiasis. Opportunistic infections and neoplasms develop because the immune system is not strong enough to kill malignant cells or bacteria and viruses.

The AIDS disorders that occur include AIDS dementia complex, neoplasms, and opportunistic infections including *Pneumocystis carinii*, tuberculosis, candidiasis, mycobacterium avium complex, and other infections. Dementia affects over 50% of people with AIDS and is caused by direct effects of the virus on brain tissue. Opportunistic infections develop because the body is unable to keep commonly occurring organisms, including fungi, bacteria, and parasites, in check. Neoplasms, including Kaposi's sarcoma, lymphomas, and cervical cancer in women, develop because the body's surveillance system is damaged.

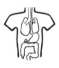

DIAGNOSTIC TESTS

The enzyme-linked immunoabsorbent assay (ELISA) and Western blot tests are used to detect the presence of HIV antibodies (seroconversion) in blood and blood products. Because ELISA and Western blot test for antibodies and not viral antigens, they cannot detect the earliest stage of the infection before antibody formation; however, they are sensitive enough to detect 99.5% of HIV-infected blood samples 12 weeks after initial infection. The Western blot test is used to confirm positive ELISA results. For persons in high-risk groups, a negative ELISA is followed by the more antibody-sensitive Western blot test. If the ELISA is negative and the Western blot is positive, the results are highly suggestive of HIV infection. False-positive results can occur in persons with conditions such as autoimmune disease, syphilis, leukemia, lymphoma, or alcohol abuse. False-negative tests can occur before antibody formation and in the end stage of the disease.

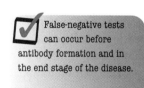

False-negative tests can occur before antibody formation and in the end stage of the disease.

OraSure HIV-1 (OraSure Technologies, Bethlehem, PA) allows for HIV testing using an oral fluid specimen instead of a blood sample. Although it is highly accurate and convenient to use, it is not as accurate as blood testing. If someone in a high-risk group has a negative test result using an oral fluid specimen, the test is repeated or a blood sample is tested instead.

The **immune complex–dissociated *p24* assay** is a test available in some research laboratories that detects the *p24* antigen, which is an indication of active HIV replication, within 2 to 6 weeks of HIV infection. It is used to confirm HIV infection before **seroconversion** (HIV antibody production) and to monitor the effectiveness of antiretroviral therapy.

Lymphocyte immunophenotyping is a test to determine the number of serum CD4 cells. A recent viral illness and immunosuppressive drugs decrease lymphocyte counts, whereas steroids can increase the counts. Laboratories are now capable of determining HIV viral load or the number of HIV viral particles in blood. By evaluating both the CD4 count and viral load, the likelihood of appropriate antiretroviral therapy is increased.

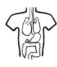

MANAGEMENT

Current research is directed at developing a vaccine against the virus. Until a safe, effective vaccine is developed, prevention of HIV infection includes avoiding direct contact with blood and blood products, semen, vaginal secretions, and breast milk of infected individuals. Educational programs that explain how the virus is transmitted are vital to stopping the spread of the disease. Because HIV infection continues to carry a stigma in many parts of the world, discussion of HIV and its modes of transmission must be culturally sensitive. Screening of donated blood and blood products for HIV is a routine practice in the United States; however, an infected blood donation before seroconversion is possible because the tests detect antibodies and not the actual virus. For that reason, autologous transfusion is suggested for planned procedures that may require a blood transfusion.

Pharmacologic approaches to HIV treatment include polytherapy to interrupt the replication process at different stages and slow the pro-

Figure 10-2 AIDS diagnostic criteria.

AIDS Diagnostic Criteria

AIDS is diagnosed based on the following criteria:
- Opportunistic infections and malignancies rarely occurring in people with healthy immune systems
  - *Pneumocystis* pneumonia, central nervous system lymphoma
- Positive HIV serology
- Infections and malignancies that commonly occur in persons with HIV
  - Pulmonary tuberculosis
  - Invasive cervical cancer
- Dementia and wasting syndrome with positive HIV serology
- Positive HIV serology and a CD4 count below 200 cells/μL
  - 80% of people with a CD4 count below 200 cells/μL develop AIDS within 3 years unless antiretroviral therapy is effective
- CD4 percentage below 14%

gression of the disease and chemotherapy to treat opportunistic infections and neoplasms. None of the antiviral medications kills the virus, and because the virus mutates readily if a dose of medication is skipped, adherence to the prescribed medication regime is essential. Opportunistic infections are treated as they develop.

PART II · QUESTIONS

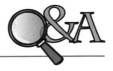

1. A nurse conducting a community health education program stresses that Lyme disease is caused by a _____.
   a. Spirochete
   b. Virus
   c. Parasite
   d. Helminth

2. When conducting a community education program related to Lyme disease, the nurse stresses that if left untreated, Lyme disease result in which of the following?
   a. Respiratory failure
   b. Acute renal failure
   c. Cardiac dysrhythmias
   d. Permanent skin lesions

3. Maria brought her 10-year-old child to the clinic. She was concerned that the child could develop Lyme disease because a deer tick was found on the child. The nurse tells Maria that infection with Lyme disease is likely if the deer tick
   a. Was large
   b. Was attached to the child's skin for at least 24 hours
   c. Caused bleeding
   d. Remained attached for at least 1 hour

4. Systemic lupus erythematosus is
   a. An acute autoimmune disease
   b. The result of hyperactivity of killer T cells
   c. A chronic multisystem inflammatory disease
   d. More common in men aged 20 to 30 than in women in that age group

5. The nurse conducting a health education program as part of a PTA meeting stresses that gastrointestinal infections are more likely to occur in people who
   a. Smoke
   b. Are lactose intolerant
   c. Take antacids
   d. Eat a spicy diet

6. During an orientation session for new hires, the nurse educator stresses that some pathogens can survive on bed rails and tables for
   a. 30 minutes to an hour
   b. Weeks
   c. 5–20 minutes
   d. 2–3 months

7. Which of the following statements about a fever is *correct?*
   a. A fever is generally harmful.
   b. Oral prednisone masks a fever.
   c. A fever suppresses the action of macrophages.
   d. A rectal fever of 99.6 °F in children indicates serious infection.

8. During an in-service in a long-term care facility, the nurse educator stresses that in the elderly (select all that apply)
   a. Infection usually produces a fever above 101° F.
   b. Changes in mental status may indicate an infection.
   c. Fatigue is a possible sign of infection.
   d. A fever 2 degrees above baseline requires immediate attention.

9. What is the most accurate test to detect HIV infection currently on the market?
   a. ELISA
   b. OraSure
   c. Western blot
   d. B-cell analysis

10. Which of the following statements about HIV is *true?*
   a. HIV infects CD8 T cells.
   b. HIV uses reverse transcriptase to convert its RNA to DNA.
   c. HIV infections can be completely eradicated by the use of antivirals.
   d. HIV infection initially causes pronounced signs and symptoms.

11. The role of histamine in the inflammatory process includes
   a. Initiating vasoconstriction to limit bleeding
   b. Coating pathogens for easier phagocytosis
   c. Promoting hyperthermia
   d. Increasing capillary permeability

12. Which of the following statements about chronic inflammation is *true?*
   a. Chronic inflammation lasts 5 to 7 days.
   b. Chronic inflammation results in granuloma formation.
   c. Chronic inflammation results from viral infections.
   d. Chronic inflammation produces copious amounts of serous exudate.

13. Granulocytes
   a. Produce antibodies
   b. Include killer T cells
   c. Contain enzymes capable of killing bacteria
   d. Arrive at the site of cell injury in approximately 24 hours

14. Macrophages
   a. Are involved in debris cleanup at the inflammatory site
   b. Are responsible for producing allergic reactions
   c. Live approximately 120 days
   d. Are immature monocytes

15. Which of the following statements about B cells is *correct?*
   a. B cells provide cell-mediated immunity.
   b. B cells produce antibodies.
   c. B cells release histamine.
   d. B cells live approximately 3 months.

16. Which of the following statements about suppressor T cells is *true?*
   a. Suppressor T cells turn off antibody production.
   b. Suppressor T cells mature in the bone marrow.
   c. Suppressor T cells are the most numerous type of T cell.
   d. Suppressor T cells release lymphokines that destroy pathogen cell walls.

17. The antibody classified as IgE is responsible for
   a. Passive immunity
   b. Protecting the lungs from infection
   c. Activating complement
   d. Allergic reactions

18. Research has indicated that chemokine receptors
   (CCR5 and CXCR4)
   a. Are found on human immunodeficiency virus particles
   b. Allow the human immunodeficiency virus to enter CD4 cells
   c. Protect HIV-positive individuals from developing opportunistic
      infections
   d. Are responsible for neoplasm development

19. The complement system
   a. Causes the release of histamine from mast cells
   b. Causes clot formation at the site of cell injury
   c. Is another name for T cells
   d. Includes bradykinin

PART II · ANSWERS

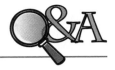

1. **The correct answer is a.** Lyme disease is caused by the spirochete *Borrelia burgdorferi,* which is carried by ticks.
2. **The correct answer is c.** Untreated Lyme disease results in severe atrioventricular block 2 to 3 months after infection.
3. **The correct answer is b.** The tick must generally remain attached to the skin for at least 24 hours for Lyme disease to occur.
4. **The correct answer is c.** SLE is an autoimmune disease caused by overactive B cells.
5. **The correct answer is c.** Antacids change the pH of gastric contents, a natural protection against pathogens.
6. **The correct answer is b.** Some pathogens can survive weeks on inanimate objects, like over-bed tables.
7. **The correct answer is b.** Immunosuppressed patients will have a low-grade fever even during a serious infectious process. Oral prednisone causes immunosuppression.
8. **The correct answers are b, c, and d.** Elders generally do not present with a high fever as a sign of infection.
9. **The correct answer is c.** The Western blot is the most sensitive test to detect HIV antibodies.
10. **The correct answer is b.** As a retrovirus, HIV carries its genetic code in RNA, which must be converted to DNA.
11. **The correct answer is d.** Histamine promotes capillary permeability, allowing leukocytes to move to the injured area.
12. **The correct answer is b.** A granuloma results from fused macrophages, which engulf large foreign particles, and is a classic sign of chronic inflammation.
13. **The correct answer is c.** Granulocytes include neutrophils, which are the first leukocytes to arrive at the site of injury and are capable of bactericidal action.
14. **The correct answer is a.** Macrophages are highly efficient at phagocytosis. They live for years in tissue and are mature monocytes.
15. **The correct answer is b.** B cells have many functions, including antibody production.

16. **The correct answer is a.** Suppressor T cells, which mature in the thymus gland, stop antibody production.
17. **The correct answer is d.** IgE binds to mast cells and causes histamine release and other mediators of allergic reactions.
18. **The correct answer is b.** Chemokine receptors (CCR5 and CXCR4) are found on CD4 cells and allow HIV particles to enter the CD4 cells; a mutation of these receptors inhibits HIV infection and if infected slows the progression of the disease.
19. **The correct answer is a.** The complement system causes the release of histamine from mast cells; the clotting cascade is responsible for fibrin and clot formation; bradykinin is part of the kinin system.

Part III

Anemias

Bernadette Madara, BC, APRN

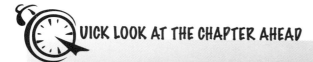

Anemias are common disorders with numerous causes. Some anemias can be easily treated, and some have lifelong life-threatening consequences. Anemias are considered to be symptomatic of an underlying disease process rather than an illness in their own right, but all anemias present with a deficiency in the number of red blood cells (RBCs) and **hemoglobin** content. Symptoms depend on the cause and rapidity with which the **anemia** develops.

11

Common Anemias

TERMS
- [ ] anemia
- [ ] hematocrit
- [ ] hemoglobin
- [ ] reticulocyte

Figure 11-1 Classification of anemias.

Classification of Anemias

By Etiology
  I. Decreased red blood cell (RBC) production
      a. Deficiency of dietary agents
      b. Bone marrow failure
      c. Decreased erythropoiesis
  II. Increased RBC destruction
      a. Hemolysis
      b. Hemorrhage

By Cell Morphology
  I. Determined according to mean corpuscular hemoglobin concentration (MCHC) and mean corpuscular volume (MCV)
      a. Cytic refers to the size of the cell
      b. Chromic refers to the color of the cell
  II. Normocytic or normochromic anemia: MCHC 31 to 35; MCV 85 to 100 (RBCs are normal in size and appearance)
      a. Acute bleeding
      b. Bone marrow failure
      c. Hemolysis
      d. Anemia of chronic disease
  III. Microcytic anemia or hypochromic microcytic anemia: MCHC < 30; MCV < 85 (RBCs are small and pale)
      a. Iron deficiency
      b. Thalassemia
      c. Sideroblastic anemia
      d. Anemia of chronic disease
  IV. Macrocytic anemia or normochromic macrocytic anemia: MCHC 31 to 35; MCV > 100 (RBCs are large and normal color)
      a. Vitamin B_{12} deficiency
      b. Folate deficiency
      c. Aplastic anemia
      d. Lead poisoning
      e. Liver disease

Anemia is diagnosed in adults if the **hematocrit** is less than 41% in males and less than 37% in females. Corresponding hemoglobin levels are below 13.5 g/dL in males and below 12 g/dL in females. Anemias are classified by the pathophysiological process

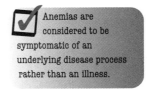

Anemias are considered to be symptomatic of an underlying disease process rather than an illness.

involved, such as decreased production of RBCs (i.e., aplastic anemia) and increased destruction of RBCs (i.e., hemolytic anemia), or by mean cell volume (i.e., microcytic anemia).

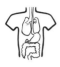

PATHOPHYSIOLOGY

Blood is composed of plasma (55%) and cells (45%). Cells include leukocytes, RBCs, and platelets. RBCs comprise one-half the total number of cells. RBCs are made in the bone marrow in response to a low oxygen level in arterial blood, which triggers the kidneys to produce the hormone erythropoietin. Erythropoietin stimulates the development of RBCs, which must pass through several stages before they enter the bloodstream. Initially, a large poorly differentiated cell called a *proerythrocyte* develops. The proerythrocyte contains no hemoglobin but is programmed, under the influence of the erythropoietin, to pass on the capacity to produce it. When proerythrocytes divide, they produce cells much smaller than themselves called *erythroblasts*. An erythroblast contains a nucleus that shrinks as the cell's cytoplasm fills with hemoglobin synthesized from the endoplasmic reticulum. When the cell is about 80% filled with hemoglobin, its nucleus is expelled and the cell is sent into the general circulation to complete its development. The newly developed, immature RBC is called a **reticulocyte.** Mature RBCs live about 120 days but cannot reproduce because they have no nucleus. When they wear out, they are sent to the spleen to be reduced to their component parts for recycling. For the process to occur as described there must be a normal stem cell pool in the bone marrow, sufficient caloric intake, and adequate supplies of erythropoietin, iron, folate, and vitamin B_{12}.

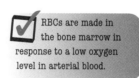

RBCs are made in the bone marrow in response to a low oxygen level in arterial blood.

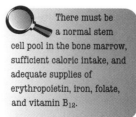

There must be a normal stem cell pool in the bone marrow, sufficient caloric intake, and adequate supplies of erythropoietin, iron, folate, and vitamin B_{12}.

Anemia is defined as a reduction below established limits of the amount of hemoglobin or volume of red blood cells (hematocrit) in a sample of peripheral venous blood. Anemias can be classified by etiology or by cell morphology (see Figure 11-1, p. 84).

IRON DEFICIENCY ANEMIA

Iron deficiency anemia is the most common anemia in the world, with an estimated 20 million individuals affected by it in the United States alone. It is most commonly seen in women of childbearing age, children younger than 2 years old, and the elderly. It occurs when the amount of iron available to make hemoglobin, which is the oxygen-carrying component of RBCs, is affected by either excessive demand for new RBCs or an inadequate supply to make hemoglobin. Adults lose approximately 1 mg/day of iron via exfoliation of skin and mucosal cells, and they absorb approximately 1 mg/day of iron from food sources to maintain a balanced state.

Iron is ingested from two food sources. Heme is from animal sources; it is broken down in the duodenum as iron and is then attached to a transport molecule, transferrin, for distribution via the bloodstream to the bone marrow and other blood-manufacturing sites as needed. Trivalent and divalent iron are from plant sources and require an acid gastric environment to make them soluble for entry into the small intestine, where they are absorbed via the brush borders. Although the average American consumes approximately 10–15 mg of iron per day, only 10% of that amount is actually absorbed.

Eighty percent of the body's iron is found in hemoglobin. The rest is stored in the liver as ferritin and is transported via transferrin to the bone marrow to make RBCs as needed. Men store about 1,000 mg and women 600 mg of iron. These iron stores are depleted before erythropoiesis is affected. Without sufficient iron, RBCs are small and contain less hemoglobin, producing a pale-colored cell. These small, pale cells cannot carry enough oxygen from the lungs to the tissues, so less energy is released from cells. Every cell in the body is affected, and the individual becomes tired, weak, and apathetic. Children deprived of iron are restless and irritable; adults appear unmotivated, are less physically active, and have trouble concentrating and doing physical work.

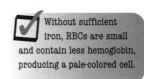

Without sufficient iron, RBCs are small and contain less hemoglobin, producing a pale-colored cell.

Children deprived of iron are restless and irritable; adults appear unmotivated, are less physically active, and have trouble concentrating and doing physical work.

Iron deficiency anemia in young people is most often a nutritional problem. A diet with too little food or not enough of the right kind of food offers too little iron to maintain stores. Approximately 25% of women in the United States have no iron stores. Excessive nutritional demands are another cause of iron deficiency anemia. Men normally need 10 mg of iron daily; all childbearing women need 15 mg daily. People absorb only 10% to 15% of the dietary iron available to them, but that amount varies according to the body's need and ability to alter absorption. Those with gastrointestinal (GI) disorders may absorb as little as 2%; a growing child may take up to 35%. In pregnancy, about 3 mg of iron is lost daily as the placenta takes most of the dietary iron for the developing fetus. Menstruating women lose 0.3 to 0.5 mg daily related to a total blood loss of 50 to 250 mL per month. Newborns rely on iron stores that last for about 6 months, and then they must begin to rely on dietary sources. It is common for an anemia to develop sometime after 6 months of age. Between the ages of 1 to 3, approximately 9% of children have iron deficiency, and 3% have iron deficiency anemia.

 Approximately 25% of women in the United States have no iron stores.

Bleeding is the most common cause of iron deficiency anemia in men, menstruating women, and the elderly. In women, a heavy menstrual flow or abnormal uterine bleeding commonly results in an iron deficiency anemia. Bleeding, usually from the GI tract, either as an acute hemorrhage or a slow chronic bleed such as occurs when taking nonsteroidal antiinflammatory drugs or with many GI disorders (i.e., peptic ulcer disease, gastritis, inflammatory bowel disease, or a malignancy), will have an iron deficiency anemia as a symptom. Aspirin used on a routine basis (i.e., as a daily anticoagulant) can cause GI blood loss even if a GI lesion cannot be detected. It also occurs postgastrectomy or with parasites, as is common in developing countries.

Bleeding is the most common cause of iron deficiency anemia in men, menstruating women, and the elderly.

Symptoms of iron deficiency anemia are not usually noted until after all iron stores are depleted and the hemoglobin falls to less than 10. All patients demonstrate signs with a hemoglobin less than 7. The elderly may complain of angina, but all anemics will be weak, dizzy, and light-headed and have shortness of breath on exertion, palpitations, a lack of endurance, and pale conjunctiva. Severe deficiency results in skin and mucosal changes such as a smooth tongue and brittle nails. Pica, a craving for specific foods, develops in many people with severe iron deficiency anemia, although the foods they crave are not necessarily high in iron.

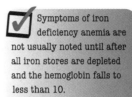

Symptoms of iron deficiency anemia are not usually noted until after all iron stores are depleted and the hemoglobin falls to less than 10.

Management

The cause for the anemia must be determined and the underlying problem corrected. Diet must include iron-rich foods, and iron supplements (see p. 89) are usually given. Patients should avoid foods that bind iron and should take vitamin C to help absorb the iron. The response to therapy is measured by the reticulocyte count, which should rise by the 10th day after treatment is initiated; the hemoglobin should approach normal in 6 to 8 weeks. Treatment is continued for 4 to 6 months because the iron stores must also be replenished.

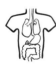

ANEMIA OF CHRONIC DISEASE

The second leading cause of anemia is commonly found with many chronic illnesses (i.e., chronic renal or liver disease, tuberculosis, diseases caused by human immunodeficiency virus infection, rheumatoid arthritis) and results from the body's inability to use iron stores and get the iron into the hemoglobin. Several problems associated with having a chronic disease state precipitate development of this anemia, such as depression, poor appetite, polypharmacy, shortened RBC survival from drug therapy, excessive radiation, or mechanical trauma (i.e., artificial heart valves).

Figure 11-2 Red blood cell terminology.

Red Blood Cell Terminology

	Normal	Increased	Decreased
Volume	Normocytic	Macrocytic	Microcytic
Hemoglobin	Normochromic	Hyperchromic	Hypochromic

Iron-Rich Foods

Meat	Spinach	Navy beans
Fish	Parsley	Lima beans
Oysters	Sauerkraut	Kidney beans
Poultry	Peaches	Soy beans
Beef liver	Black-eyed peas	Green beans

Consume vitamin C in same meal to maximize absorption. Teas and foods and/or drugs containing calcium decrease absorption.

Folic Acid–Rich Foods

Brewers yeast	Spinach	Pinto beans
Beef liver	Asparagus	Navy beans
Parsley	Turnip greens	Black-eyed peas
Beets	Broccoli	Lima beans

Common Iron Preparations

Optimally 50 to 60 mg/d of elemental iron should be taken daily until serum ferritin levels exceed 50 µg/L.

Preparation	Elemental Iron/Tablet	Dosing/Day
Ferrous sulfate (most economical)	65 mg	325 mg/tid to qid
Ferrous gluconate	37 mg	320 mg/tid to qid
Ferrous fumarate	106 mg	325 mg/bid to tid
Ferrous fumarate	66 mg	200 mg/tid to qid

Management

Management is directed at the underlying illness and includes adequate caloric intake, good nutrition, and nutritional and iron supplements as needed.

Table 11-1 Laboratory Tests Used To Evaluate RBC and Function

Tests	Significance	Critical Values
MCV	Mean corpuscular volume • Volume occupied by a single RBC • Measured in cubic micrometers of the mean volume	Normocytic (normal value) • 82–98 fL Microcytic (smaller than normal) • 50–82 fL • i.e., Iron deficiency anemia Macrocytic (larger than normal) • 100–150 fL • i.e., anemia related to a vitamin B_{12} deficiency
MCHC	Mean corpuscular hemoglobin concentration • Measures the average concentration of hemoglobin in RBCs	Normal • 32–36 g/dL • Decreased value (below 30 g/dL) → hypochromic anemia • Increased values (37 g/dL) → normal in newborns • Cannot increase more than 37 g/dL due to size of RBCs
MCH	Mean corpuscular hemoglobin • Measures the average weight of hemoglobin per RBC • Calculated value • Average weight of a RBC is measured in picograms of hemoglobin	Normal • 26–34 pg/cell • Increased value → macrocytic anemia and normally higher in newborns • Decreased value → microcytic anemia
RWD	Red cell size distribution • There is normally a slight variation in the size of each RBC • Large variations in RBC size can help diagnose the type of anemia	Normal • 11.5–14.5 coefficient of variation • Increased value → iron deficiency anemia • Decreased value → no known cause

Each of these anemias is due to some type of genetic disorder affecting the production of red blood cells (RBCs). Thalassemias may be of the α or β or major or minor types. Thalassemia comes from the Greek word **thalassa** meaning "sea" and **Haima** meaning "blood" because of the prevalence of this disorder in people of Greek and Italian descent (Mediterranean area).

Sickle cell anemias are found in 1 in 400 African-Americans, with 8% having the sickle cell trait. Both have asymptomatic carrier states and active states that can be fatal. Pernicious anemia is actually an autoimmune disorder found in adults over 60 with a strong familial tendency for developing it.

12

Thalassemia, Sickle Cell Anemia, and Pernicious Anemia

TERMS
- [ ] achlorhydria
- [ ] allogenic
- [ ] α thalassemia
- [ ] β thalassemia (Cooley's anemia)
- [ ] chelating agent
- [ ] hemoglobin F
- [ ] indirect bilirubin
- [ ] intrinsic factor
- [ ] pernicious anemia
- [ ] RBC sickling
- [ ] polyneuropathies
- [ ] proprioception
- [ ] Schilling test
- [ ] thalassemia
- [ ] thalassemia major (Cooley's anemia)
- [ ] thalassemia minor

Figure 12-1 Common laboratory tests associated with anemias.

Common Laboratory Tests Associated with Anemias

- Blood indices—Tests done to determine the characteristics of red blood cells (RBCs) and their hemoglobin; help determine the type of anemia present; consist of mean corpuscular volume (MCV) (volume of the RBC), MCH (weight of hemoglobin in each RBC), mean corpuscular hemoglobin concentration (MCHC) (amount of hemoglobin in a cell compared to its size), RBC, hemoglobin, and hematocrit.
- Complete blood count (CBC)—Broad-spectrum test evaluating different cellular components of blood, including hemoglobin, hematocrit, RBCs, and blood cell indices. Normal values vary by age and gender.
- Fetal hemoglobin (HbF)—Fetal hemoglobin is present during fetal development and remains up to 6 months of age; test can differentiate between thalassemia and other disorders.
- Hematocrit (Hct)—Percentage of RBCs in a volume of whole blood; ratio of RBCs to whole blood.
- Hemoglobin (Hb)—The oxygen-carrying component of RBCs made up of two amino acids: heme and globin.
- Hemoglobin electrophoresis—Process by which hemolyzed RBCs are matched against standards for >350 varieties of hemoglobin to identify normal and abnormal types; HbS is present in sickle cell anemia and increased amounts of HbA2 are diagnostic for thalassemia.
- Mean corpuscular volume (MCV)—The average size of the RBCs.
- Mean corpuscular hemoglobin concentration (MCHC)—The amount of hemoglobin contained in RBCs.
- Red blood cell (RBC)—Formed in the red bone marrow; lives about 120 days; transports oxygen to tissues bound to the hemoglobin inside the cell; passes through multiple developmental stages as it matures; mature cells have no nucleus.
- Red cell distribution width (RDW)—Determines the relative size and variability of RBCs.
- RBC morphology—Examination of RBCs under a microscope to compare their size, shape, color, developmental stage, structure, and content.
- Reticulocyte count—A measure of bone marrow function and its ability to produce new RBCs.
- Schilling test—Measures 24-hour urinary excretion of an oral dose of a radiolabeled substance to determine whether intrinsic factor needed for vitamin B_{12} absorption is present.
- Serum ferritin—Index of body's store of iron.
- Sickle cell test—Screening test used to identify HbS responsible for RBCs assuming a sickle shape when under reduced oxygen tension.
- Total iron binding capacity (TIBC)—The maximum amount of iron that can be bound to transferrin.
- Transferrin—A glycoprotein that transports iron from the intestine to the liver for storage and from the liver to sites engaged in hemoglobin synthesis.

Vitamin B_{12}–Rich Foods

Animal sources of all types: beef, poultry, shellfish, eggs, cheese, and milk.

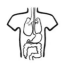

THALASSEMIA

Pathophysiology

Thalassemia is a hereditary disorder leading to anemia because of defective hemoglobin synthesis. α Thalassemia is more common in southeast Asia and China, whereas β thalassemia is more common in the Mediter-

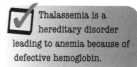

Thalassemia is a hereditary disorder leading to anemia because of defective hemoglobin.

ranean area (Italy and Greece) and is also seen in people of Chinese, Asian, or black heritage. Hemoglobin A is normally synthesized by a combination of two α chains located on chromosome 16 and two β chains found on chromosome 11. **α Thalassemias** are due to a genetic defect that causes the α chains to be too short. **β Thalassemias** are due to a mutation of chromosome 11, resulting in reduced or absent β chain synthesis. An individual heterozygous for the thalassemia gene has a condition called **thalassemia minor,** which produces a mild, chronic, hemolytic anemia with microcytic and hypochromic RBCs. A person with thalassemia minor tends to produce extra RBCs to compensate for the anemia.

If two people, each having thalassemia minor, pass the defective gene on to their offspring, the child will have **thalassemia major (Cooley's anemia).** In β thalassemia, excess α chains are produced, but these chains tend to become attached to the RBC membrane, damaging them and forming toxic substances. Some chromosome 11 mutations result in no β chain formation, while other mutations allow for a limited number of β chain formations. Approximately 5% of children with thalassemia major continue to produce fetal hemoglobin, and when given the drug hydroxyurea the amount of fetal hemoglobin produced is increased. Children born with this disorder are usually normal at birth but develop a severe anemia after 6 months of age when hemoglobin F synthesis declines and hemoglobin A synthesis increases. They then require blood transfusions. They experience growth failure, developmental problems,

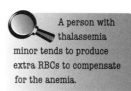

A person with thalassemia minor tends to produce extra RBCs to compensate for the anemia.

Approximately 5% of children with thalassemia major continue to produce fetal hemoglobin, and when given the drug hydroxyurea the amount of fetal hemoglobin produced is increased.

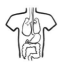

hepatosplenomegaly, jaundice, and bony deformities. The numerous transfusions produce an overload of iron, which causes heart failure, cirrhosis, and endocrinopathies that, in turn, cause the child's death by age 20 to 30.

> Children born with this disorder are usually normal at birth but develop a severe anemia after 6 months of age when hemoglobin F synthesis declines and hemoglobin A synthesis increases.

Management

Those with thalassemia minor have a chronic hemolytic anemia but require no treatment except in times of great or prolonged stress, when they may require transfusions. Patients should be aware of their status and receive genetic counseling. Those with thalassemia major should have a regular transfusion schedule and folate supplements. A persistently enlarged spleen may be removed. Deferoxamine is routinely given as an iron **chelating agent.** Children who have not yet experienced an episode of iron overload with resulting organ toxicity may be candidates for an **allogenic** bone marrow transplant.

SICKLE CELL ANEMIA

Pathophysiology

Sickle cell anemia is a genetic defect occurring at the sixth amino acid position on the β globin chain of the hemoglobin molecule. This defect leads to the amino acid valine being substituted for the amino acid glutamine. As a result, neither the hemoglobin molecule nor the RBCs form properly. When oxygen tension is reduced, as occurs in the venous system, **RBC sickling** takes place, in which the cells assume a crescent shape. Sickling also occurs when RBCs become dehydrated.

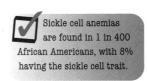
Sickle cell anemias are found in 1 in 400 African Americans, with 8% having the sickle cell trait.

The sickle cells clump in capillaries and arterioles, obstructing blood flow and depriving tissues of oxygen. All organs, especially the heart and kidneys, are affected. These defective RBCs are inflexible, oddly shaped, and have a fragile cell membrane. They are able to revert to a normal shape until repeated sickling damages their membrane beyond repair, thereby shortening their life span and leading to the development of severe, chronic, hemolytic anemia. The rapid destruction of RBCs stimulates the production of reticulocytes at a rate that leaves little time for them to mature, so many nucleated reticulocytes can be seen on microscopy. The hematocrit is usually between 20% and 30%, and sickled cells account for up to 50% of all RBCs. The white blood cell count is high, at 12,000 to 15,000, and **indirect bilirubin** levels are also high.

 The sickle cells clump in capillaries and arterioles, obstructing blood flow and depriving tissues of oxygen.

There are various types of hemoglobin, and each is synthesized by a specific gene. Heterozygous carriers of the sickle cell gene are said to have *sickle cell trait,* meaning they have RBCs that contain both hemoglobin S and hemoglobin A. These individuals do not have symptoms unless engaged in vigorous exercise in a high altitude climate. *Sickle cell anemia* occurs when there is a homozygous state and the RBCs do not contain any hemoglobin A.

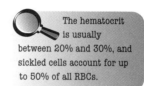
The hematocrit is usually between 20% and 30%, and sickled cells account for up to 50% of all RBCs.

Newborns with sickle cell anemia are often asymptomatic, with the first symptoms developing after 6 months of age because **hemoglobin F** protects the cell from the sickling process. Infants are noted to be pale and may have symmetrical swelling of their hands and feet. As they grow, they have an increased susceptibility to infection, especially pneumonia, and sepsis; delayed sexual maturity; and multiorgan problems throughout childhood and adolescence.

They experience a variety of crises, including vaso-occlusive or painful crisis, which is the most common. The crisis may be spontaneous or may be caused by tissue hypoxia, dehydration, and infection. It may last hours to days, producing a low-grade fever and acute pain, especially in the back and chest. Vascular occlusion may result in tissue necrosis and organ damage, including stroke. These episodes are not associated with increased destruction of RBCs. Other types of crisis include aplastic crisis, which is

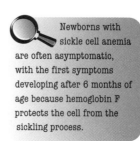
Newborns with sickle cell anemia are often asymptomatic, with the first symptoms developing after 6 months of age because hemoglobin F protects the cell from the sickling process.

Table 12-1 Consequences of Blood Vessel Occlusion

Area of Occlusion	Result
Bone	Susceptibility to osteomyelitis due to staph
Papillae of renal medulla	Gross hematuria
	Renal tubular concentrating defects
Eye	Retinopathy
	Blindness
Sinus	Stroke
Spleen	Hyposplenism
	Susceptibility to infection
Liver	Jaundice
	Hepatomegaly
Miscellaneous	Enlarged heart
	Slow-healing leg ulcers

caused by a severe infection, causing RBC production to be suppressed; hyperhemolytic crisis with accelerated destruction of RBCs; and sequestration crisis, when a large number of sickled cells collect in the spleen. Patients may complain of fever, headache, and severe pain in the arms, legs, abdomen, and back in a crisis state.

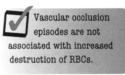 Vascular occlusion episodes are not associated with increased destruction of RBCs.

 The crisis may be spontaneous or may be caused by tissue hypoxia, dehydration, and infection.

Management

Genetic counseling is essential for those with sickle cell trait, but no other care is required. For those with sickle cell disease, the goal is to minimize infections, minimize crises, and manage the crises that occur with hydration, analgesics, and bed rest. Cytoxic agents such as hydroxyurea have been shown to increase hemoglobin F levels. A bone marrow transplant may offer hope for a cure. Currently, people with sickle cell disease rarely live beyond age 50.

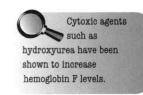 Cytoxic agents such as hydroxyurea have been shown to increase hemoglobin F levels.

Figure 12-2 Normal blood. Note the number and consistency of the cells.

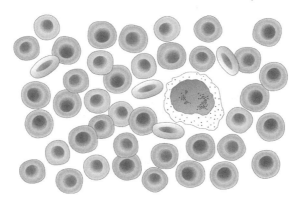

Figure 12-3 Sickle cell anemia. Note the reduced numbers of cells and abnormal shapes.

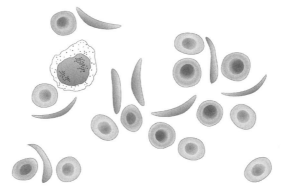

Figure 12-4 Thalassemia. Note the reduced numbers and unusual shapes.

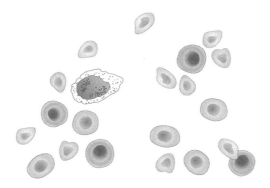

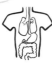

PERNICIOUS ANEMIA

Pathophysiology

A vitamin B_{12} deficiency results in pernicious anemia. One of the causes of **pernicious anemia** is an autoimmune disease that causes autoantibodies to form against **intrinsic factor** and the parietal cell binding sites for vitamin B_{12}. Risk factors for developing vitamin B_{12} deficiency also include a strict vegetarian diet because all vitamin B_{12} comes from foods of animal origin and vegans do not consume any dairy, fish, or meat products. People who have had a gastrectomy develop a vitamin B_{12} deficiency because removal of the stomach eliminates intrinsic factor production. Surgical resection of the ileum removes receptor sites responsible for absorbing vitamin B_{12}, as does destruction of part of the ileum because of severe Crohn's disease.

Diagnosis is made from gastric analysis, **Schilling test,** and blood studies.

A vitamin B_{12} deficiency results in pernicious anemia.

Table 12-2 Schilling Test

24 hr urine test—measures urinary excretion of radioactive B_{12} Indirect test of intrinsic factor deficiency	Used to diagnose pernicious anemia and malabsorption syndrome Tests body's ability to absorb vitamin B_{12} from the GI tract

Stage 1: (without intrinsic factor)
• Fasting for 12 hrs prior to test and for 3 hrs after the vitamin is given
• Oral dose of radioactive vitamin B_{12} (tasteless capsule)
• IM injection of vitamin B_{12} (2 hrs after oral dose)
  • Saturates liver and serum protein-binding sites
  • Allows radioactive vitamin B_{12} to be excreted
	Stage 2: (with intrinsic factor)
	• Same procedure
	• Done only if stage 1 yields abnormal results

Expected result: absorption and excretion of 10% or more of the administered dose	Absorption of less than 5% is abnormal and absorption of 5% to 9.9% is considered borderline
	• Absence of intrinsic factor
	• Defective absorption in the ileum
	  • Stage 2 test done
	  • Intrinsic factor given
	  • Rules out malabsorption factor

An autoimmune reaction results in atrophy of the parietal cells, leading to **achlorhydria** and lack of the glycoprotein intrinsic factor. Normally, vitamin B_{12} binds with intrinsic factor in the stomach and is finally absorbed in the terminal ileum by cells that have receptors for the B_{12} intrinsic factor complex. Once absorbed, it travels to the liver, where it is stored. A vitamin B_{12} deficiency does not become apparent for approximately 3 years after absorption ceases because the liver stores 2,000 to 5,000 µg of vitamin B_{12} and daily losses are only 3–5 µg/day.

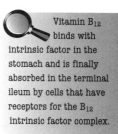

Vitamin B_{12} binds with intrinsic factor in the stomach and is finally absorbed in the terminal ileum by cells that have receptors for the B_{12} intrinsic factor complex.

A vitamin B_{12} deficiency does not become apparent for approximately 3 years after absorption ceases.

Vitamin B_{12}, which contains cobalt and is also called cobalamin, has many important roles in the body, including myelin formation,

Table 12-3 Signs and Symptoms of a Vitamin B_{12} Deficiency

Megaloblastic anemia (larger than normal red blood cells)	**Hematocrit as low as 10–15% with severe anemia**
Leukopenia	Thrombocytopenia
Glossitis	Anorexia
Diarrhea	Paresthesia
Balance problems	Dementia
Neuropsychiatric changes	Pale skin color
Mild icterus (jaundice)	Mean corpuscular volume elevated (110–140 fL)
Anisocytosis (red cells of unequal size)	Poikilocytosis (red cells of abnormal shape)
Hyperpigmented neutrophils	Reduced reticulocyte count
Low vitamin B_{12} serum level (below 170 pg/mL) (normal level, above 240 pg/mL)	Necessary for rapid synthesis of DNA during cell division
Fatigue	Shortness of breath
Necessary for the metabolism of fatty acids responsible for maintenance of the myelin sheath	

gastrointestinal digestion and absorption functions, and DNA and protein synthesis. Although all cells of the body are affected, the chief signs are neurological and hematological in nature. Patients present with neurological complaints such as problems with balance and **proprioception, polyneuropathies,** and possible cognitive changes.

Blood tests show a megaloblastic anemia because cells produced in the bone marrow stop maturing in the time when erythroblasts are changing into reticulocytes and the cells are large (i.e., macrocytic). They are also irregularly shaped, still contain a nucleus, and have a fragile cell membrane. They contain some hemoglobin and can bind some oxygen, but they lyse easily and need to be constantly replenished, hence the anemia. The anemia develops slowly, and patients adjust to the fatigue and chronic hypoxia. Although hemoglobin levels are low, hematocrit levels may be normal because the large-sized cells take up a lot of space and volume.

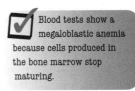

Blood tests show a megaloblastic anemia because cells produced in the bone marrow stop maturing.

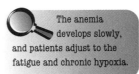

The anemia develops slowly, and patients adjust to the fatigue and chronic hypoxia.

Management

Cobalamin (vitamin B_{12}) is given intramuscularly daily for a week, then weekly for a month, and then monthly for the rest of the person's life. Oral cobalamin of 1,000 µg/day may be used in place of the monthly intramuscular cobalamin if the person still produces intrinsic factor. Central nervous symptoms can be reversed if cobalamin therapy is begun within 6 months of symptom onset.

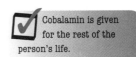

Cobalamin is given for the rest of the person's life.

PART III • QUESTIONS

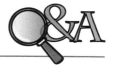

1. Which of the following statements concerning vitamin B_{12} is *correct?*
   a. Vitamin B_{12} is absorbed in the stomach.
   b. Vitamin B_{12} requires extrinsic factor for absorption.
   c. Vitamin B_{12} excess is stored in parietal cells for later use.
   d. Vitamin B_{12} contains cobalt.

2. The nurse reviewing lab results recognizes that the reticulocyte count represents the
   a. Rate at which RBCs are being recycled and broken down
   b. Amount of iron stored in the liver
   c. Rate of RBC production
   d. Amount of transferrin available to transport iron

3. Which anemia is associated with depression, polypharmacy, and poor appetite?
   a. Iron deficiency
   b. Anemia of chronic disease
   c. Thalassemia
   d. Folic acid deficiency

4. When parents, each having the sickle cell trait, have a child, and one parent passes on the sickle cell gene, the child will
   a. have sickle cell disease
   b. carry the sickle cell trait
   c. not have a sickle cell defect
   d. die in utero

5. What treatment is required for pernicious anemia that results from a gastrectomy?
   a. Iron by mouth daily for 6 months
   b. Oral cobalamin daily
   c. Folate supplements daily for life
   d. Vitamin B_{12} injections monthly for life

6. What does an individual with thalassemia minor experience?
   a. Premature death
   b. Mental retardation
   c. Mild chronic hemolytic anemia
   d. Growth failure and bony deformities

7. Individuals with sickle cell anemia are susceptible to all of the following *except*
   a. Infection
   b. Delayed sexual maturity
   c. Organ damage
   d. Premature aging

8. The clinic nurse reviewing the chart of Adam, a 6-month-old, notes that a diagnosis of thalassemia minor has been made. The nurse knows that another term for thalassemia minor is
   a. Cooley's anemia
   b. Megaloblastic anemia
   c. Pernicious anemia
   d. Hemolytic anemia

9. The nurse conducting an in-service at the hematology clinic stresses that infants with thalassemia major
   a. Are born with severe anemia
   b. Begin to show signs of the disorder after 6 months of age
   c. Have high levels of hemoglobin F until they are 24 months of age
   d. Have a normal life expectancy

10. Events that may lead to a sickle cell crisis include (select all that apply)
    a. Dehydration
    b. Infection
    c. Fever
    d. Overhydration

11. Which of the following events lead to pernicious anemia? (Select all that apply.)
    a. Gastrectomy
    b. Ileum resection
    c. Vegan diet
    d. Autoimmune disease

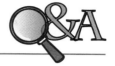

PART III • ANSWERS

1. **The correct answer is d.** Vitamin B_{12} is absorbed in the ileum and requires intrinsic factor manufactured by parietal cells in the stomach for absorption. Excess amounts are stored in the liver.

2. **The correct answer is c.** New, not fully matured RBCs are called *reticulocytes.* They are produced in the bone marrow and sent into circulation. Their amount indicates how fast or slow the bone marrow is making new RBCs and is a first indicator that therapy for iron deficiency anemia is working.

3. **The correct answer is b.** People with chronic illnesses, in addition to the underlying chronic condition itself, often suffer from the problems listed, making it difficult for them to take in and use sufficient iron to meet body requirements.

4. **The correct answer is b.** This is a heterozygous situation; with only one gene passed on, the child has the trait and will be essentially asymptomatic.

5. **The correct answer is d.** Pernicious anemia is an autoimmune disease in which the individual can no longer absorb vitamin B_{12} from the gut and needs to have it supplemented monthly for life.

6. **The correct answer is c.** Those with thalassemia minor experience a persistent mild anemia that they compensate for with increased RBC production. The other choices are all sequelae of thalassemia major, which is a severe, life-threatening disorder.

7. **The correct answer is d.** Currently, individuals with sickle cell anemia rarely live beyond the age of 50 because of damage to major organs during childhood and adolescence and because of difficulty mounting a response to infections.

8. **The correct answer is a.**

9. **The correct answer is b.** Children born with this disorder are usually normal at birth but develop a severe anemia after 6 months of age when hemoglobin F synthesis declines and hemoglobin A synthesis increases. Their life expectancy is 20–30 years.

10. **The correct answers are a, b, and c.**

11. **All the answers are correct.** A gastrectomy removes the source of intrinsic factor. A resection of the ileum removes receptor sites for vitamin B_{12} absorption. A vegan diet is devoid of animal products, including meat, fish, and dairy—all sources of vitamin B_{12}. Autoimmune disease causes autoantibodies to form against intrinsic factor and the parietal cell binding sites for vitamin B_{12}.

Part IV

Nervous System

Vanessa Pomarico-Denino, MSN, APRN

The nervous system is composed of complex interconnections that allow every system in the body to work in a synchronized way. It is responsible for the regulation of the activities of the body's internal organs and also for the body's ability to interact with the external environment. It regulates many activities through a complex network of structures that transmits electrical and chemical signals.

13

The Nervous System

TERMS
- ☐ **autonomic nervous system (ANS)**
- ☐ **central nervous system (CNS)**
- ☐ **neurotransmitters**
- ☐ **parasympathetic nervous system (ANS-P)**
- ☐ **peripheral nervous system (PNS)**
- ☐ **somatic nervous system (SNS)**
- ☐ **sympathetic nervous system (ANS-S)**

Figure 13-1 Brain anatomy and physiology: Functions and manifestations of dysfunction.

Brain Anatomy and Physiology: Functions and Manifestations of Dysfunction

Brainstem

- Medulla—Relay/crossing motor fibers; control and coordination of respiratory, vasomotor, cardiac, and reflex centers (e.g., coughing, swallowing, vomiting, gagging); cranial nerves (CN) IX, X, XI, and XII
  Signs and symptoms (S&S)—Plegia/paralysis ipsilateral; pupils dilate/fixed; decrease/loss of consciousness (LOC), abnormal extensor movement; ataxic, clustered breathing, hiccups; deficits CN IX to XII, absent cough, gag
- Pons—Relay center between medulla and higher centers; respiratory center; CN V, VI, VII, and VIII
  S&S—Pinpoint pupils; semicomatose "locked-in"; abnormal extensor movement, hyperventilation, apneustic breathing (prolonged inhalation); deficits CN VI and VII
- Midbrain—Relay, contains visual and auditory reflexes: bodies for CN III and IV at level of tentorium
  S&S—Ptosis ipsilateral eyelid; pupils midposition and sluggish; LOC varies; abnormal extensor movements; hyperventilation

Cerebellum—Coordination and control of voluntary movements

S&S—Tremors, nystagmus, and ataxia

Diencephalon (superior to brainstem)

- Thalamus coordinates and regulates activity of cerebral cortex by integrating afferent input; contributes to affective expression
  S&S—Altered LOC, loss of perception, and contralateral spontaneous pain
- Hypothalamus—Integration ANS and endocrine function (tropic hormones, oxytocin, ADH); temperature; with limbic system, regulates emotional and behavioral patterns of sexual arousal, feeding, satiety, and thirst centers; diurnal rhythms/sleep
  Reticular formation—Small areas interspersed in brainstem and diencephalon
- Reticular activating system; arousal—maintains consciousness and awakens from sleep, receives incoming stimuli, and arouses the cerebral cortex

Cerebral Cortex

Analyzes sensory data; memory, learns new information, forms thoughts, and makes decisions
- Frontal lobe—intellect, personality, recent memory, voluntary movement, motor speech
  S&S—Impaired recent memory and intellect, flat emotion, emotional lability, lack of inhibition, contralateral plegia/paresis, and expressive aphasia
- Parietal lobe—Sensory discrimination, body orientation
  S&S—Inability to discriminate sensory stimulation, body neglect, disorientation of space, inability to write
- Occipital lobe—visual perception, visual interpretation
  S&S—Loss of vision and loss of ability to recognize objects in opposite visual field
- Temporal lobe—Auditory receptive area, receptive speech, expressed behavior, memory
  S&S—Hearing deficits, agitation, childish behavior, and receptive aphasia

- Limbic system (with hypothalamus)—Sex, rage, fear, emotions; biological rhythms; smell; and recent memory
  S&S—Loss of smell, agitation, loss of control of emotions, and loss of recent memory
- Basal ganglia—Extrapyramidal (i.e., regulation of automatic movement, balance, postural, and reflexes)
  S&S—Movement disorders (e.g., chorea), tremors (rest and intention), increased muscle tone, difficulty initiating movements, Parkinson's disease

Functions of Peripheral Adrenergic Receptor Subtypes

Receptor Subtype	Location	Response to Receptor Activation
Alpha₁ Epinephrine Norepinephrine	Eye	Contraction of the radial muscle of the iris causes mydriasis

Dopamine	Arterioles
	  Skin
	  Viscera
	  Mucous membranes
		Constriction

	Veins	Contraction
	Sex organs, male	Ejaculation
	Bladder neck and prostatic capsule	Contraction
Alpha₂* Epinephrine Norepinephrine	Presynaptic nerve terminals	Inhibition of transmitter release
Beta₁ Epinephrine Norepinephrine	Heart	Increased rate Increased force of contraction Increased arial ventricular conduction velocity
Dopamine	Kidney	Renin release

Beta₂	Arterioles
	  Heart
	  Lung
	  Skeletal muscle
		Dilation

	Bronchi	Dilation]
	Uterus	Relaxation
	Liver	Glycogenolysis
	Skeletal muscle	Enhanced contraction, glycogenolysis
Dopamine	Kidney	Dilation of kidney vasculature

*Note: Alpha₂ receptors in the central nervous system are postsynaptic.

(continued)

Figure 13-1 *Continued*

Functions of Peripheral Cholinergic Receptor Subtypes

Receptor	Subtype Location	Response to Receptor Activation
Nicotinic$_N$	All autonomic nervous system ganglia and adrenal medulla	Stimulation of parasympathetic and sympathetic postganglionic nerves and release of epinephrine from the adrenal medulla
Nicotinic$_M$	Neuromuscular junction	Contraction of skeletal muscle
Muscarinic	All parasympathetic target organs:	
	Eye	Contraction of the ciliary muscle focuses the lens for near vision
		Contraction of the iris sphincter muscle causes miosis (decreased pupil diameter)
	Heart	Decreased rate
	Lung	Constriction of bronchi
		Promotion of secretions
	Bladder	Voiding
	GI tract	Salivation
		Increased gastric secretions
		Increased intestinal tone and motility
		Defecation
	Sweat glands*	Generalized sweating
	Sex organs	Erection
	Blood vessels†	Vasodilation

*Although sweating is due primarily to stimulation of muscarinic receptors by acetylcholine, the nerves that supply acetylcholine to sweat glands belong to the sympathetic nervous system rather than the parasympathetic nervous system.
†Cholinergic receptors on blood vessels are not associated with the nervous system.

Reprinted with permission from Lehne, R. A., Moore, L. A., Crosby, L. J., & Hamilton, D. (2007). *Pharmacology for nursing care* (6th ed.). Philadelphia, PA: W. B. Saunders.

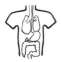

NEURONS AND THE ORGANIZATION OF THE NERVOUS SYSTEM

The basic structures of the nervous system, called *neurons*, are arranged into **the central nervous system (CNS)** (the brain and spinal cord) and the **peripheral nervous system (PNS),** which is further divided into the **somatic nervous system (SNS)** and the **autonomic nervous system (ANS).** The PNS contains the cranial nerves and the spinal nerves. The pathways of the PNS are divided into afferent pathways, which carry the sensory impulses toward the CNS, and efferent pathways, which innervate muscles or effector organs by carrying impulses away from the CNS. The ANS is further subdivided into the **sympathetic nervous system (ANS-S)** and the **parasympathetic nervous system (ANS-P).**

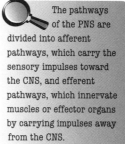

The pathways of the PNS are divided into afferent pathways, which carry the sensory impulses toward the CNS, and efferent pathways, which innervate muscles or effector organs by carrying impulses away from the CNS.

Neurons, the building blocks of nerve cells, are divided into motor, sensory, and association neurons. They have three components—the body, the dendrite, and the axon—all of which form synapses or connections with other cells. Most cell bodies are found in the CNS or organized into groups, called *ganglia,* in the PNS. Dendrites are extensions that carry electrical impulses toward the cell body and axons carry impulses away. Axons may be covered with a myelin sheath, which is a segmented layer of lipid. A thin neurilemma or sheath of Schwann underlies the myelin sheath. The myelin sheath and neurilemma have interruptions at regular intervals, which are called the *nodes of Ranvier.* Myelin insulates the axons, allowing impulses to pass quickly. Neurons use glucose for energy production. They do not store glucose, nor do they need insulin for transport of glucose into the cell. Mature nerve cells cannot divide, and injury may produce permanent loss of function. In the PNS, axon repair may occur if the neurilemma is intact.

Impulses are transmitted across synapses, which are spaces between neurons, by chemicals called **neurotransmitters.** The neurotransmitters are stored in the presynaptic neurons. The postsynaptic neurons have receptors that bind the neurotransmitters; therefore transmission of impulses is unidirectional. Binding of the neurotransmitter changes the permeability of the postsynaptic neuron and may either excite (depolarize) or inhibit (hyperpolarize) the postsynaptic neuron (see Figure 13-1, p. 109, for a list of receptors).

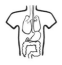

THE BRAIN

The three major divisions of the brain are the forebrain, the midbrain, and the hindbrain. The forebrain includes the cerebral hemispheres, limbic system, basal ganglia, thalamus, and hypothalamus. The cerebral cortex is composed of the following four lobes: frontal, parietal, temporal, and occipital. The midbrain, at the level of the tentorial notch, has the corpora quadrigemina (involved with movements associated with vision and hearing), part of the basal ganglia (substantia nigra), nuclei of the cranial nerves III and IV, efferent spinal tracts, and the cerebral aqueduct connecting the third and forth ventricles. The hindbrain, which is below the tentorial membrane, includes the pons, the medulla, and the cerebellum. It also has the nuclei for cranial nerves V to XII. The midbrain and hindbrain together constitute the brainstem. The reticular formation is a collection of cell bodies within the brainstem, which contains portions of vital reflexes such as cardiovascular and respiratory. It is essential for maintaining wakefulness; thus it is referred to as the *reticular activating system*. The brainstem continues as the spinal cord, which exits the skull at the foramen of Monro.

The brain is protected by the skull bones, meninges, cerebrospinal fluid (CSF), and four ventricles. The meninges are made up of the following three membranes: the dura mater, the arachnoid, and the pia mater. The dura mater is the double-layered outermost membrane. The inner layer forms rigid plates that protect and separate brain structures. The falx cerebri separates the two hemispheres, and the tentorium cerebelli separates the cerebellum and lower brainstem from the cerebral structures. Venous sinuses are between the two layers of the dura mater.

> ✓ The brain is protected by the skull bones, meninges, cerebrospinal fluid (CSF), and four ventricles. The meninges are made up of the following three membranes: the dura mater, the arachnoid, and the pia mater.

The arachnoid membrane is the meningeal layer underlying the dura mater and the space between is the subdural space. The pia mater is the inner meninges. The subarachnoid space is between the arachnoid and the pia mater. CSF circulates in the subarachnoid space and ventricles and is formed and reabsorbed in the ventricles.

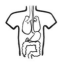

THE SPINAL CORD

The spinal cord is also protected by the vertebrae, meninges, and CSF. It extends from the foramen magnum and the first cervical vertebra to the second lumbar vertebra. Spinal nerves that continue below that level comprise the cauda equina. The filum terminale continues to the second sacral vertebrae and is composed of non-neural tissues and the pia mater. The spinal cord functions essentially as a large cable, carrying sensory information to and motor information from the brain. It also provides neurons and synapse networks within the spinal cord that produce involuntary reflex responses to sensory stimulation. CSF acts as a protective fluid cushion for the CNS, and its total volume is 125 mL.

A cross-section of the spinal cord reveals an inner core of gray matter that can be divided into three regions, each with a specific functional characteristic. The posterior/dorsal horn contains interneurons and primarily afferent/sensory neurons whose cell bodies lie in the dorsal root ganglion. The lateral horn contains cell bodies involved with the ANS, and the anterior/ventral horn contains cells bodies for motor/efferent nerves that leave the spinal cord by way of spinal nerves. Ascending/sensory and descending/motor pathways/tracts are grouped into anterior, lateral, and posterior columns. The spinal tract may or may not cross to the opposite side at different levels.

Neural circuits within the spinal cord form reflex arcs that display specific motor responses to stimuli. An afferent sensory neuron and an efferent motor neuron are needed for a reflex arc. Upper motor neurons are efferent neurons housed entirely within the CNS that influence and modify spinal reflexes. Lower motor neurons influence muscles. Their cell bodies lie in the spinal cord, but their processes extend out to the PNS.

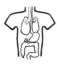

THE AUTONOMIC NERVOUS SYSTEM

The ANS regulates activity and maintains a steady state among visceral organs. Its main functions are regulation of the heart; regulation of secretory glands such as salivary, sweat, gastric, and bronchial; and regulation of the smooth muscles such as bronchial, blood vessels, urogenital organs, and gastrointestinal organs. There are components of the ANS in both the CNS and PNS, afferent sensory neurons and efferent motor neurons. The two divisions of the ANS are the ANS-S (adrenergic nervous system) and the ANS-P (cholinergic nervous system). Some organs are innervated by both the ANS-S and

The two divisions of the ANS are the ANS-S (adrenergic nervous system) and the ANS-P (cholinergic nervous system). Some organs are innervated by both the ANS-S and ANS-P with opposing actions, some by both with complementary actions, and some by only one or the other.

ANS-P with opposing actions, some by both with complementary actions, and some by only one or the other.

In both the ANS-S and ANS-P, there are two neurons in the pathway leading from the spinal cord, a preganglionic and a postganglionic neuron. The postganglionic neurons go to the effector organ. The effector organs have receptors for the neurotransmitters released by the postganglionic neurons. The adrenal medulla is a special feature of the ANS-S. Though not a neuron itself, it functions like a postganglionic neuron, releasing epinephrine. The ANS uses four neurotransmitters: Norepinephrine is released by most postganglionic sympathetic neurons; epinephrine is released from the adrenal medulla; acetylcholine is released from all preganglionic neurons of both the ANS-S and ANS-P, all postganglionic neurons of the ANS-P, and all motor neurons to skeletal muscles; and dopamine is released centrally and can stimulate receptors of the ANS-S. Different receptors on effector organs determine the specific activities regulated (see p. 110).

Full consciousness is a state of awareness of oneself and one's environment and the ability to respond or interact with the environment. Coma is a state of total lack of awareness and wakefulness accompanied by the inability to respond to vigorous stimulation. Between these two extremes, there is a full spectrum of different levels of awareness and responsiveness. Unconsciousness itself is not a diagnosis or disease but is a manifestation of various pathological processes. There are many causes of unconsciousness, including structural and metabolic alterations or diseases.

The rigid cranial cavity holds brain tissue, blood, and cerebrospinal fluid (CSF). The volume of these three components and the intracranial pressure (ICP) they create are normally in equilibrium. Increased ICP is a life-threatening situation that results from an increase in any or all of these components. Increased ICP is a common factor in many pathological conditions affecting the brain due to masses, head injury, infection, vascular insults, toxic and metabolic conditions such as fluid and electrolyte imbalances, and hypoxia. Regardless of cause, increased ICP affects cerebral blood flow, produces compression and distortion of structures, and shifts content. If left untreated, increased ICP causes decompensation of neurological function, leading to death.

14

Altered Level of Consciousness and Increased Intracranial Pressure

TERMS
- [ ] autoregulation
- [ ] Cushing's reflex
- [ ] Cushing's triad
- [ ] decerebrate posturing
- [ ] decorticate posturing
- [ ] Monro-Kellie hypothesis

Figure 14-1 Glasgow coma scale.

Parameter	Score	Response
Eye opening	Spontaneous	4
	To voice	3
	To pain	2
	No response	1
Best verbal response	Oriented, converses	5
	Disoriented, converses	4
	Inappropriate words	3
	Incomprehensible sounds	2
	No response or intubated	1
Best motor response	Follows commands	6
	Localizes response (pushes away stimulus)	5
	Withdraws	4
	Abnormal flexion (decorticate)	3
	Abnormal extension (decerebrate)	2
	No response	1

Highest score = 15; lowest score = 3

Terms and Descriptive Behaviors for Levels of Consciousness

- Alert—Fully awake; aware of self and environment; appropriate, spontaneous response to stimuli.
- Confusion—Disoriented to person, time, and place (progresses from time to person to place); has difficulty following commands; may be agitated or irritable; may hallucinate.
- Delirium-disoriented to person, place and time; often agitated and uncooperative.
- Lethargy—Orientated to time, person, and place but somnolent; speech and thought processes slowed.
- Obtundation—decreased alertness accompanied by psychomotor retardation; can be aroused only with repeated verbal or tactile stimulation.
- Stupor—Awakens only to vigorous stimulation such as shaking; responds appropriately to painful stimuli; verbal responses are incomprehensible.
- Coma—Cannot be aroused; does not respond to verbal or tactile stimulation; brainstem reflexes may or may not be intact; may exhibit decerebrate or decorticate posturing.
- Light coma—Can be aroused; no spontaneous movement; withdraws appropriately to painful stimuli; brainstem reflexes (pupillary responses, gag, and corneal reflexes) are intact.
- Deep coma—Cannot be aroused; unresponsive to painful stimuli; absent brainstem reflexes; decerebrate posturing.

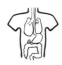

ALTERED LEVEL OF CONSCIOUSNESS

Pathophysiology

There are two primary components of consciousness: arousal and content of thought. Arousal refers to a state of wakefulness that is a function of the upper brainstem and, in particular, the reticular activating system (RAS). Content of thought refers to the ability to think, reason, feel, and react to stimuli with purpose. These activities are mediated by the cerebral hemispheres. A functioning brainstem can maintain wakefulness even without a functioning cerebrum, which is a condition referred to as *persistent vegetative state*. Disruptions in arousal, content, or both can alter the level of consciousness (LOC). Other LOCs include confusion, delirium, stupor, and coma (including irreversible coma and brain death).

The etiology includes any condition that widely disrupts the functioning of both cerebral hemispheres or depresses or destroys the upper brain stem. Supratentorial mass lesions, such as a hematoma, interrupt consciousness by compressing and shifting cerebral contents, causing direct compression of the brainstem RAS or herniation through the falx cerebri or tentorial notch. Infratentorial mass lesions can also disrupt the RAS through compression or herniation. Metabolic problems or diffuse cerebral disorders can disturb cerebral metabolism. Metabolic conditions that disrupt consciousness include uremia, liver failure, diabetes, hypoglycemia, toxins such as alcohol, and drug overdose. Encephalitis and seizures can diffusely affect the cerebral cortex.

Complications that may result from decreased consciousness may be related to decreased mobility or loss of reflexes, such as asphyxiation with loss of gag reflex or corneal injury with loss of blink.

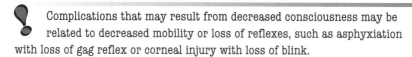

Complications that may result from decreased consciousness may be related to decreased mobility or loss of reflexes, such as asphyxiation with loss of gag reflex or corneal injury with loss of blink.

Manifestations

Full consciousness requires the individual to be awake and spontaneously responding to stimuli in the environment in an appropriate manner. The individual is oriented and able to follow commands to move. These abilities, which include spontaneous eye opening and verbal and motor responses to verbal and pain stimuli, diminish with decreasing consciousness and are commonly evaluated and quantified using the Glasgow coma scale (see Figure 14-1, p. 116). Labels are often used to identify different LOCs; however, there is no universal agreement on the meaning of the labels. Objective descriptions of behaviors are better used to differentiate various levels of altered consciousness (see p. 116 for commonly used labels and descriptive behaviors). Bowel and bladder continence, spontaneous blinking, gagging, and swallowing reflexes are lost as unconsciousness deepens.

Treatment

Primary treatment deals with the specific etiology of the unconsciousness. It is also directed at protecting the individual and maintaining body functions. Treatment may include intubation and mechanical ventilation, airway maintenance, intravenous fluid administration, feeding tube, and urinary catheterization.

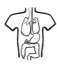

INCREASED INTRACRANIAL PRESSURE

Pathophysiology

A modified **Monro-Kellie hypothesis,** which explains the relatively constant intracranial volume and pressure, theorizes if the volume added to the cranial vault equals the volume removed, then the pressure remains relatively constant. Other factors that influence ICP are blood pressure, venous pressure, intrathoracic pressure, posture, temperature, and blood gases. Normal ICP is 60 to 200 mm H_2O or 4 to 15 mm Hg. Nonsustained elevation fluctuations occur constantly with change of position, coughing, or sneezing. Mechanisms such as increased absorption and decreased production of CSF, displacement into spinal subarachnoid space, and collapse of veins and sinuses that diminish blood volume compensate for elevations.

Compensatory changes have limits, however, and in sustained pathological conditions of uncontrolled increased ICP, compression of brain tissue, decreased cerebral perfusion, and cerebral herniation cause serious problems as the volume and pressure increase.

The brain has two compensatory mechanisms to maintain perfusion to ischemic tissues. **Autoregulation** is an effort to maintain blood supply by dilating vessels, thus increasing the blood flow but also allowing fluid to leak out, which increases the ICP. The other compensatory mechanism is an increased systolic blood pressure (widening the pulse pressure) to maintain cerebral perfusion pressure (CPP), which is the pressure needed to ensure perfusion. (Note: CPP equals the mean arterial blood pressure minus ICP [CPP = mean arterial blood pressure – ICP].) Normal CPP is 70 to 100 mm Hg. A CPP of less than 50 mm Hg causes irreversible brain dysfunction. This increase in systolic blood pressure to overcome the increased ICP is called **Cushing's reflex.**

In supratentorial lesions, as ICP increases, brain tissue is shifted down laterally under the falx cerebri or down centrally toward the tentorial notch, through which it may herniate. The midbrain and upper brainstem are in this area; thus, portions of RAS, bodies of some cranial nerves, including the third cranial nerve (controls pupillary function), and some portions of the respiratory centers are located here. Compression of this area can cause changes in LOC, abnormal pupillary function, and changes in respiratory pattern. Further transfer of pressure toward the brainstem, with ensuing ischemia, can interfere with vital cardiovascular and respiratory centers with slowing of the pulse and respiration. The slowing of the pulse and respirations combined with the elevation of the systolic pressure is referred to as **Cushing's triad.** Infratentorial lesions may herniate up through the tentorium or down through the foramen magnum, compressing the respiratory centers (see above).

Two other potential complications are diabetes insipidus and syndrome of inappropriate secretion of antidiuretic hormone as a result of posterior pituitary dysfunction.

Manifestations

Early recognition of increased ICP is important in terms of prognosis. The manifestations of increased ICP can vary depending on the cause, the location, and the rapidity with which it develops. Focal signs related to the location of the lesion may also be present. Manifestations include the following:

- Change in the LOC
- Changes in vital signs (Cushing's triad), including temperature regulation

Figure 14-2 Decorticate and decerebrate posturing. (A) Decorticate response. Flexion of arms, wrists, and fingers with adduction in upper extremities. Extension, internal rotation, and plantar flexion in lower extremities. (B) Decerebrate response. All four extremities in rigid extension with hyperpronation of forearms and plantar extension of feet. (C) Decorticate response on the left side of the body and decerebrate response on the right side of the body.

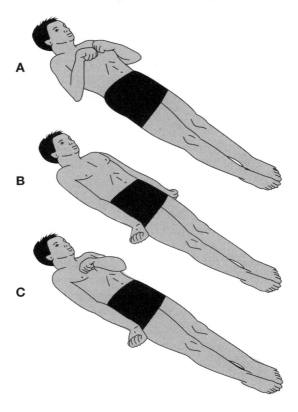

- Altered respiratory pattern (see p. 000)
- Ocular signs, including ipsilateral/bilateral pupillary dilation, sluggish to fixed pupil reflexes, papilledema, inability to look up, and ptosis of eyelid
- Decreased motor function, including **decorticate and decerebrate posturing** (see Figure 14-2 above)
- Headache

- Vomiting (often projectile)
- Fluid and electrolyte disturbances, if diabetes insipidus or syndrome of inappropriate secretion of antidiuretic hormone occurs

ICP can be directly monitored by catheters placed in brain tissue or the ventricles.

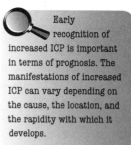

Early recognition of increased ICP is important in terms of prognosis. The manifestations of increased ICP can vary depending on the cause, the location, and the rapidity with which it develops.

Treatment

Treatment directed at reducing the cerebral edema includes osmotic and loop diuretics and corticosteroids. Careful ventriculostomy drainage of CSF may be used in patients refractory to other methods of controlling ICP. Barbiturates or pharmacological paralyzing agents are sometimes used to reduce brain metabolism.

There are different causes for disruption in the electrical activity of the brain, which results in seizures. Not all seizures are due to epilepsy but may occur as a result of trauma, infection, or tumors. Seizures may also be a result of imbalances in fluid and electrolytes, certain drugs, or withdrawal from alcohol or barbiturates.

Overview: A seizure is a result of a sudden, uncontrolled electrical discharge of cerebral neurons that interrupts normal function. The neuronal activity may involve a restricted area of the cortex or the entire cortex. Frequently, seizures are a manifestation of a variety of underlying conditions or they may occur spontaneously without apparent cause. Meningitis is an acute inflammation of the meninges surrounding the brain and spinal cord. Infectious processes, mainly bacteria, are the most common cause, although viruses and other organisms can be causative. Meningitis is classified as either aseptic or septic.

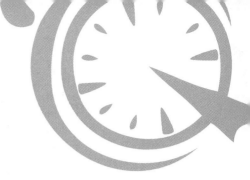

15

Seizures and Infections of the Nervous System

TERMS
☐ aura
☐ aseptic meningitis
☐ bacterial meningitis
☐ Brudzinski's sign
☐ epilepsy
☐ Kernig's sign
☐ status epilepticus

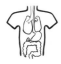

SEIZURES

Epilepsy is a condition of recurrent seizures for which there is no underlying or correctable cause. Seizures resulting from systemic and metabolic disturbances are not considered epileptic if the seizures cease when the underlying problem is corrected.

Seizure is not a disease entity unto itself; rather, it is a syndrome resulting from congenital or biochemical disorders, trauma, cerebral lesions, or toxicity that affects the brain in a variety of ways. Seizures generally last a short time and rarely cause permanent damage. Some seizures are preceded by an **aura** or a prodrome, which is an indication of an impending seizure.

> ✓ Seizures generally last a short time and rarely cause permanent damage. Some seizures are preceded by an aura or a prodrome, which is an indication of an impending seizure.

Status epilepticus are seizures that last longer than 20 minutes or the experience of subsequent seizures before the individual has fully regained consciousness from a preceding seizure. It is a medical emergency commonly due to the abrupt withdrawal of antiseizure medications. Without intervention, brain damage may occur.

More than 2 million people in the United States have epilepsy, which is one of the most common chronic neurological disorders. Seizures occur before the age of 20 in 75% of individuals. They decline through adolescence, plateau in middle age, and rise among the elderly.

Improvements in diagnostic technology, such as magnetic resonance imaging or computed tomography, have led to earlier diagnosis and treatment of head injuries, tumors, and brain infections, saving those whose condition often led to seizures. The death rate for those with epilepsy is two to four times the nonepileptic population. Ten percent of the deaths are due directly to the seizure, and 5% are due to fatal accidents during the seizure.

Seizures have different etiologies often related to an individual's age. Seizures in infancy commonly result from birth injury or congenital defects, trauma, or infection. Idiopathic and fever-related seizures most often occur in childhood. In middle-aged adults, seizures commonly result from mass lesions such as trauma and tumors.

Metabolic disturbances that precipitate seizures include acidosis, electrolyte disturbances, hypoglycemia, hypoxia, alcohol and barbiturate withdrawal, dehydration, and water intoxication. Extracranial disorders associated with seizures include heart, lung, liver, and kidney disease; diabetes; and hypertension. Cerebral inflammation that occurs with infection or injury and structural lesions such as tumors or scars can cause seizures. Cerebrovascular disorders are a common cause of seizures in the elderly.

Seizures may also be precipitated by environmental stimuli including loud noise or music, odors, or blinking lights. Hormonal fluctuations in women contribute to seizure activity.

> Seizures may also be precipitated by environmental stimuli including loud noise or music, odors, or blinking lights. Hormonal fluctuations in women contribute to seizure activity.

Pathophysiology

Normally, neurons discharge when an excitatory stimulus of sufficient magnitude alters membrane permeability, initiating an action potential. Inhibitory neurotransmitters prevent excitation. Mechanisms postulated as responsible for excessive firing of neurons in seizures include altered membrane ion channels, altered extracellular electrolytes, or imbalanced excitatory and inhibitory neurotransmitters. Some neurons are hypersensitive or remain in a partial state of depolarization. A genetic link has not been found for most seizures. In recurring epilepsy, abnormal neurons undergo spontaneous depolarization. The firing may spread by physiological pathways to involve adjacent or distant areas or the whole brain.

Manifestations

Cerebral neurons control motor, sensory, autonomic, and psychic functions and are involved with conscious awareness. The clinical manifestations of a seizure reflect the functions of the neurons that are abnormally discharging. The International Classification of Epileptic Seizures is a commonly used classification system based on location and manifestations (Figure 15-1).

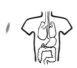

INFECTIOUS MENINGITIS

Aseptic meningitis, a noncontagious, relatively benign, self-limiting form, refers to viral meningitis or cases of meningeal irritation from a

Figure 15-1 International Classification of Epileptic Seizures.

International Classification of Epileptic Seizures

I. Partial Seizures (Focal Seizures)—Initially, only a restricted area of one hemisphere is activated; subdivided into simple partial and complex partial. Originate from cortex.
   a. Simple Partial (consciousness is preserved, may become generalized)
      1. With motor signs—involves precentral gyrus/primary motor area; usually clonic movements
        — without "jacksonian march," focal motor activity does not extend into adjacent areas
        — with "jacksonian march," focal motor activity extend into adjacent areas, same side
        — adversive—turning of hand, eyes opposite to irritative focus
      2. With somatosensory signs (e.g., paresthesias [tingling, burning]) or special sensory symptoms (visual, hearing, gustatory, olfactory) involves postcentral gyrus/primary sensory area.
      3. With autonomic symptoms or signs (e.g., sweating, flushing, pupil dilation, abnormal epigastric sensations).
      4. With psychic symptoms (usually accompanied by impairment of consciousness) affective disturbance, illusions, hallucinations, "déjà vu."
      5. Adversive—Head, eyes turn to opposite side of irritative focus, involves frontal lobe, anterior to primary motor area, may generalize.
   b. Complex Partial (formerly Temporal Lobe or Psychomotor Seizures)—Impairment of consciousness.
      1. Simple Partial onset followed by impaired consciousness, with or without automatisms (i.e., lip smacking, grimacing, patting, picking).
      2. Impaired consciousness from the beginning with or without automatisms.
   c. Partial Seizures, Secondarily Generalized—Begin in unilateral hemisphere then spread bilaterally; unconsciousness appears, generalized symptoms are produced.
II. Generalized Seizures—Begin with epileptic activity over entire cortex. Bilateral and multifocal. They originate from deep in the cortex. There is loss of consciousness and no aura.
   a. Absence seizures (formerly petit mal)—Children 4 years old until puberty; abrupt cessation of activity; momentary unconsciousness; eyes vacant and roll or stare, lips droop; sometimes mild tonic, clonic, or atonic activity; abrupt onset and termination.
   b. Myoclonic—Sudden, uncontrolled, shock-like jerking movement, single or successive; consciousness thought to be preserved.
   c. Tonic—Sudden sustained tone, frequently extensor or flexor posturing; may be accompanied by a shrill cry.
   d. Clonic—Repetitive, relatively symmetrical, bilateral, synchronous, rhythmic jerking with diminishing frequency.
   e. Tonic-Clonic (formerly grand mal)—Occasionally has a prodromal period, though usually without warning
      1. Tonic phase begins with sudden loss of consciousness, brief body flexion, body stiffness, opisthotonos posture, jaw snaps shut, shrill cry as respiratory muscles stiffen, bladder and, less often, bowel may evacuate, apneic, pupils dilated, and unresponsive. Tonic phase lasts less than 1 minute, average 10–15 seconds.
      2. Clonic phase is characterized by flexion spasms of the whole body alternating with relaxation, strenuous hyperventilation, face contorted, eyes roll, excessive salivation, profuse sweating, rapid pulse; tongue may be bitten. Clonic activity subsides over about 30 seconds.
      3. Usually stupor or coma follows for 5 minutes, with quiet breathing, limpness, pupils responsive. The entire seizure lasts 2 to 5 minutes.

f. Postictal—May be confused, disoriented, and have headache, muscle aches, and fatigue. He or she may not remember the event.
g. Atonic ("drop attack")—Sudden brief loss of muscle tone, mild to dramatic head nod to fall.

Subcategories include

- Idiopathic—Most common, no obvious underlying cause or pathophysiological alteration except presumed genetic predisposition
- Symptomatic—Occurs as a result of a cerebral disorder
- Cryptogenic—Suspect symptomatic despite absence of proof of cause

nonbacterial source such as blood in the subarachnoid space. Septic meningitis, which is also called *purulent meningitis* or *community acquired meningitis,* refers to **bacterial meningitis** (usually accompanied by an underlying encephalitis). Bacterial meningitis is contagious through respiratory droplets and is the most common and most deadly form. Individuals who acquire the organism and do not develop the disease can become carriers.

Bacterial meningitis is contagious through respiratory droplets and is the most common and most deadly form.

Risk factors for meningitis include extremes of age, debilitation, splenectomy, sickle cell disease, alcoholism, liver disease, upper respiratory infections, sinusitis, otitis media, pneumonia, diabetes, immunosuppression, ventricular shunt, cerebrospinal fluid (CSF) fistula, lumbar puncture, and neurosurgical procedures.

Meningitis usually occurs in fall, winter, or early spring secondary to respiratory illnesses.

Pathophysiology

The main viruses involved in meningitis are the mumps, enteroviruses, herpes type 1, adenovirus, and California virus. Pathological organisms causing bacterial meningitis vary with age—group B streptococci, *Escherichia coli,* and *Listeria* in newborns; *Neisseria meningitidis* (meningococcus) in ages 2 through adolescence; *Haemophilus influenzae* in infants and school-aged children (usually after an otitis or upper respiratory infection); *Streptococcus pneumo-*

niae (pneumococcal) in those 4 years of age and older; staphylococcal and gram-negative bacteria after surgery or trauma; and gram-negative organisms in the elderly and those who are immunosuppressed. The incidence of *H. influenzae* meningitis has decreased since the development of the Hib vaccine.

Infections generally originate in three ways: through the bloodstream (bacteremia) as a consequence of other infections, commonly infections of the nasopharynx, lungs, or skin; contiguous extension (such as otitis, sinusitis); and direct inoculation through trauma, lumbar puncture, or cranial surgery. The infection then extends to the meninges, CSF, and quickly to the brain tissue. Once the infection has a portal of entry, it spreads quickly throughout the CSF and brain.

Acute inflammation causes meningeal irritation, disrupts the blood–brain barrier, and, in bacterial meningitis, causes white blood cells and protein to infiltrate the CSF. Edema and obstruction can cause increased intracranial pressure (ICP), reduced cerebral blood flow, ischemia, and death.

> Acute inflammation causes meningeal irritation, disrupts the blood–brain barrier, and, in bacterial meningitis, causes white blood cells and protein to infiltrate the CSF. Edema and obstruction can cause increased intracranial pressure, reduced cerebral blood flow, ischemia, and death.

Complications include visual or hearing impairment, seizures, paralysis, hydrocephalus, and septic shock.

Manifestations

Symptoms may include fever, a progressively worsening headache often accompanied by nausea and vomiting, stiff neck, rash (with meningococcal meningitis), somnolence or irritability, photophobia, seizures, blurred vision, numbness, and weakness.

Examination may reveal fever, decreased level of consciousness, nuchal rigidity, **Brudzinski's** and **Kernig's signs,** cranial nerve palsies, focal neurological deficits, and rashes.

Treatment

Meningitis is treated with appropriate antibiotics and antiviral agents. Management of increased ICP is crucial. Vaccinations exist for meningococcal, pneumococcal, and *H. influenzae* meningitis.

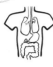

ENCEPHALITIS

Pathophysiology

The most common viruses that cause encephalitis are the arthropod-borne arboviruses and the herpes simplex type 1 virus. The arthropod-borne viruses occur in epidemics that vary by geographical region. Encephalitis may also be caused by bacterial infections, rickettsia, parasites, or fungal infections. It can also occur as a secondary complication in the presence of mononucleosis, rabies, and less commonly with malaria, typhus, or postviral infection due to rubella or rubeola. Of late, it has had an increased incidence from arthropod-borne (mosquito) infections. It can result from attenuated virus vaccines such as mumps, measles, and rubella vaccine. Toxoplasmosis, cytomegalovirus, and herpes simplex virus encephalitis are common opportunistic infections in AIDS.

Encephalitis can range from a mild self-limiting infection to a life-threatening disorder. Meningeal involvement occurs in all encephalitides. Large, degenerative injuries are found in arthropod-borne viral encephalitis that causes widespread nerve cell degeneration, edema, and areas of necrosis.

Manifestations

Manifestations may be similar to meningitis but with a more gradual onset. The manifestations are high fever, delirium or confusion progressing to unconsciousness, seizures, cranial nerve palsies, paresis and paralysis, involuntary movements, and abnormal reflexes. Signs of increased ICP may be present.

Treatment

Treatment is supportive, with control of ICP being paramount.

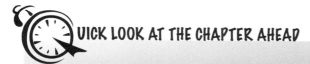
Any trauma to the head (skull, scalp, or brain) increases the risk of damage to the underlying structures and the potential for permanent damage or death. Some initial injuries are very apparent, while the extent of other injuries may not be obvious for several days after the incident.

16

Trauma to the Nervous System

TERMS
- [ ] autonomic hyperreflexia
- [ ] concussion
- [ ] contusion
- [ ] coup-countrecoup injury
- [ ] diffuse axonal injury
- [ ] spinal shock

Figure 16-1 Types of head injury.

Scalp Injuries

Abrasion, contusion, laceration, hematoma; bleed profusely, portal of entry if dura involved

Skull Fractures (with or without brain damage)

Types of Fractures
- Linear—May cross blood vessels
- Comminuted
- Depressed
- Basilar
- Open—Potential for brain infection if dura is torn
- Closed—No tear in dura
- Fractures at base of skull tend to traverse paranasal sinuses of frontal bone or middle ear; thus they may produce hemorrhage from nose, ears, and pharynx, and blood may appear under conjunctiva, behind tympanic membrane, periorbital ecchymosis/edema, Battle's sign (i.e., ecchymosis over mastoid).
- Basal skull fracture suspected when cerebrospinal fluid (CSF) leaks from ears (i.e., CSF otorrhea) or nose (i.e., CSF rhinorrhea).
- Check CSF; if clear, check for glucose (present in CSF) and if blood, check for halo; potential for infection; if leakage of CSF, keep ears/nose clean, do not blow nose/sneeze, DO NOT PACK, do not perform nasal suctioning.

Brain Injury (seemingly minor injury can cause serious brain damage)

Concussion
- Temporary loss of neurological function without apparent structural damage, generally involves brief decrease in loss of consciousness (LOC), can produce bizarre behavior (frontal lobe) or temporary amnesia (temporal lobe), can produce postconcussion syndrome (headache, dizzy, lethargy, irritability, anxiety, personality/behavioral changes, memory/attention deficit)
- Emergency department discharge instructions—Observe for difficulty awakening, difficulty speaking, confusion, severe headache, vomiting, one-sided weakness

Contusion
- Brain is bruised, possible surface hemorrhage
- Unconscious for period of time
- Manifestations depend on extent of injury and cerebral edema if widespread; poor outcome (brain damage/death) if residual headache, vertigo, impaired mental function, seizures persist

Diffuse Axonal Injury
- No lucid interval, immediate coma, abnormal posturing, global cerebral edema

Laceration
- Intracranial hemorrhage—Manifestations depend on location and speed; if rapid, may be fatal
- Epidural injury involves middle meningeal artery, temporal and basilar fractures, decrease LOC—lucid interval—then decreasing LOC with rapid deterioration, extreme emergency
- Subdural more frequently venous bleed
- Acute subdural hematomas are associated with major head injury, develop over 24 to 48 hours, and are signs of a rapidly developing mass and increasing intracranial pressure (ICP)

- Subacute subdural hematoma is less severe; manifestations appear within 48 hours to 2 weeks
- Chronic subdural hematoma is from a seemingly minor head injury, sometimes forgotten, in the elderly due to atrophy; may present like stroke; may occur 3 weeks to months after injury; clot absorbs fluid and expands slowly
- Intracerebral hemorrhage or hematoma is common when force has been over a small area (e.g., gunshot or stab wound)

Complications
- Cerebral edema/increased ICP (swelling peaks at 48 to 72 hours), impaired LOC, impaired ventilation, diabetes insipidus, syndrome of inappropriate secretion of antidiuretic hormone (impaired fluid balance), CSF fistulas, infections, and seizures

Spinal Cord Injury Syndromes

Syndrome	Area/Cause of Injury	Characteristics
Central cord syndrome	Injury or edema in central cord area, usually cervical	Motor deficits (>upper extremities) Sensory loss varies (>upper extremities) Bowel/bladder function is variable
Anterior cord syndrome	Injuries caused by the following: Hyperflexion Fractures/dislocations Disc herniation Injury to anterior spinal artery	Pain, temperature, motor loss below the level of lesion Light touch, vibration, position sensations intact
Brown-Séquard's syndrome (lateral cord syndrome)	Transection or lesion of one-half of the spinal cord Usually penetrating injury or acute ruptured disc	Ipsilateral paresis or paralysis Ipsilateral loss and touch, pressure, and vibration sensations Contralateral loss of pain and temperature sensations

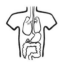

HEAD TRAUMA

Head injury includes injury to the scalp, skull, or brain. The major risk in head injury is damage to the brain from bleeding, swelling, and increasing intracranial pressure (ICP), with the potential for disability or death.

Two million head injuries occur each year in the United States, and approximately 75,000 to 100,000 patients die of the injury. Seventy thousand to 90,000 injuries are severe enough to cause permanent brain dysfunction. Most deaths are immediate from direct trauma, massive hemorrhage, and shock. Deaths may occur within a few hours from progressive bleeding or within weeks from multisystem failure.

The major causes of head injury are due to motor vehicle accidents (50%), falls (21%), assaults (12%), and sports injuries (10%). Firearms-related head injuries are increasing. Two-thirds of head injuries are in individuals younger than 30 years old, with males outnumbering females 3:1. The second highest incidence is among the elderly.

The incidence of head injuries has been reduced due to recent safety guidelines and public awareness of the importance of wearing helmets during sports, installation of air bags in automobiles, and use of passive seat restraints.

Pathophysiology

The brain is protected from external injuries by hair, skin, and the skull. Damage to the brain occurs as a result of compression of the skull from impact, which compromises integrity of the bone. The amount of damage depends on the force of the injury.

> Head injuries are divided into two categories: primary or direct injuries (damage is caused by the impact) and secondary injuries that result in brain swelling, infection, and hypoxia of the cerebral tissue.

Head injuries are divided into two categories: primary or direct injuries (damage is caused by the impact) and secondary injuries that result in brain swelling, infection, and hypoxia of the cerebral tissue. Head injuries are also referred to as *closed* or *blunt trauma* and *open* or *penetrating trauma*.

Mechanisms of trauma include deformation, acceleration-deceleration as seen in **coup-countercoup injury,** and **diffuse axonal injury.** The injuries may be insignificant or may lead to poor outcomes. Factors predictive of poor outcomes include intracranial hematoma, increasing age, abnormal motor signs, impaired or absent eye movements or pupil reflexes, early sustained hypotension, hypoxemia/hypercapnia, and ICP > 20 mm Hg. Scalp injuries such as abrasions, contusions, lacerations, and hematomas often bleed profusely, but most are benign and only significant if associated with meningeal tears.

Skull fractures occur with or without brain injury. The major complications of skull fractures are intracranial infections, bleeding and hematomas, meningeal tears, brain tissue damage, and increased ICP. The location of a fracture may be significant, as a basilar fracture generally crosses the paranasal sinuses in the frontal bone or the middle ear in the temporal bone, causing meningeal tears that result in cerebrospinal fluid (CSF) fistulas, increasing the risk of infection. In addition, blood may collect around the eyes or ears.

Injury to the brain can result in alteration of brain cell function or structural damage. **Concussion** involves a brief period of loss of consciousness due to temporarily altered function of brain cells. It may cause altered behavior or temporary amnesia, which is referred to as *postconcussion syndrome*, with headache, dizziness, irritability, and alterations in memory, attention span, and personality that can last for months. It may also be the beginning of a more serious and progressive problem such as intracranial bleeding.

Contusion, or bruising of brain tissue, results in a longer period of unconsciousness. It often involves a coup-countercoup injury. Its significance depends on the extent of the injury and the amount of cerebral edema. It is most often found in the frontal lobes and the inferior orbital surfaces

Diffuse axonal injury results in axonal swelling and disconnection that takes 12 to 24 hours to develop. It results in global cerebral edema, loss of consciousness, increased ICP, and decerebrate or decorticate posturing.

Secondary complications may occur with major primary head trauma. Hemorrhaging and hematomas (epidural, subdural, and intracerebral) may develop at various rates, creating an expanding, space-occupying mass that causes increasing ICP. Subdural hematomas can develop 48 hours to 2 weeks after the initial injury; they increase the ICP and cause compression of vessels. Temporary seizures may occur due to early inflammation. Later, seizures result from scarring of the damaged brain tissue. CSF fistulas that occur may be a factor in intracranial infections. Damage to the posterior pituitary can result in increased production of antidiuretic hormone, potentially causing syndrome of inappropriate antidiuretic hormone, or decreased production of antidiuretic hormone, resulting in diabetes insipidus.

 Subdural hematomas can develop 48 hours to 2 weeks after the initial injury; they increase the ICP and cause compression of vessels.

Manifestations

Indications of serious head trauma include signs of increasing ICP, such as altered or loss of consciousness, hemiplegia on the contralateral side, dilated pupil on the ipsilateral side, and alterations in ventilation and vital signs. CSF rhinorrhea or otorrhea may be evident. (CSF tests positive for glucose or will show a "halo" sign when blood is present). Blood behind the eardrum, also known as hemotympanum; periorbital ecchymosis or "raccoon eyes"; or blood over the mastoid (Battle's sign) all are indicative of basilar fractures. Seizure activity and indications of infection may be evident. Changes in the volume or tonicity of the urine or serum sodium levels indicate syndrome of inappropriate antidiuretic hormone and diabetes insipidus.

Treatment

Computed tomography or magnetic resonance imaging of the brain is used to diagnose the extent of injury. Treatment is directed at preserving brain homeostasis and preventing secondary complications. Cardiorespiratory function is stabilized to maintain cerebral blood flow. Hemorrhaging and increasing ICP are aggressively treated and often require surgery. Antibiotics and anticonvulsants may be used prophylactically or acutely.

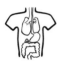

SPINAL CORD INJURY

Spinal cord injuries (SCI) result from vertebral injuries commonly involving cervical vertebrae 5, 6, and 7; thoracic vertebra 12; and lumbar vertebra 1. Partial to complete disruption of the neurons or nerve tracts can occur, resulting in loss of motor, sensory, and reflex activity and bowel and bladder control. Complications include **spinal shock, autonomic hyperreflexia,** and respiratory failure.

Approximately 10,000 to 20,000 serious SCIs occur each year in the United States. Males between the ages of 15 to 30 who experience motor vehicle accidents (55%), sports injuries (18%), and penetrating injuries from stab and gunshot wounds (15%) are at greatest risk. A high correlation exists between SCI and substance abuse. Accidental falls in the elderly account for 21% of SCIs.

Pathophysiology

There are two types of SCI: primary and secondary neurological injury. Primary injury is irreversible and occurs as a result of compression or shear associated with fracture or dislocation of the vertebrae. They occur at the time of the mechanical injury. Secondary injury begins after the primary injury due to the progression of tissue destruction in the neurons, vessel trauma, and hemorrhage causing ischemia and necrosis.

Acceleration, deceleration, or deformation forces compress, pull, or shear tissue or fracture bones. Structures may become displaced and slide into each other. The dura of the brain is rarely lacerated or transected, except in penetrating injuries. After an injury, however, hemorrhages, edema, and metabolic products cause ischemia, which in turn causes necrotic destruction of the spinal cord. After 48 hours, necrosis is complete, and the function of any nerves that arise in or pass through the area is lost. Edema extends the level of injury for up to a week, and it is at that time when the exact extent of damage can be determined.

High cervical or thoracic injuries initially cause spinal shock, lasting 7 to 10 days, and are characterized by decreased reflexes and flaccid paralysis below the level of injury, loss of bowel and bladder function, and loss of sympathetic stimulation (hypotension, bradycardia, loss of sweating). Spasticity, reflex emptying of the bladder, and hyperreflexia indicate the end of spinal shock. Autonomic hyperreflexia, most likely with lesions at T6 or above, is associated with massive uncompensated cardiovascular response to stimulation. The resulting hypertension and cardiac stimulation may cause cerebral vascular accident or death.

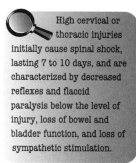
High cervical or thoracic injuries initially cause spinal shock, lasting 7 to 10 days, and are characterized by decreased reflexes and flaccid paralysis below the level of injury, loss of bowel and bladder function, and loss of sympathetic stimulation.

The degree of injury may be complete or partial. Complete cervical injuries lead to quadriplegia, and complete thoracic and lumber injuries lead to paraplegia. Three syndromes, related to which nerve tracts are damaged, are associated with incomplete

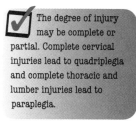
The degree of injury may be complete or partial. Complete cervical injuries lead to quadriplegia and complete thoracic and lumber injuries lead to paraplegia.

lesions: central (cervical) cord syndrome, anterior cord syndrome, and Brown-Séquard's syndrome (lateral cord syndrome) (see p. 131).

Manifestations

Manifestations are related to the level and degree of injury. Loss of voluntary motor and sensory function, spasticity, and hyperreflexia occur below the level of injury. Cervical injury above C4 results in loss of respiratory muscle function/ventilation. With injuries below C4, diaphragmatic breathing or hypoventilation occurs, and loss of abdominal muscle function decreases one's ability to cough. Injuries above T5 decrease influence of sympathetic stimulation of the cardiovascular system, causing bradycardia and hypotension. The bladder becomes distended as a result of urinary retention and bladder atony during spinal shock and then empties reflexively, causing incontinence. With cord injury above T5, the primary gastrointestinal problem is hypomotility with distention and potential for development of an ileus. Gallstones, constipation, and fecal impaction may also become problematic. Immobility and spasticity cause contractures and decubitus. Deep vein thrombosis and pulmonary emboli are common.

Treatment

Diagnosis is based on physical examination, computed tomography or magnetic resonance imaging, and immobilization of spine. Treatment is aimed at maintaining neurological function. Decompression and surgical fixation may be necessary. Corticosteroids may be used to decrease inflammation. Respiratory, nutrition, skin, and elimination status need to be addressed. Prompt treatment of autonomic hyperreflexia involves removing the stimulus, elevating the head of the bed, and using antihypertensive medication.

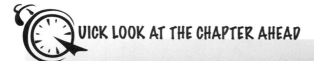

Cerebrovascular accident (CVA), also called **stroke** or **brain attack**, is a focal neurological disorder that develops suddenly because of a pathological process involving the blood vessels to the brain. A CVA may result in disruption of motor, sensory, cognitive, and emotional function that can range from minor to severe disability and death.

17

Cerebrovascular Accident

TERMS
- [ ] ataxia
- [ ] dysarthria
- [ ] dysphagia
- [ ] hemiparesis
- [ ] hemiplegia

The two major types of stroke are ischemic stroke (75%), which results from vessel occlusion due to atherosclerosis, thrombosis, or embolism, and hemorrhagic stroke (15%), which results from bleeding into the brain tissue (intracerebral) or into the subarachnoid space due to hypertension, tumor, vascular malformations, or bleeding disorders due to anticoagulant therapy. Lacunar strokes, also known as a small vessel stroke, occur in smaller arteries and are associated with hypertension and diabetes mellitus. They are more likely to cause motor and sensory deficits.

> CVA, also called **stroke** or **brain attack**, is a focal neurological disorder that develops suddenly because of a pathological process involving the blood vessels to the brain. A CVA may result in disruption of motor, sensory, cognitive, and emotional function that can range from minor to severe disability and death.

   CVA remains the third leading cause of death and is the major cause of disability in the United States, despite a general decline. What has probably contributed to the decline is an increased awareness of risk

Table 17-1 Types of Strokes

Stroke	Cause	Course of Progression
Thrombotic or central	Atherosclerosis Arteritis Increased coagulation	Sudden or slow progression, minutes to hours
Embolic	Obstruction of vessel causing ischemia Atrial fibrillation or rheumatic heart disease Recent myocardial infarction Valve replacement Air or fat emboli	Sudden onset of hemiplegia
Hemorrhagic	Hypertension Trauma Ruptured aneurysm Vascular malformations Anticoagulation	Sudden onset of vomiting while active Headache Contralateral hemiplegia Coma leading to death
Lacunar	Occlusion of smaller branches Large cerebral arteries Hypertension, embolism	"Lacunar syndrome" includes pure motor and sensory hemiplegia and dysarthria

factors, improved prophylactic measures such as therapeutic life-style changes, improvements in pharmaceutical therapies, and surveillance of those at risk.

The risk of CVA increases with a correlating number of risk factors. The incidence of ischemic CVA, the most common type, increases with age until age 75; however, the incidence of subarachnoid hemorrhage is higher in young adults. The overall incidence in men is higher than women, although the incidence in women increases after menopause. CVAs tend to have a familial component. The incidence of CVA among African Americans is twice that of whites, with greater morbidity and mortality. The higher occurrence of CVAs among African Americans may be due to their increased incidence of hypertension, which is the most important modifiable risk factor for all types. Smoking increases the risk two to five times, but risk declines to normal 4 to 5 years after smoking cessation. Obesity, high dietary saturated fat, sedentary life-style, excessive alcohol consumption, diabetes, dyslipidemia, atherosclerosis, and recent myocardial infarction are all risk factors. A history of CVA is considered a risk factor for development of future CVAs. Atrial fibrillation and valvular disorders, hypercoagulability states such as oral contraception (especially in women who smoke), sickle cell disease, and polycythemia are risk factors for embolic stroke.

Risk factors for hemorrhagic CVAs include hypertension, smoking, sickle cell disease, coagulopathies, iatrogenic anticoagulation, aneurysms, arteriovenous malformations, and alcohol, cocaine, and amphetamine abuse.

PATHOPHYSIOLOGY

Ischemic CVAs usually result from blockage of a major artery by a thrombus forming on an atherosclerotic plaque, which is known as an *atherothrombotic stroke*. Rupture of a plaque that has been developing for years leads to clot formation. Dehydration, shock, hypotension, and vasospasm can increase the risk of thrombogenesis.

Thrombotic strokes are usually subdivided into *transient ischemic attack* (TIA), *stroke-in-evolution*, and *completed stroke*. TIAs probably represent microemboli from atherosclerotic plaque in extracerebral arteries, causing intermittent occlusion of vessels and temporary neurological deficits. TIAs may be prodromal (symptoms that precede onset and serve as a warning of an impending stroke). Symptoms of thrombotic strokes typically progress slowly over hours to days and, at this stage, are *strokes-in-evolution*. A completed stroke is a stroke that has reached its maximum destruction. The extent of the neurological damage may depend on collateral circulation. Thrombi can also develop in smaller arteries and are called *lacunar strokes*, in which the prognosis for recovery is usually good.

Ischemic strokes also develop from emboli originating in the heart (resulting from atrial fibrillation, myocardial infarction with aneurysm, valvular disease, or congestive heart failure) and can move into and block cerebral arteries, causing a *cardioembolic stroke*. Cardioembolic strokes generally have a rapid occurrence without prodromal symptoms.

These obstructive processes lead to ischemia and infarction. An area of central necrosis is surrounded by an area of diminished perfusion, the ischemic penumbra. The extent of damage depends on the rapidity of development, size of the lesion, and amount of collateral circulation. Spontaneous or therapeutic reperfusion can limit the size of the infarction.

Hemorrhagic strokes result from bleeding into the brain parenchyma or the subarachnoid space and can last from minutes to days. Intracerebral hemorrhage is most common in people with hypertension and atherosclerosis because the degenerative changes from these processes weaken the vessel wall, and the pressure causes rupture. In individuals less than 40 years old, aneurysms and arteriovenous malformations are responsible for the vessel rupture. The bleeding is usually arterial, occurs with activity, and is without prodromal symptoms.

Subarachnoid hemorrhages usually result from aneurysms or malformations of vessels in the circle of Willis that either suddenly rupture or slowly leak. There may be prodromal symptoms because of the pressure the aneurysm puts on surrounding structures.

Subarachnoid hemorrhages usually result from aneurysms or malformations of vessels in the circle of Willis that either suddenly rupture or slowly leak. There may be prodromal symptoms because of the pressure the aneurysm puts on surrounding structures.

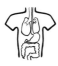

MANIFESTATIONS

The specific nature of the neurological deficit resulting from a CVA reflects the specific region of the brain perfused by the involved vessel and the amount of collateral circulation (see Figure 17-1, p. 142 for areas of brain related to behaviors). Manifestations include motor deficits, communication deficits, affective changes, intellectual deficits, and altered spatial-perceptual function. Typically, signs and symptoms peak within 72 hours as the edema in the area increases. After resolution of the edema, usually within 2 weeks, the signs and symptoms decrease. Typical manifestations are briefly discussed here.

Motor deficits on the contralateral side of the body occur if the CVA affects the motor cortex or pyramidal tracts and may involve voluntary movement, integration, tone, and reflexes. Contralateral weakness such as **hemiparesis** or **hemiplegia, ataxia, dysarthria,** and **dysphagia** may occur. Initial hyporeflexia progresses to hyperreflexia.

In most cases, communication deficits occur with a lesion in the left hemisphere, which is dominant for language. CVAs affecting Broca's motor speech area result in an inability to form words, verbally or in writing, that are understandable (expressive aphasia). CVAs of Wernicke's area impair the ability to comprehend the spoken or written language (receptive aphasia). Massive strokes may affect both expressive and receptive language (global aphasia).

A CVA of the right brain most often results in deficits of spatial-perceptual orientation. With lesions of the parietal area, the individual may have disturbances in visual-spatial relationships. He or she may deny sensory input from one side of his or her body. With lesions of the optic pathways, he or she may experience homonymous hemianopsia, which is blindness in corresponding halves of the visual fields of both eyes on the same side as any motor loss. Sensory losses may involve any modality or the inability to interpret visual, tactile, or auditory stimuli. This is known as agnosia. Paresthesias (numbness, tingling, burning) may occur on the side opposite the lesion.

 A CVA of the right brain most often results in deficits of spatial-perceptual orientation.

Figure 17-1 Neurologic deficits of stroke: Manifestations.

Neurologic Deficit	Manifestation
Visual Field Deficits	
Homonymous hemianopsia (loss of half of the visual feild)	• Unaware of persons or objects on side of visual loss • Neglect on one side of the body • Dificulty judging distances
Loss of peripheral vision	• Difficulty seeing at night • Unaware of objects or the borders of objects
Diplopia	• Double vision
Motor Deficits	
Hemiparesis	• Weakness of the face, arm, and leg on the same side (due to a lesion in the opposite hemiphere)
Hemiplegia	• Paralysis of the face, arm, and leg on the same side (due to a lesion in the opposite hemisphere)
Ataxia	• Staggering, unsteady gait • Unable to keep feet together; needs a broad base to stand
Dysarthria	• Difficulty forming words
Dysphagia	• Difficulty swallowing
Sensory Deficits	
Paresthesia (occurs on the side opposite of the lesion)	• Numbness and tingling of body parts • Difficulty with proprioception
Verbal Deficits	
Expressive aphasia	• Unable to form words that are understandable; may be able to speak in single-word responses
Receptive aphasia	• Unable to comprehend the spoken word; can speak but may not make sense
Global aphasia	• Combination of both receptive and expressive aphasia
Cognitive Deficits	
	• Short- and long-term memory loss • Decreased attention span • Impaired ability to concentrate • Poor abstract reasoning

Reproduced with permission from Smeltzer, S.C., & Bare, B.G. (1999). *Brunner and Suddarth's textbook of medical-surgical nursing* (9th ed.). Philidelphia, PA: Lippincott, Williams & Wilkins.

Damage to the frontal lobe may result in cognitive impairment, such as diminished learning capacity, memory attention span, or other intellectual functions. The individual may be prone to inappropriate outbursts because he or she is unable to control his or her emotions.

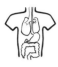

TREATMENT

A computed tomography or magnetic resonance imaging is primarily used to diagnose a CVA. If used with contrast medium and angiography within 24 hours of the onset of symptoms, it can indicate the location and size of the CVA and differentiate between an infarction and a hemorrhage. Other diagnostic tests used are positron emission tomography, digital subtraction angiography, and carotid ultrasound. Laboratory profiles include complete blood count, erythrocyte sedimentation rate, prothrombin time/partial thromboplastin time, electrolytes, liver function tests, and a lipid profile.

Measures to prevent stroke include prevention of thrombosis with daily use of platelet aggregation inhibitors and surgical procedures such as endarterectomy and angioplasty to clear vessels.

Acute care includes control of arterial blood pressure and intracranial pressure. Thrombolytic, anticoagulant, and antiplatelet drugs may be used in ischemic strokes. Surgical decompression may be needed in hemorrhagic stroke, and antifibrinolytic drugs may be needed to prevent rebleeding. Aneurysms and arteriovenous malformations may be surgically repaired.

Parkinson's disease is a common degenerative disorder of the basal ganglia involving the dopaminergic (dopamine-secreting) substantia nigra pathway. It is a slowly progressive disease generally diagnosed in late middle-aged and elderly persons. Parkinsonism is a term applied to the resulting movement disorders, such as poverty of movement, stiffness, tremors, and altered posture. Multiple sclerosis (MS) is a chronic progressive disease diffusely affecting neurons of the central nervous system. It is an acquired primary demyelinating disorder. Without myelin, nerve impulses slow down.

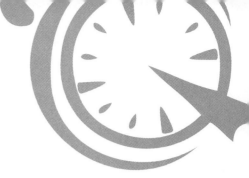

18

Degenerative Disorders of the Nervous System

TERMS
- [ ] akinesia
- [ ] festinating gait
- [ ] hypokinesia/ bradykinesia

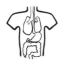

PARKINSON'S DISEASE

Parkinson's disease is an idiopathic primary disease. Secondary parkinsonism is caused by disorders from trauma, postencephalitic parkinsonism infection, neoplasm, and toxins. Drug-induced parkinsonism is caused by some drugs such as reserpine, methyldopa, haloperidol, and phenothiazine and is usually reversible.

Parkinson's disease is one of the most prevalent of the primary central nervous system problems and a major cause of disability in individuals over the age of 65. An estimated 500,000 individuals in the United States are affected. Men and women are affected equally. African Americans are rarely affected.

Pathophysiology

The pathology of Parkinson's disease is associated with the loss of dopamine-producing cells in the substantia nigra in the midbrain, causing depletion of dopamine in the basal ganglia. The basal ganglia include the extrapyramidal system, which influences coordination, muscle tone, initiation, and completion of movement. It is thought that aging may predispose to this damage. A significant reduction in dopamine receptors in the basal ganglia has also been found. Dopamine is an inhibitory neurotransmitter that is necessary for the normal functioning of the extrapyramidal motor system. The depletion of dopaminergic activity leaves a relative excess of cholinergic activity. Acetylcholine is an excitatory neurotransmitter. It is postulated that an imbalance between inhibitory dopaminergic activity and excitatory cholinergic activity causes abnormalities in movement commonly associated with Parkinson's disease.

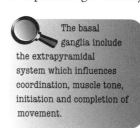

The basal ganglia include the extrapyramidal system which influences coordination, muscle tone, initiation and completion of movement.

Manifestations

The classic manifestations of Parkinson's disease are tremors, rigidity, **akinesia,** and postural abnormalities. These manifestations may develop alone or in combination, but all four are usually present as the disease progresses. The onset of the disease is insidious, with a gradual progression and long course. It is usually 15 to 20 years before it produces invalidism. Cognitive-affective symptoms may also be a part of the disease and manifest as deterioration in memory or problem solving.

Initially, only a mild tremor, slight limp, and decreased arm swing may be evident. The tremor is usually the first manifestation. Initially, tremors are asymmetrical and later become symmetrical. They involve the arm more than the leg. The hand tremor is described as "pin rolling." Tremors occur at rest, disappear with movement, and are aggravated with stress.

The first symptom of rigidity may be painful muscle cramps in the toes or hands. The rigidity has a jerky quality to it and is often called *cogwheel rigidity*. It causes sore, achy, tired muscles and slow movement.

Akinesia may be the most crippling of all manifestations. All striated muscles are affected—trunk, ocular, and facial (including muscles of chewing, swallowing, blinking, expression, speaking) and swinging of the arms. A mask-like expression is common. Akinetic movements include **hypokinesia/bradykinesia.** The facial expression looks blank, and speech is slow and monotonous.

The individual with Parkinson's disease has a flexed leaning-forward posture. Equilibrium is off, and the individual has a shuffling gait (short accelerating steps), known as **festinating gait,** in an attempt to remain upright.

Because of the connection of the basal ganglia to the hypothalamus, there may also be autonomic and neuroendocrine manifestations. Autonomic and neuroendocrine manifestations include inappropriate diaphoresis, heat intolerance, excessive salivation, orthostatic hypotension, gastric retention, constipation, urinary retention, and seborrheic dermatitis.

> Autonomic and neuroendocrine manifestations include inappropriate diaphoresis, heat intolerance, excessive salivation, orthostatic hypotension, gastric retention, constipation, urinary retention, and seborrheic dermatitis.

Fifty percent of individuals with Parkinson's disease have endogenous depression. In the early stages of the disease, mental status is preserved, but 30% of those affected develop dementia later.

Diagnosis and Treatment

Diagnosis of Parkinson's disease is based on clinical presentation and findings. It is important to exclude causes of secondary parkinsonism. Although there are no definitive diagnostic tests, computed tomography or magnetic resonance imaging may reveal the pigmented cells of the substantia nigra progressively degenerating, resulting in dopamine depletion. A trial of levodopa (L-dopa) is recommended to determine a therapeutic response.

There is no cure for Parkinson's disease, so therapy is directed toward controlling symptoms. Pharmacological agents attempt to correct the imbalance of neuroreceptors by either enhancing the supply of dopamine with dopaminergic drugs or decreasing the supply of acetylcholine with anticholinergic drugs. Current research is being directed at stem cell therapy, pallidotomy, thalamotomy, and deep brain stimulation. Deep brain stimulation is currently the primary surgical intervention for those afflicted with Parkinson's disease. Supportive therapies include targeted exercises to improve balance and to maintain coordination.

MULTIPLE SCLEROSIS

Multiple scleriosis (MS) is the most prevalent central nervous system demyelinating disorder and a leading cause of neurological disability in young adults. The onset of MS is usually between the ages of 20 and 50 years. It is a relatively common disorder with approximately 250,000 to 350,000 individuals in the United States diagnosed with the disease annually. It is more prevalent in temperate climates than it is in the tropics. The ratio of males to females is 1:2. It occurs in all races but is more prevalent in whites. Fifteen percent of affected individuals have a relative with the disease.

Pathophysiology

MS is an acquired disease, and its cause is unknown. Most theories suggest that MS is related to infectious (viral) or immunological disease, but susceptibility to MS appears to be inherited. MS is characterized by chronic inflammation, demyelination, and scarring scattered diffusely in the central nervous system. The primary pathological mechanism is an immune-mediated inflammatory process that damages myelin-producing cells, causing demyelinization of the white matter of the

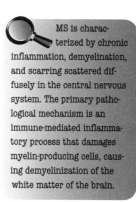
MS is characterized by chronic inflammation, demyelination, and scarring scattered diffusely in the central nervous system. The primary pathological mechanism is an immune-mediated inflammatory process that damages myelin-producing cells, causing demyelinization of the white matter of the brain.

brain. Suggested possible precipitating factors include infection, physical injury, stress, excessive fatigue, pregnancy, and poor state of health.

The onset of the disease is often insidious and gradual. Early in the disease the myelin sheath is damaged, but the nerve fiber is preserved and can transmit impulses. This is thought to be caused by an autoimmune reaction, which instigates the initial inflammatory reaction. Once the inflammation resolves, diffuse lesions and plaques form along the sheath, causing demyelinization. The plaques form in the early stages of the disease and progress to coalescing plaques and scarring of the axons, which cause loss of motor function. In the early stages of the disease the individual may complain of some weakness. The myelin can regenerate, symptoms disappear, and a remission occurs. As the disease continues, however, the myelin sheath is destroyed and is replaced by diffuse lesions and sclerotic plaques in multiple regions of the brain. Eventually, the neurons are destroyed. Without myelin, nerve impulses slow down and with nerve destruction they are totally blocked. Because of the scattered nature of the lesions, the loss of function varies.

Manifestations

The course and type of manifestations of MS vary among individuals. A classification scheme has been developed that identifies the various courses that the disease may take. Usually, individuals with MS initially have a predominant syndrome or grouping of manifestations depending on the area involved. Fifty percent of the individuals develop multiple manifestations, depending on the individual and the progression of the disease.

Common manifestations include motor, sensory, cerebellar, and emotional problems. Motor symptoms include weakness or paralysis of the limbs, trunk, or head; diplopia; scanning speech; and spasticity of muscles. Sensory symptoms include numbness, tingling, and other paresthesias; patchy blindness; blurred vision; red–green color deficiencies; decreased pupillary reflex; optic neuritis; vertigo; tinnitus; and decreased hearing. Cerebellar symptoms include nystagmus, ataxia, dysarthria (difficulty pronouncing words), and dysphagia.

Decreased intestinal motility results in constipation. The individual may develop a spastic bladder (frequency, urgency, dribbling, incontinence) or a flaccid bladder (retention) depending on the location of the lesion. Sexual dysfunction such as erectile problems, decreased libido, or painful intercourse may occur, although MS has no apparent effects on pregnancy.

Intellectual function is generally preserved, although there may be some problems with memory, attention, and word finding. Emotional stability may be affected. Mood alterations are common, with depression occurring more than euphoria.

Diagnosis and Treatment

Diagnosis is usually based on symptomatology and neurological episodes reported by the patient. Magnetic resonance imaging with gadolinium may reveal plaques, although the use of gadolinium is contraindicated in those with certain diseases, including kidney disease. Cerebrospinal fluid immunoglobulin G electrophoresis is also helpful in determining the presence of leukocytes and protein, which are associated with the disease.

Drug therapy is aimed at treating the disease process and providing symptomatic relief. Adrenocorticotropic hormone, glucocorticoids, and immunosuppressive drugs are used in treating acute episodes. Muscle relaxants are used for reducing spasticity. Physical and speech therapy may also be helpful.

PART IV · QUESTIONS

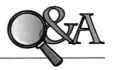

1. What is the role of myelin that surrounds the axon of the neuron?
   a. Protection from injury
   b. Nourish the cell body
   c. Provide energy
   d. Speed transmission of impulse

2. Where do motor fibers originating in the precentral gyrus cross to the other side of the body?
   a. At the level of the spinal segment at which they emerge from the spinal cord
   b. At the level of the medulla
   c. One or two segments above the level at which they emerge
   d. One or two segments below the level at which they emerge

3. From what area of the brain do the cell bodies of the third cranial nerve originate?
   a. Medulla
   b. Cerebellum
   c. Midbrain
   d. Frontal lobe

4. Which of the following statements regarding the autonomic nervous system is *correct?*
   a. Acetylcholine is the neurotransmitter of the sympathetic nervous system.
   b. β_1 Receptors are found in the myocardium.
   c. Stimulation of α_1 receptors causes vasodilation of the arterioles.
   d. Pupil dilation is a result of parasympathetic stimulation.

5. Which of the following is the earliest compensatory mechanism for increasing intracranial pressure?
   a. Increased systemic blood pressure due to systemic arterial vasoconstriction
   b. Displacement of cerebrospinal fluid (CSF) into the spinal column
   c. Vasodilation of intracranial arteries
   d. Herniation of brain tissue

6. The nurse is caring for a patient who sustained a head injury in a motor vehicle accident. In her assessment of the patient, the nurse should keep in mind that one of the earliest signs of increased intracranial pressure in a supratentorial lesion is what?
   a. Pupillary changes
   b. Changes in the level of consciousness
   c. Respiratory pattern alterations
   d. Widened pulse pressure and tachycardia

7. Which of the following changes in vital signs occurs in the late decompensation stage of increased intracranial pressure?
   a. Rapid respirations
   b. Slow pulse
   c. Widening pulse pressure
   d. Rapid pulse

8. What does a loss of consciousness during a seizure indicate?
   a. An infection is causing the seizure
   b. That the locus of seizure activity is in the frontal lobe
   c. That the seizure activity involves both hemispheres of the brain
   d. The individual has status epilepticus

9. The individual with bacterial meningitis may present with which of the following manifestations?
   a. Decreased body temperature
   b. Decreased blood pressure
   c. Edema of the eyelids
   d. Stiff neck

10. Clinical manifestations of bacterial meningitis include which of the following?
   a. Fever, swollen tongue, and diminished level of consciousness
   b. Photophobia, elevated blood pressure, and skin rash
   c. Fever, stiff neck, and diminished level of consciousness
   d. Diminished level of consciousness, nausea, and low body temperature (hypothermia)

11. Which of the following is included among the complications of meningitis?
   a. Septic shock, hearing loss, and hydrocephalus
   b. Chronic pain, cardiac dysrhythmias, and seizures
   c. Visual loss, paralysis, and arthritis
   d. Seizures, hydrocephalus, and arthritis

12. In what way do subdural hematomas differ from epidural hematomas?
  a. Subdural hematomas result from arterial damage, thus bleeding forcefully and occurring rapidly.
  b. Subdural hematomas exhibit a classic picture of momentary loss of consciousness, lucid interval, and rapid deterioration.
  c. Subdural hematomas should be suspected if the individual has a fracture that crosses the middle meningeal artery.
  d. Subdural hematomas may develop weeks to months after a head injury.

13. The patient who sustained a head injury now has clear fluid dripping from his nose that tests positive for glucose. The nurse suspects that the patient has which of the following complications of head injury?
  a. Meningitis
  b. Syndrome of inappropriate secretion of antidiuretic hormone
  c. CSF fistula
  d. Damage to the hypothalamus

14. Which of the following statements regarding spinal shock following a spinal cord injury is *correct?*
  a. It results in a massive, uncompensated cardiovascular response to stimulation.
  b. It results in decreased reflexes and flaccid paralysis.
  c. It may cause death or stroke.
  d. It may occur approximately 7 to 10 days after the injury.

15. Respiratory muscle function is disrupted with spinal cord injuries above which level of the spinal cord?
  a. C4
  b. C13
  c. T1
  d. T5

16. Which of the following is a risk factor for embolic stroke?
  a. Atherosclerosis
  b. Atrial fibrillation
  c. Hypertension
  d. Smoking

17. A stroke that involves the left hemisphere may have which of the following consequences?
    a. Paralysis on the right side and loss of hearing
    b. Loss of sweating and communication problems
    c. Paralysis on the left side and loss of gag reflex
    d. Paralysis on the right and communication problems

18. A cerebrovascular accident causing damage to which area of the brain would result in cognitive impairment?
    a. Temporal lobe
    b. Parietal lobe
    c. Frontal lobe
    d. Occipital lobe

19. Which of the following pathophysiological mechanisms explains the movement disorder seen in Parkinson's disease?
    a. Deficit of dopamine
    b. Excess of dopamine
    c. Deficit of acetylcholine
    d. Excess of acetylcholine

20. Which of the following is correct regarding characteristics of multiple sclerosis?
    a. It occurs most commonly in the elderly.
    b. It results from a deficit of myelin.
    c. It always has a rapidly deteriorating course.
    d. It results in motor rigidity.

21. A patient is disoriented to where she is. She is most likely
    a. Confused
    b. Delirious
    c. Obtundated
    d. Stuporous

22. Seizures are most likely to be precipitated by attendance at which of the following events?
    a. A movie
    b. Reading a book
    c. Attending a laser show concert
    d. Dinner at a restaurant

23. Which of the following symptoms is common with a spinal cord injury above T5?
    a. Bradycardia and hypotension
    b. Hypermotility and ileus
    c. Loss of respiratory function
    d. All of the above

24. _____ affects the trunk, eyes, face, and swinging of arms in those with Parkinson's.
    a. Hypokinesia
    b. Bradykinesia
    c. Hyperkinesias
    d. Akinesia

25. Symptoms of MS include which of the following?
    a. Insidious onset
    b. Weakness
    c. Intermittent symptoms
    d. All of the above

PART IV · ANSWERS

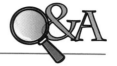

1. **The correct answer is d.** The myelin sheath insulates the axon and is interrupted periodically at the nodes of Ranvier, which enables the impulse to "jump" more quickly.

2. **The correct answer is b.** Motor fibers cross at the level of the medulla; thus, the left hemisphere controls all the activities on the right side of the body and vice versa.

3. **The correct answer is c.** The midbrain is at the level of the tentorial notch; thus, third cranial nerve function/pupillary function is compromised with herniation through the tentorial notch with increased intracranial pressure.

4. **The correct answer is b.** β_1 Receptors on the heart are stimulated by the sympathetic nervous system, resulting in increased impulse formation, conduction, and myocardial contraction. Acetylcholine is the neurotransmitter of the parasympathetic nervous system. Stimulation of α_1 receptors causes vasoconstriction. Pupillary dilation is a result of sympathetic stimulation.

5. **The correct answer is b.** Movement of CSF is easiest to accomplish; thus, it is the earliest compensatory mechanism mobilized. According to the Monro-Kellie hypothesis, when one of the components of the cranium (i.e., brain tissue, blood, and CSF) expand, another component must contract to maintain the normal level of intracranial pressure. The other mechanisms mentioned occur at stages when the earlier mechanisms are exceeded.

6. **The correct answer is b.** The cerebral cortex and the reticular activating system are involved in consciousness, and these areas are the first to be affected by increased intracranial pressure. The other functions are regulated in the brainstem at a lower level and, therefore, are not affected until later.

7. **The correct answer is b.** As the severity of the increased cranial pressure increases, the perfusion to the vital center in the brainstem diminishes, functions of the cardiovascular and the respiratory system slow down, and regulation of blood pressure is disrupted. The pulse rate slows, the respiratory rate slows, and the pulse pressure narrows as the systolic blood pressure falls.

8. **The correct answer is c.** A pathological process must involve both cerebral hemispheres for a loss of consciousness to occur.

9. **The correct answer is d.** Irritation of the meninges due to inflammation causes stiff neck or nuchal rigidity.

10. **The correct answer is c.** The infection causes the fever, meningeal irritation causes the stiff neck, and increased intracranial pressure can alter the level of consciousness. Photophobia, petechial skin rash, and nausea are other manifestations; however, the tongue does not swell, the body temperature does not become hypothermic, and the blood pressure is unaffected.

11. **The correct answer is a.** The organisms can enter the bloodstream and cause septicemia, damage to the eighth cranial nerve can cause hearing loss, and scarring can block the ventricles, leading to hydrocephalus. Irritation of brain tissue and scarring can cause seizures. Other cranial nerves can be damaged, leading to visual impairment. Damage to motor pathways can cause paralysis. Cardiac dysrhythmias, chronic pain, and arthritis are not complications of meningitis.

12. **The correct answer is d.** Subdural hematomas are a result of venous bleeding. The breakdown products of the clot absorb fluid slowly, becoming an expanding mass, so it may take weeks to develop. Epidural hemorrhaging occurs more rapidly because it results from arterial tears, most often involving the middle meningeal artery.

13. **The correct answer is c.** CSF normally contains glucose. An individual with fractures involving the sinuses may develop dural tears that allow CSF to leak, thus increasing the risk of infection.

14. **The correct answer is b.** For 7 to 10 days after the spinal cord injury, edema in the area of injury suppresses function of the spinal nerves, resulting in decreased reflexes and paralysis. The other choices apply to autonomic hyperreflexia, a condition that may begin after the period of spinal shock when the peripheral autonomic nerves have recovered.

15. **The correct answer is a.** The nerves that innervated the muscles for respiratory ventilation emerge from the spinal cord at this level. There is no C13. Nerves innervating respiratory muscles emerge above the thoracic area.

16. **The correct answer is b.** Stasis of blood in the heart due to atrial "quivering" with atrial fibrillation causes mural clots to form that, if released, travel through the arterial system to the brain and obstruct blood vessels. The other factors mentioned cause stroke through ischemia and vasoconstriction.

17. **The correct answer is d.** The left brain is involved with language. Motor tracts cross to the contralateral side in the medulla; thus, motor loss would be on the side opposite the cerebrovascular accident.

18. **The correct answer is c.** The frontal lobe is responsible for cognitive functions. The other answers do not apply.

19. **The correct answer is a.** Dopamine is an inhibitory neurotransmitter. Acetylcholine is an excitatory neurohormone both necessary for the proper functioning of the extrapyramidal motor system. A deficit in the production of dopamine in Parkinson's disease leads to imbalance and the motor problems that are seen.

20. **The correct answer is b.** A deficit of myelin explains the motor weakness that occurs.

21. **The correct answer is b.** Patients who are delirious are disoriented to person, place, and time as well as agitated and uncooperative.

22. **The correct answer is c.** Bright flashing lights and loud noise or music may precipitate a seizure.

23. **The correct answer is a.** Injuries above T5 decrease influence of sympathetic stimulation of the cardiovascular system.

24. **The correct answer is d.** Akinesia is the poverty of movement and is the most crippling of all the manifestations of Parkinson's disease.

25. **The correct Answer is d.** All of the answers are characteristic of MS.

Part V

Endocrine System

Vanessa Pomarico-Denino, MSN, APRN

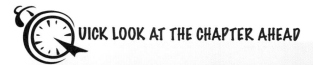
Hormones maintain and regulate body systems and act on specific target cells, regulating physiological function. They are secreted in any of three patterns—diurnal, pulsatile, or cyclical—or in patterns that are dependent on the levels of circulating substrates, such as electrolytes or minerals. Hormones bind onto specific receptor sites, not on cells or tissue. Generally, hormones are metabolized in the liver and excreted by the kidneys. Hormone release can be regulated by chemical factors, endocrine or hormonal factors, and/or neural factors. Feedback systems function to keep hormone levels within physiological ranges. The complexity of the feedback systems of the endocrine glands contributes to the difficulty in timely diagnosis of endocrine disorders. Any dysfunction of a particular gland causes decreased release of hormones that may produce adverse effects on specific body systems.

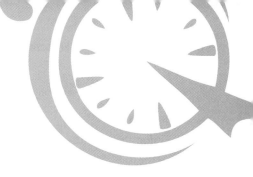

19

Anatomy and Physiology of the Endocrine System

TERMS
- ☐ affinity
- ☐ down-regulation
- ☐ endocrine glands
- ☐ exocrine glands
- ☐ iatrogenic
- ☐ negative feedback mechanism
- ☐ positive feedback mechanism
- ☐ up-regulation

Figure 19-1 Anatomy and physiology of the endocrine system.

Definitions

- **Endocrine glands**—Ductless glands that secrete hormone directly into the circulation (e.g., adrenal, thyroid).
- **Exocrine glands**—Secrete hormone to ephithelial surface either directly or through a duct (e.g., sweat, salivary).

Common Abbreviations

TRH—Thyroid-releasing hormone
TSH—Thyroid-stimulating hormone
CRH—Corticotropin-releasing hormone

T_4—Thyroxine
T_3—Triiodothyronine
PTH—Parathyroid hormone

Relationship Between Hypothalamic, Pituitary, and Selected Endocrine Glands and Hormones

TRH from hypothalamus
CRH from hypothalamus

TSH from anterior pituitary
ACTH from pituitary

T_3 and T_4 from thyroid
Cortisol and aldosterone from adrenal cortex

Effects of Aging

- Increased amount of connective tissue
- Structural changes (nodules)
- Variable changes in hormone secretion
- Decreased sensitivity of target organs
- Decreased receptor binding

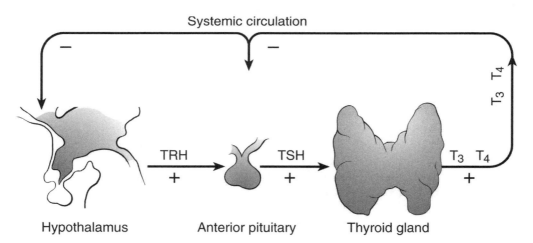

The **negative feedback mechanism** is the most common feedback system in hormonal regulation. For example, reduced levels of circulating thyroid hormone stimulate the release of thyroid-stimulating hormone (TSH) from the anterior pituitary, which in turn causes the thyroid gland to secrete additional thyroxine. Conversely, if circulating levels of thyroxine are too high, the anterior pituitary decreases production of TSH, thereby reducing the level of thyroid hormone in the blood. **Positive feedback mechanisms** are less common and occur when the release of hormone from the target organ stimulates the **endocrine gland** to secrete additional hormone.

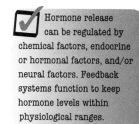

Hormone release can be regulated by chemical factors, endocrine or hormonal factors, and/or neural factors. Feedback systems function to keep hormone levels within physiological ranges.

Hormones are divided into four categories: (1) steroids (such as androgens, glucocorticoids, or thyroid hormones), which are lipid soluble; (2) protein or polypeptides (such as insulin), which are water soluble; (3) amines and amino acids (such as epinephrine), which are water soluble; or (4) fatty acid derivatives (such as prostaglandins or thromboxane). Those that are lipid soluble diffuse through the walls of the capillaries. Thyroid hormones and adrenal hormones are among the lipid-soluble hormones and are bound to proteins for transport in the blood. Conditions that affect the amount of protein available to act as a carrier can affect the concentration of hormone available for bodily functions. Additionally, the amount of receptor sites directly affects the cells' sensitivity to the hormone. Lipid-soluble hormones are metabolized more slowly than water-soluble hormones. Metabolism can also take place through degradation of the hormone by the target cell after being bound to the receptors. In some instances, metabolism increases hormonal activity, as in the case of the metabolism of the thyroid hormone thyroxine to triiodothyronine, which is a more biologically active form. Hormones that are water soluble, such as epinephrine, generally circulate in free or unbound form and enter capillaries through pores in their walls.

Target cells are cells with specific receptors appropriate for, or responsive to, a particular hormone and are the only cells affected by that particular hormone. Some receptors, which are proteins, are located on the cell membrane; others are intracellular. The receptors for lipid-soluble hormones are intracellular. The sensitivity of a target cell is related to the number of receptors it contains. If concentrations of a hormone are low, the target cells increase their number of receptors. This is known as **up-regulation.** Likewise, if concentrations are high, target cells decrease their number of receptors, which is known as **down-regulation.** This process allows the cells to adjust their sensitivity to the concentration of circulating hormone, thereby facilitating homeostasis. Another process known as permissiveness increases the number of receptors in target cells for other hormones. For example, thyroid hormone increases the number of receptors on adipose tissue, which are the target cells for epinephrine. The physiological effect of this increase is that greater amounts of fatty acids are released for cellular metabolism than would normally occur in the absence of thyroid hormone.

Plasma concentrations of hormones depend on the rate of synthesis and release of the hormone as well as its rate of metabolism and excretion. Failure of the end organ to respond to the hormone when hormone levels are normal or elevated indicates end-organ resistance, which can occur to both endogenous and exogenous hormones. Ectopic hormone production is usually caused by a malignant tumor such as certain lung tumors that produce antidiuretic hormone. Medical treatment can also result in endocrine disorders such as cushingoid syndrome, which occurs when glucocorticoids are used to treat autoimmune disorders, or hypothyroidism after thyroidectomy. These disorders are termed **iatrogenic.**

Affinity is the ability of the receptor sites to bind with the hormone. The amount of hormone required to elicit a response depends on the degree of affinity: the higher the affinity, the less hormone needed to elicit a response. Cross-specificity or cross-sensitivity may occur between hormones if their structures are similar. For example, some hypothalamic hormones may affect the secretion of more than one hormone from the anterior pituitary. Which hormone takes precedence at a given time is to some degree dependent on the concentration of the hormone in the body, as are the types of clinical manifestations seen in patients. For example, thyroid-releasing hormone stimulates both TSH and prolactin; therefore, the effects of both of these hormones may be seen in patients. An example of this would

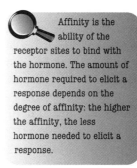

Affinity is the ability of the receptor sites to bind with the hormone. The amount of hormone required to elicit a response depends on the degree of affinity: the higher the affinity, the less hormone needed to elicit a response.

be when thyroid hormone replacement causes gynecomastia. If hormones are administered exogenously, the effects seen may not reflect the actions of the hormones at physiological levels. Certain medications can also act as agonists or antagonists of hormones, thereby increasing or decreasing the desired effects.

The hypothalamic–pituitary axis is an important dimension of the physiology of the endocrine system. It produces various releasing/inhibitory hormones and tropic hormones that affect the function of various glands and body processes. Releasing/inhibitory hormones are produced and secreted by the hypothalamus (thyroid-releasing hormone and corticotropin-releasing hormone), and tropic hormones are produced and secreted by the pituitary (TSH and adrenocorticotropic hormone). Tropic hormones, in turn, cause the release of hormones from other glands, which act on target cells in particular organs. There are both neural (posterior pituitary) and vascular (anterior pituitary) connections between the hypothalamus and the pituitary.

Endocrine pathology can result from hyposecretion, hypersecretion, or altered responsiveness of the target cells. These can occur because of altered function anywhere along the hypothalamic–pituitary axis or in the target gland itself. Therefore, diagnosis of specific disorders depends on the complex mechanisms among these organs. Primary disease is of the endocrine gland itself, and secondary disease is a consequence of abnormalities of the pituitary or other ectopic sources. For example, hypothyroidism could be caused by decreased secretion of thyroid hormone (primary disease) or by decreased concentrations of TSH (secondary disease). Therefore, accurate diagnosis requires determination of highly specific levels of hormones. Endocrine disorders may also be referred to as functional if caused by nonendocrine disease. Hyporesponsiveness of the target organ is usually a result of receptor deficiency such as insulin resistance with diabetes.

EFFECTS OF AGING

It is difficult to establish the precise relationship between normal aging and endocrine function due to the complexities of the endocrine system and the many other factors that contribute to its function. For example, changes in organ function and metabolism, excretion, nutrition, medication use, and various acute and chronic diseases can all influence endocrine function, particularly in the elderly. This helps explain how drug toxicity occurs with relative ease in the elderly, as well as those with renal and liver disease. It also explains the need for control of polypharmacy, careful dosing, and conscientious monitoring of drug regimens in the elderly.

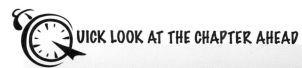

The thyroid gland, located anteriorly to the trachea at the lower part of the neck, is a highly vascular gland responsible for regulation of many physiological functions of the body. Any imbalance in the hormones produced by this gland can cause multiple system dysfunction. These imbalances can easily be corrected through the use of medications or surgery.

20

The Thyroid Gland

TERMS
- [ ] cretinism
- [ ] exophthalmus
- [ ] goiter
- [ ] myxedema
- [ ] thyroid-stimulating hormone (TSH)
- [ ] thyroid storm
- [ ] thyrotoxicosis
- [ ] thyrotropin-releasing hormone (TRH)
- [ ] thyroxine (T₄)
- [ ] triiodothyronine (T₃)

Figure 20-1 Thyroid gland.

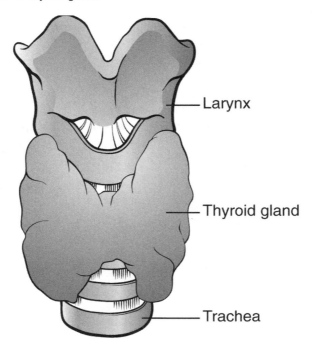

— Larynx

— Thyroid gland

— Trachea

Anterior View

Additional Effects of Aging on the Thyroid
- Decrease in serum T_3
- Decrease in calcitonin
- Decrease in production and clearance of T_3 and T_4

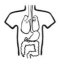

PATHOPHYSIOLOGY

The thyroid gland is located in the anterior aspect of the neck just below the larynx and contains follicular and nonfollicular cells. The thyroid gland produces **thyroxine (T_4)** and **triiodothyronine (T_3),** which control metabolism, and calcitonin, which lowers serum calcium levels by opposing bone resorption (inhibition of osteoclastic activity) and promotes formation of osteoblasts. The follicular cells synthesize and secrete some of the thyroid hormones, and the nonfollicular cells

Figure 20-2 Primary diagnostic tests for thyroid conditions.

Primary Diagnostic Tests for Thyroid Conditions

- TSH, TRH
- Free and total T_4 (thyroxine)
- Total and free T_3 and (triiodothyronine)
- Thyroxine binding globulin (TBG)
- Thyroid ultrasound or radioactive iodine uptake
- Thyroid-stimulating immunoglobulins
- Iodine, iodide
- Thyroid antibodies (antiperoxidase and antithyroglobulin)

Causes of Hypothyroidism

- Hashimoto's thyroiditis
- Iodine deficiency
- Defects in TSH or TRH production
- Congenital
- Iatrogenic—Surgery, irradiation, medications (such as lithium), foods (such as cabbage)

Causes of Hyperthyroidism

- Graves' disease
- Increased use of thyroid medications
- Use of other medications (such as amiodarone, lithium, interferon)
- Increased ingestion of iodides

Table 20-1 Manifestations of Thyroid Disease

Hypothyroidism	Hyperthyroidism
• Intolerance to cold	• Heart palpitations
• Unexplained weight gain	• Heat intolerance
• Dysphagia	• Anxiety
• Fatigue	• Dyspnea on exertion
• Decreased concentration	• Unintentional weight loss
• Constipation	• Diarrhea
• Thinning of hair and eyebrows	• Increased perspiration
• Menstrual irregularities (especially menorrhagia)	• Menstrual irregularities (especially amenorrhea)
• Dry skin	

(C cells) secrete various polypeptides including calcitonin, which is also called *thyrocalcitonin.* The follicular cells also contain a gelatinous substance called *thyroglobulin.* If iodine, which is necessary for the formation of T_4 and T_3, is deficient, inadequate amounts of T_4 and T_3 are produced. If the thyroid does not produce enough hormones to inhibit **thyroid-stimulating hormone (TSH),** the thyroid produces additional thyroglobulin, which is not affected by iodine, in an effort to increase circulating levels of thyroid hormone. This results in hypertrophy of the thyroid gland known as **goiter.** An enlarged thyroid gland can occur with either hypothyroidism or hyperthyroidism, although it is not necessarily indicative of thyroid dysfunction. If the thyroid is enlarged but not associated with identifiable clinical manifestations, it is referred to as a nontoxic goiter. Thyroid nodules may be malignant and are usually solitary nodules that are less than 1 cm or may be benign with multiple nodularities (multinodular goiter). Nodules may also be due to inflammation, as seen with Hashimoto thyroiditis, or may be cystic in nature. Nodules may be palpable or discovered on ultrasound.

An enlarged thyroid gland can occur with either hypothyroidism or hyperthyroidism, although it is not necessarily indicative of thyroid dysfunction.

   TSH is synthesized and stored in the anterior pituitary. Once released, it binds to receptors located on cell membranes of the thyroid gland. This causes a release of stored thyroid hormones, increases iodine uptake and oxidation, increases thyroid hormone syntheses, and increases the synthesis and secretion of prostaglandins by the thyroid. Thyroid hormone is regulated through a negative feedback loop involving the hypothalamus, anterior pituitary, and thyroid gland. TRH is synthesized and stored in the hypothalamus. It is released and travels to the anterior pituitary through vascular channels where it stimulates the release of TSH. Thyroid hormones thus produced have a negative feedback effect and inhibit **thyrotropin-releasing hormone (TRH)** and TSH, which in turn decreases thyroid hormone synthesis and secretion. Normally, the thyroid gland produces 90% of T_4 and 10% of T_3. T_4 is converted to T_3 in body tissues. Of all the thyroid hormones, T_3 has the greatest metabolic effect. Ninety percent of these hormones are bound to protein for transport to body tissue. T_4 and T_3 have a diurnal variation that peaks in the late evening. Their secretion is influenced by gender, pregnancy, nutrition, and levels of selected hormones or chemicals. TRH is increased with exposure to cold, stress, and decreased levels of T_4. T_3 may be elevated in those taking oral contraceptives or who are pregnant.

> TSH is synthesized and stored in the anterior pituitary. Once released, it binds to receptors located on cell membranes of the thyroid gland. This causes a release of stored thyroid hormones, increases iodine uptake and oxidation, increases thyroid hormone syntheses, and increases the synthesis and secretion of prostaglandins by the thyroid.

In addition to TSH, the thyroid gland is also stimulated to produce thyroid hormone as a result of low iodide levels and drugs that interfere with uptake of iodide. Because there is a high concentration gradient of iodine between the thyroid gland and the blood, iodide is moved into the follicular cells of the gland via active transport, where it is oxidized and becomes iodine. Thyroglobulin, a glucoprotein, is also necessary for the formation of the T_3 and T_4.

The thyroid hormones regulate protein, fat, and carbohydrate metabolism; metabolic rate; and therefore the production of body heat. Because of its influence on cellular function, thyroid hormones play a role in the function of other body systems such as cardiac, respiratory, gastrointestinal, musculoskeletal, humoral, and neurological. They also influence growth and development and the effectiveness of growth hormone. In the United States, iodine is added to salt and flour, so iodine deficiency is less common here than in some other countries.

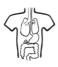

EFFECTS OF AGING

Atrophy and fibrosis with nodule formation and an increase in inflammatory infiltrates are normal changes in the thyroid gland due to aging. Because of the multiple factors that can affect endocrine function in the elderly, it is difficult to determine how much of an effect the changes in the gland itself have on the physiological function of the thyroid. However, research seems to indicate that there is a decrease in T_4 secretion and turnover, a decline in serum T_3 levels, an increase in hypothyroidism, variation in TSH secretion, and decreased responsiveness of plasma TSH concentrations to exogenous TRH administration, particularly in men.

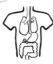

HYPOTHYROIDISM

In primary hypothyroidism, decreased thyroid hormone levels cause an increase in TSH levels, resulting in hypertrophy of the thyroid or goiter. Secondary hypothyroidism is most commonly caused by failure of the pituitary to produce sufficient amounts of TSH. Hypothyroidism is caused by a deficiency in thyroid hormone and may be classified as congenital or acquired as well as primary or secondary.

There are several types of hypothyroidism: acute (caused by a bacterial infection of the thyroid), subacute (inflammation of the thyroid, most likely caused by a viral infection), painless (similar to autoimmune), postpartum (which can occur up to 6 months after giving birth), and autoimmune (also known as Hashimoto) thyroiditis. Another form of hypothyroid is acquired hypothyroidism, or **myxedema,** which if left untreated can lead to myxedema coma that is associated with a high mortality rate. It is a medical emergency.

The most common cause of acquired primary hypothyroidism is autoimmune thyroiditis, in which antibodies destroy thyroid tissue. Infiltration of lymphocytes contributes to enlargement of the gland and formation of nodules. Cellular destruction caused by inflammation can initially release large amounts of T_4 and T_3, temporarily causing symptoms of hyperthyroidism. Ultimately, hormone production is decreased, causing increased secretion of TSH by the anterior pituitary in an effort to increase the amount of circulating thyroid hormone. As the disease progresses, the thyroid gland atrophies and becomes fibrotic and hypothyroidism results. Anemia is often associated with hypothyroidism due to a decrease in erythropoiesis.

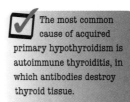

The most common cause of acquired primary hypothyroidism is autoimmune thyroiditis, in which antibodies destroy thyroid tissue.

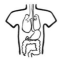

HYPERTHYROIDISM

Thyrotoxicosis is a broad term that may be assigned to any condition resulting in excess thyroid hormone regardless of cause. Iatrogenic thyrotoxicosis can be caused by ingestion of excessive thyroid hormone or iodine preparations. Hyperthyroidism is a form of thyrotoxicosis in which excess hormones are secreted by the thyroid gland. It can be caused by increased synthesis and secretion of T_4 and T_3; follicular cell destruction, which causes a release of stored T_4 and T_3; or thyroid cancer. Stimulation of thyrotropin receptors by TSH or stimulation of thyrotropin receptor antibodies (TRAb) can also result in elevated T_4 and T_3 levels. Stimulation of thyrotropin receptors by TRAb is the mechanism underlying Graves' disease, the most common cause of hyperthyroidism.

Graves' disease is an autoimmune process in which the negative feedback mechanism is ineffective in lowering circulating levels of thyroid hormone. It is often triggered by stress or viral infections. It is reported that thyroid autoantibodies are found in more than 95% of subjects with Graves' disease. Immunoglobulins bind to TSH receptors, ultimately causing thyroid hypertrophy. This condition is more common in women and increases with puberty, pregnancy, and menopause. Ocular manifestations are associated with sympathetic nervous system hyperactivity and infiltrative changes involving the orbital contents with associated enlargement of orbital muscles known as **exophthalmus.**

Arrhythmias are commonly associated with hyperthyroidism. There is also increased cardiovascular and metabolic sensitivity to catecholamines. This is most likely due to an increase in the number and reactivity of β- and α-adrenergic receptors.

> Hyperthyroidism is a form of thyrotoxicosis in which excess hormones are secreted by the thyroid gland. It can be caused by increased synthesis and secretion of T_4 and T_3; follicular cell destruction, which causes a release of stored T_4 and T_3; or thyroid cancer.

Enlargement of the thyroid from an increased number of follicular cells is a compensatory mechanism and is normal during puberty, pregnancy, or with some infectious disorders. If the gland does not revert to its normal size when the need for excess thyroid hormone subsides, hyperthyroidism may result. This is often referred to as toxic multinodular goiter. Thyrotoxic crisis is rare but can be fatal if not treated within 48 hours. It occurs most commonly in undiagnosed persons, after thyroid surgery, or in those under extreme physical or emotional stress.

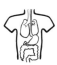

MANAGEMENT

The goal of management with any thyroid disease is to produce an euthyroid state. Once treatment is begun, the goiter usually regresses.

Primary hypothyroidism is treated with oral medications. If the deficiency is caused by a nonthyroid disorder, that condition needs to be identified and appropriately managed. Thyroid replacement doses in the elderly should be lower than those in other adults, starting at no more than one-half of the normal adult dose, with adjustments being made as indicated. Increasing dosages is based on laboratory results. Dosages are generally not increased more frequently than 4 weeks.

It is thought that peripheral metabolism of thyroid hormone decreases with age. Signs of thyroid disease are more difficult to detect in the elderly. Extreme care must be taken in treating those with angina or myocardial infarction. Early detection and treatment of congenital hypothyroidism, or **cretinism**, is essential for normal central nervous system development and to prevent mental retardation. Treatment of hyperthyroidism consists of the use of antithyroid medications such as methimazole or β-adrenergic antagonists to reduce cardiovascular insult. Although the size of the goiter may decrease with treatment, exophthalmos ordinarily does not. Long-term treatment (18 months) is necessary and frequent monitoring is important. Relapse after treatment may occur.

Management of thyroid nodules includes ultrasound-guided fine-needle aspiration to determine whether the nodule is benign or malignant. Benign nodules are monitored with serial TSH and ultrasound for stability of size. Malignancies are treated with radioiodine therapy or surgery. Radioactive iodine is the treatment of choice for most adults and is often used for ablation. Treatment commonly results in hypothyroidism, which then requires lifelong replacement and management. Surgical removal increases the risk of secondary hypoparathyroidism and is less commonly used. **Thyroid storm** is a life-threatening form of thyrotoxicosis and must be treated promptly and aggressively.

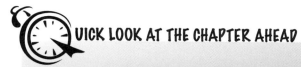

The parathyroid glands are comprised of four glands in the posterior aspect of the thyroid gland. These four glands are responsible for the production of parathyroid hormone, which regulates calcium and phosphorus levels in the body. Elevated levels of parathyroid hormone can have potentially life-threatening consequences if there is no intervention.

21

The Parathyroid Gland

TERMS
- ☐ bone remodeling
- ☐ calcitonin
- ☐ Chvostek's sign
- ☐ hyperparathyroidism
- ☐ hypoparathyroidism
- ☐ osteoblasts
- ☐ osteoclasts
- ☐ parathyroid hormone (PTH)
- ☐ secondary hyperparathyroidism
- ☐ Trousseau's sign

Figure 21-1 Primary diagnostic tests for parathyroid conditions.

Primary Diagnostic Tests for Parathyroid Conditions

Parathyroid hormone (PTH), Ca, PO_4, HCO_3, Mg, Cl, pH, UA, for Ca, x-ray/bone density, cAMP (cyclic adenosine monophosphate levels), 1 to 25 vitamin D levels

Causes of Hyperparathyroidism

- Chronic renal failure
- Familial tendency
- Malabsorption of vitamin D and calcium
- Certain drugs (e.g., phenytoin, laxatives, phenobarbital)

Physical Examination Signs

- Chvostek's sign—Ipsilateral contraction of facial muscles elicited by tapping facial nerve anterior to the ear.
- Trousseau's sign—Carpal spasm related to ischemia of nerves in upper arm during inflation of blood pressure cuff (wait 3 to 5 minutes) above systolic pressure.

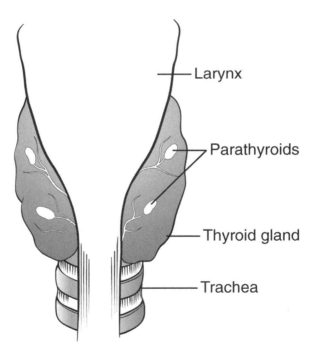

Posterior View

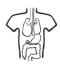

PATHOPHYSIOLOGY

The parathyroid glands are located behind the upper and lower poles of the thyroid, which is anterior to the larynx. There are commonly four parathyroid glands, although there can be as few as two or as many as six. The parathyroid glands produce **parathyroid hormone (PTH)**, which maintains calcium homeostasis. PTH is primarily regulated by the serum level of ionized calcium. If serum calcium is low, PTH is released. If it is high, PTH is suppressed. PTH is not part of the hypothalamic–pituitary feedback mechanism, so marked increases or decreases can have severe consequences. Magnesium and phosphate levels also influence PTH secretion in that hyperphosphatemia leads to hypocalcemia, which in turn influences PTH secretion. The relationship among these three minerals is complex. **Calcitonin**, pro-

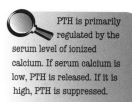

PTH is primarily regulated by the serum level of ionized calcium. If serum calcium is low, PTH is released. If it is high, PTH is suppressed.

duced by the thyroid, also plays a role in controlling serum calcium levels by increasing bone formation by **osteoblasts** and decreasing bone breakdown by **osteoclasts**. Its effect is to decrease serum calcium levels and conserve bone matrix.

PTH is the most important hormone in the regulation of serum calcium levels. It is secreted in response to lowered serum calcium levels and acts directly on bone (the body's primary reservoir of calcium) by causing release of calcium from the bone and on the kidneys. PTH causes bone resorption or breakdown of osteoclasts, thereby increasing serum calcium levels. If PTH release is chronically stimulated, it results in **bone remodeling**. PTH also acts in the proximal and distal tubules of the kidneys to increase reabsorption of calcium and decrease reabsorption of phosphorus, thereby increasing serum levels of calcium and phosphate. In addition, it influences tubular reabsorption of bicarbonate and stimulates the synthesis of biologically active vitamin D. Vitamin D facilitates calcium and phosphorus transport through the intestinal wall. Elevated levels of serum magnesium inhibit the secretion of PTH.

PTH also acts in the proximal and distal tubules of the kidneys to increase reabsorption of calcium and decrease reabsorption of phosphorus, thereby increasing serum levels of calcium and phosphate.

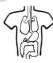

EFFECTS OF AGING

With aging, the level of PTH increases. In addition, intestinal adaptation to variations in calcium intake is reduced, leading to a decrease in intestinal absorption. There may also be an impaired renal response to decreased calcium intake and decreased levels of circulating vitamin D. Dietary intake of calcium also tends to decrease with aging. All these factors may contribute to changes in calcium metabolism apparent in the elderly, although there is insufficient evidence to explain the changes more fully.

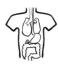

HYPERPARATHYROIDISM

Hyperparathyroidism is a consequence of increased secretion of PTH and is classified as either primary or secondary. In primary hyperparathyroidism, the normal feedback mechanism fails to inhibit PTH secretion in response to elevated serum levels of ionized calcium. Primary hyperparathyroidism is usually due to adenoma but can also be due to cancer or hyperplasia. Decreased synthesis of vitamin D and renal phosphate retention promote hyperplasia of the parathyroid gland, and as a result, increased secretion and synthesis of PTH occurs. **Secondary hyperparathyroidism** is an increased level of PTH as a result of chronic disease or a condition that causes hypocalcemia and is commonly seen in those with chronic renal failure. Hypocalcemia stimulates PTH secretion as well as renal and gastrointestinal calcium absorption, which ultimately leads to hyperparathyroidism (as the parathyroid responds to increased demand for hormone) and hypercalcemia. Bone turnover is accelerated in hyperparathyroidism. **Chvostek's sign** and **Trousseau's sign** are used to assess patients for hypocalcemia.

Primary hyperparathyroidism is usually due to adenoma but can also be due to cancer or hyperplasia.

Hypercalcemia affects many body systems because of the role it plays in cellular and/or tissue function throughout the body. For example,

bone resorption puts one at risk for fractures; hypercalcemia can produce renal calculi and cause metabolic acidosis because it
alters renal tubular function. Chronic hypercalcemia is also associated with insulin resistance. Extreme levels of hypercalcemia are
rarely of parathyroid origin; rather, they are

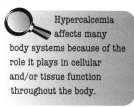

Hypercalcemia affects many body systems because of the role it plays in cellular and/or tissue function throughout the body.

associated with ectopic sources from elsewhere in the body such as
metastatic tumors. Mild hyperparathyroidism may be asymptomatic
and discovered through routine blood chemistries. It predisposes one to
fractures and renal stones.

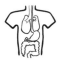

HYPOPARATHYROIDISM

Hypoparathyroidism is the result of decreased secretion of PTH due to
decreased tissue responsiveness, autoimmune destruction, or, more
commonly, damage to the parathyroid glands during surgery. It can also
be a consequence of hypomagnesemia associated with a variety of
chronic illnesses or drugs. Lack of circulating PTH depresses serum calcium levels, increases phosphate levels, and impairs calcium resorption
from bone, causing hypocalcemia. Calcium is necessary for the formation of bone and teeth but also is needed for blood clotting, hormone
secretion, and muscle contraction. The most serious consequence of
hypocalcemia is lowering of the threshold for neuromuscular excitation;
therefore, neuromuscular irritability, spasm, hyperreflexia, and convulsions may occur. Phosphate retention also impairs vitamin D conversion
to its active form, which further exacerbates depression of serum calcium levels. In primary hypoparathyroidism, calcium levels are
decreased and phosphate levels are increased, whereas PTH levels are
usually normal.

Lack of circulating PTH depresses serum calcium levels, increases
phosphate levels, and impairs calcium resorption from bone, causing
hypocalcemia.

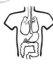

MANAGEMENT

The goal of management in hyperparathyroidism is to reduce hypercalcemia through the use of hydration, diuretics, and other drugs that decrease resorption of bone. Definitive treatment is surgical excision of hyperplastic glands. In hypoparathyroidism, vitamin D and calcium replacements (1–3 g) are prescribed. Drugs to decrease phosphate absorption from the gastrointestinal tract are used if phosphate levels are significantly elevated.

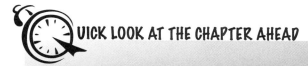

The adrenal glands are responsible for a variety of physiological functions. This pair of organs is located behind the peritoneum, and each gland is responsible for different functions, including secretion of catecholamines, blood glucose regulation and maintaining fluid and electrolyte balance.

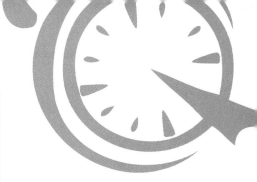

22

Adrenal Physiology

TERMS
- ☐ Addison's disease
- ☐ cortex
- ☐ Cushing's syndrome
- ☐ diurnal rhythm
- ☐ gluconeogenesis
- ☐ hyperaldosteronism
- ☐ lipogenesis
- ☐ medulla

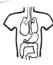

PHYSIOLOGY

The adrenal glands are located on the upper poles of the kidneys and are composed of two parts: the outer part, called the **cortex,** and the inner part, called the **medulla.** The cortex comprises 80% of the gland and secretes several steroid hormones: the mineralocorticoids (aldosterone), androgens, and glucocorticoids (cortisol). The medulla makes up the remaining volume (20%) and secretes epinephrine, norepinephrine, and dopamine and is innervated by the parasympathetic and sympathetic nervous systems.

The hormones of the adrenal cortex are synthesized from cholesterol and acetate. Most corticosteroids (steroids) are produced in response to stimulation of the cortex by adrenocorticotropic hormone (ACTH) from the anterior pituitary, which in turn is stimulated by corticotropin-releasing hormone (CRH) in the hypothalamus. The secretion of ACTH is regulated by three factors: negative feedback, diurnal rhythms, and stress. Negative feedback due to high levels of cortisol or exogenous glucocorticoids suppresses CRH and ACTH. Secretion peaks 3 to 5 hours after sleep begins and declines throughout the day. This is referred to as **diurnal rhythm.** This pattern is reversed in those who work the night shift. ACTH secretion and cortisol levels are also increased in response to psychological or physical stress. In addition, the adrenals produce small amounts of androgens that are converted in peripheral tissues to estrogen and testosterone. Because of the cyclical pattern of glucocorticoids, it is important to obtain a morning cortisol level to accurately measure levels.

The glucocorticoids, such as cortisol, have metabolic, antiinflammatory, and growth-suppressing effects that include immune responses and antibody production. They increase blood glucose levels by promoting **gluconeogenesis** in the liver, decreasing cellular uptake of glucose, and stimulating protein catabolism in addition to inhibiting protein synthesis. They also promote **lipogenesis** and increase blood cholesterol. These hormones inhibit immune and inflammatory responses by suppressing the mediators of these responses and by depressing the action of T lymphocytes and macrophages. The glu-

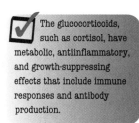

The glucocorticoids, such as cortisol, have metabolic, antiinflammatory, and growth-suppressing effects that include immune responses and antibody production.

Figure 22-1 Additional actions and effects of glucocorticoids.

Additional Actions and Effects of Glucocorticoids

Gluconeogenesis	Increased circulating red blood cells
Increased appetite	Mood changes
Increased fat deposition	Increased uric acid secretion
Decreased growth hormone	Decreased serum calcium levels
Melanocyte stimulation	Decreased secretion/synthesis of adrenocorticotropic hormone (ACTH)

Additional Stimuli to Adrenal Medullary Secretion

Hypoglycemia	Hypoxia
Hypercapnia	Acidosis
Hemorrhage	Glucagon
Nicotine	Pilocarpine
Histamine	Angiotensin II

Common Diagnostic Tests

Radioimmunoassay	Urine catecholamines
Dexamethasone suppression test	Computed tomography
Complete blood count	Blood chemistry
Serum and urinary electrolytes/hormones	Enzyme-linked immunosorbent assays

Signs and Symptoms of Hypercorticalism

Weight gain	"Moon face"	"Buffalo hump"
Truncal obesity	Glycogenesis	Sodium and water retention
Glucose intolerance	Gluconeogenesis	Insulin resistance
Polyuria	Overt diabetes mellitus	Protein/muscle wasting
Pathological fractures	Weakness	Osteoporosis
Kyphosis	Renal stones	Thinning of skin
Capillary fragility	Ecchymosis	Purple striae
Hyperpigmentation	Vasoconstriction	Hypertension
Poor wound healing	Fungal infections	Decreased immune response
Increased susceptibility to infection	Altered mental status	Emotional lability
Euphoria	Hirsutism	Psychosis
Menstrual irregularities		Acne

cocorticoids produce a variety of additional effects because of the presence of receptors on extraadrenal tissues (Figure 22-1). In addition, they potentiate the effects of catecholamines, thyroid hormone, and growth hormone on adipose tissue. Cortisol is necessary for maintenance of life and protection from emotional and behavioral stress.

Figure 22-2 Sympathetic nervous system (SNS) and adrenal medullary (AM) response to stress.

Sympathetic Nervous System (SNS) and Adrenal Medullary (AM) Response to Stress

Stressor	SNS Stimulation	AM Stimulation
	Epinephrine	Norepinephrine (SNS fibers)
	Glycogenolysis	Tachycardia
	Gluconeogenesis	Vasoconstriction
	Lipolysis	Tachypnea
	Bronchodilation	

Effects of Aging on Adrenals

- Decreased aldosterone secretion
- Increased sensitivity to antidiuretic hormone (ADH) in the brain
- Decreased sensitivity to ADH in the kidney
- Decreased production of cortisol and aldosterone
- Decreased cortisol secretion (basal level is unchanged because degradation rate is unchanged)

Mineralocorticoids are steroids that maintain normal salt and water balance by promoting sodium retention and potassium loss. Aldosterone is the most potent of these, and its primary role is to conserve sodium (Na^+) and to increase the excretion of potassium (K^+) and hydrogen ions. Its synthesis and secretion are regulated primarily by the renin-angiotensin system (as opposed to ACTH control) in response to decreases in blood volume, renal circulation, and potassium levels. High levels of aldosterone promote Na^+ retention but may also result in alkalosis and hypokalemia.

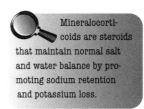

Mineralocorticoids are steroids that maintain normal salt and water balance by promoting sodium retention and potassium loss.

The adrenal glands produce small amounts of androgens. Under normal circumstances, these play a minor role in the development and maintenance of secondary sex characteristics. The amount of estrogen converted peripherally from the androgens (androstenedione) is minimal and is physiologically unimportant; however, it becomes the major source of endogenous estrogen in postmenopausal women. Weak androgens are converted in peripheral tissues to stronger ones, such as testosterone, and thus have some androgenic effect. Certain conditions, such as obesity and aging, increase peripheral conversion of androgens, leading to more obvious effects such as hirsutism or acne.

The catecholamines include epinephrine (adrenaline) and norepinephrine. These are the main products secreted by the adrenal medulla. Epinephrine comprises approximately 75% to 85% of catecholamines secreted by the adrenal medulla. Epinephrine is significantly more potent than norepinephrine in producing direct metabolic effects. The catecholamines are synthesized from the amino acid phenylalanine. Their secretion is increased by ACTH and the glucocorticoids and is affected by a variety of other stimuli (see Figure 22-2). Catecholamines bind to receptors throughout the body, accounting for the widespread effects of their secretion in response to stressors and the stress response known as "fight or flight."

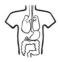

EFFECTS OF AGING

Metabolic clearance of cortisol decreases in response to declines in liver and kidney function. There is also a decrease in the amount of cortisol used by the body as a function of lower lean body mass associated with aging. Diurnal variations and feedback mechanisms remain intact. Adrenal androgens decrease to 50% to 75% of young adult levels.

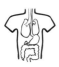

ADRENAL DYSFUNCTION

Hyperfunction of the adrenals can result in **Cushing's syndrome,** virilization and/or feminization due to an imbalance in androgens and estrogen, and **hyperaldosteronism.** Hypofunction leads to **Addison's disease.**

Cushing's Syndrome and Disease

There are three types of Cushing's syndrome: ACTH dependent (hypersecretion of ACTH or pituitary form), ACTH independent (hypersecretion of adrenal cortisol due to an adrenal tumor), and steroid induced. Cushing's syndrome is due to excess circulating cortisol from adrenal cortical disease or exogenous steroid administration, whereas Cushing's disease is caused by excessive secretion of ACTH by the anterior pituitary. Cushing's disease is more common in adults and in females. Cushing's syndrome is more common in adults between the ages of 30 and

50 and in elderly adults, particularly men. Adrenal tumors are more common in children.

Hypercortisolism is usually caused by Cushing's disease (75–80%) but may also result from ACTH or cortisol-secreting tumors. Most persons with Cushing's disease have a pituitary microadenoma and a loss of normal feedback mechanisms to control CRH and ACTH secretion. A variety of ectopic tumors can produce CRH and ACTH that are not affected by the normal feedback mechanisms. Cortisol-secreting tumors suppress CRH and ACTH, leading to atrophy of normal adrenal cortical tissue. With these conditions, diurnal activity is lost, as is the body's ability to increase ACTH and cortisol production under stress.

Addison's Disease

Hypocorticalism, or adrenal insufficiency, involves either inadequate stimulation of the adrenal glands by CRH and ACTH as a result of secondary hypocorticalism or inability of the adrenals to produce and secrete adrenocortical hormone, known as primary hypocorticalism or Addison's disease. Idiopathic or organ-specific autoimmune causation is most common. More than 90% of adrenal tissue must be destroyed before manifestations become evident. Addison's disease is often associated with other autoimmune disorders, and a genetic predisposition is suggested in come cases.

Secondary hypocorticalism is due to low levels of ACTH from a variety of disorders or exogenous administration of glucocorticoids. Abrupt withdrawal of these medications can be life threatening. Manifestations involve a number of body systems; hypoglycemia, hyperkalemia, hypotension, and possibly hyperpigmentation will be most evident. Acute adrenal insufficiency is an emergency.

Management

For both Cushing's syndrome and Addison's disease treatment is essential. It is directly related to the cause and can include drugs, radiation, and/or surgery.

Hyperaldosteronism

Hyperaldosteronism is caused by either a primary adrenal disorder, such as an adrenal tumor, or extraadrenal stimulation, a secondary adrenal disorder due to extraadrenal stimulation from excessive angiotensin II. Pathophysiological alterations are manifestations of fluid and electrolyte changes, which include Na^+ and H_2O retention, hypokalemia, hypokalemic alkalosis, and hypertension.

Hypersecretion of adrenal androgens can be caused by a tumor, Cushing's syndrome, or other pathology. Manifestations include feminization, virilization, early sexual development, and bone aging and depend on age, gender, and which hormone is secreted.

Management

The goal of management of these disorders is to normalize hormone levels. This is accomplished by surgery or drugs, depending on the particular disease and its cause. Sometimes dietary modification is indicated.

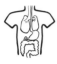

ADRENAL MEDULLA DISORDERS

The adrenal medulla secretes two important catecholamines—epinephrine and norepinephrine. These hormones bind to receptors in the sympathetic nervous system to prolong and enhance the effects of sympathetic stimulation. Hypofunction of the adrenal medulla does not produce any known physiological problems. Hyperfunction, however, can be life threatening. Pheochromocytoma (an uncommon disorder) is caused by an adrenal medullary tumor, which causes hypersecretion of catecholamines. Manifestations are those associated with sustained catecholamine release, including persistent hypertension, tachycardia, headaches, diaphoresis, hypermetabolism, glucose intolerance, and palpitations.

Management

The usual management is surgical excision of the adrenal gland with medications used to stabilize the patient preoperatively and to normalize hormone levels if needed postoperatively. Surgery is considered curative.

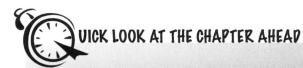

Diabetes mellitus (DM) is a group of heterogeneous disorders characterized by abnormalities in glucose homeostasis, resulting in chronic hyperglycemia. Hyperglycemia is caused by a decrease in the secretion or activity of insulin and destruction of pancreatic beta cells. This alteration in insulin results in disordered metabolism of carbohydrates, fats, and proteins, which may lead to acute, life-threatening complications or chronic complications, including vascular and neurological deficits.

23

Diabetes Mellitus

TERMS

- [ ] **glomerulosclerosis (Kimmelstiel-Wilson disease)**
- [ ] **hyperglycemic hypertonic nonketotic syndrome**
- [ ] **hyperinsulinemia**
- [ ] **polydipsia**
- [ ] **polyuria**

Figure 23-1 Comparison of Type 1 and Type 2 diabetes mellitus.

Comparison of Type 1 and Type 2 Diabetes Mellitus

I. Type 1 (Juvenile Diabetes Mellitus [DM]; Ketosis Prone)
  A. Etiology
    1. Genetic susceptibility (HLA-DR3)
    2. Environmental exposure to virus/infection leading to immune destruction of beta cells
    3. Family history of autoimmune disease
    4. Islet cells antibodies
    5. Insulin antibodies
    6. Absence of C peptide
    7. Ten percent of DM, <20 years old, and of European ancestry
  B. Manifestations
    1. Symptomatic
      a. Onset is usually sudden and severe
      b. Early stage—Polyuria, polydipsia, polyphagia; weight loss; normal or increased appetite; blurred vision; fatigue/weakness; nausea/vomiting; vaginal itch, infection; skin rashes; ketones in blood/urine
      c. Advanced disease (long-term complications)—Loss of appetite, bloating, dehydration, diabetic ketoacidosis, neurogenic/microvascular paresthesias, visual impairment, constipation, nocturnal diarrhea, nocturia, neurogenic bladder, impotence, nephropathy, foot deformity, silent myocardial infarction, cold extremities
    2. Physical Examination
      a. Early—Thin, decreased weight; ill appearance; orthostatic hypotension
      b. Advanced disease—Skin ulcers, "shin spots," hair loss; poor eyes: retinopathy, cataracts, glaucoma; cardiovascular: cool pale extremities, diminished peripheral pulses, decreased capillary refill, pretibial edema; neurological: sensory loss, absent reflexes, deficits of extraocular movement
II. Type 2 (Adult Onset; Ketosis Resistant)
  A. Etiology
    1. Strong genetic link—familial pattern
    2. Insulin resistance, decreased insulin receptors in target cells
    3. Postreceptor defect impairing glucose uptake into cells
    4. Insulin resistance → hyperinsulinemia → diminished insulin production
    5. Relationship to obesity, unknown genetic link, or increased demand
    6. Eighty percent to 90% of DM, >40 years old, overweight, sedentary, family history
  B. Manifestations
    1. Symptomatic
      a. Onset is usually insidious
      b. Early stage—Polyuria, polydipsia, polyphagia; blurred vision; fatigue; sores that heal slowly; recurrent infections (vaginal *Monilia,* urinary tract infections, furuncles, poor dentition); and spontaneous abortion
      c. Advanced disease (long-term complications)—Similar to type 1 but macrovascular problems are more prominent; dyslipidemia, atherosclerosis; hypertension; arterial insufficiency; coronary artery disease; and hyperosmolar hyperglycemic nonketotic coma
    2. Physical Examination
      a. Early—Usually obese; hypertension
      b. Advanced disease—Similar to Type 1

Criteria for Diagnosis of Diabetes

Diabetes Mellitus
- A fasting plasma glucose (FPG) > 126 mg/dL on more than one occasion, a random PG of >200 with symptoms, or a PG value in the 2-hour sample (2hPG) of the standard oral glucose tolerance test (OGTT) of >200 mg/dL PG

Impaired Fasting Plasma Glucose (IFG) (prediabetes)
- A fasting plasma glucose of 100 to 125 mg/dL

Impaired Glucose Tolerance (IGT)
- A 2hPG on standard OGTT ≥ 140 mg/dL but ≤200 mg/dL

Normoglycemia
- FPG < 110 mg/dL, random PG < 140 mg/dL, or 2hPG on standard OGTT < 140 mg/dL

Note: Individuals with IGT and IFG are at increased risk for progressing to diabetes mellitus.

Normal Actions of Insulin

- Facilitates glucose transport into cells (except neurons and hepatic cells)
- Facilitates glycogenesis (the synthesis of glycogen from glucose for storage in liver and skeletal muscles)
- Facilitates lipogenesis (the storage of excessive glucose as lipid in adipose tissue)
- Inhibits glycogenolysis (the breakdown of glycogen stores that is facilitated by glucagon and epinephrine)
- Inhibits gluconeogenesis (the formation of glucose from breakdown of protein and lipids that is facilitated by cortisol and glucagon)

Hyperglycemic Hypertonic Nonketotic Syndrome (HHNK) versus Diabetic Ketoacidosis (DKA)

HHNK
- Severe hyperglycemia
- Severe osmotic diuresis
- Severe hypovolemia (tachycardia, hypotension, shock)
- Severe dehydration (dry mucous membranes, poor turgor)
- Oliguria/anuria
- Neurological abnormalities (altered sensorium, somnolence, coma, seizures, paresis, aphasia)
- Lactic acidosis
- Minimal or absent ketosis

DKA
- Hyperglycemia (polyuria, polydipsia, blurred vision)
- Dehydration/hypovolemia (weakness, tachycardia, hypotension)
- Ketoacidosis (acetone breath, Kussmaul's breathing [deep/rapid], nausea, vomiting, abdominal pain)
- Headache

Table 23-1 Risk Factors for Diabetes Mellitus

First degree relative with DM	History of gestational DM
HDL < 35	Birth of infant > 9 lbs
Triglyceride > 250	Hypertension
BMI > 25 kg/m²	Impaired glucose tolerance
PCOS	Physical inactivity
History of vascular disease	

BMI, body mass index; HDL, high-density lipoprotein; PCOS, polycystic ovary disease.

Table 23-2 Screening Guidelines for Diabetes Mellitus

Prediabetes:
Screen if ≥45 years of age and/or body mass index ≥ 25 kg/m²
OR
If ≤45 years of age and overweight plus one risk factor
Screen those with one or more risk factors every 3 years

DM affects 16 million Americans (6%), with one-third undiagnosed. The number is expected to double in the next decade. African Americans, Hispanics, and Native Americans are particularly vulnerable to the disease and its complications. It is the seventh leading cause of death in the United States and is a significant contributing factor in deaths from other causes. Life expectancy is reduced by about 15 years, and quality of life is impacted. It is the leading cause of end-stage renal disease, blindness, and nontraumatic lower extremity amputations. Approximately 80% of diabetics have cardiovascular complications. The economic cost is estimated to be $102 billion per year.

The American Diabetes Association identifies four types of DM: Type 1 (absolute insulin deficiency, ketosis prone), Type 2 (insulin resistant, nonketosis prone), gestational (glucose intolerance first recognized

The American Diabetes Association identifies four types of DM: Type 1 (absolute insulin deficiency, ketosis prone), Type 2 (insulin resistant, nonketosis prone), gestational (glucose intolerance first recognized during pregnancy, usually the third trimester), and "other specific types" (due to gestational diabetes or less common secondary conditions such as pancreatic disorders, drug related).

during pregnancy, usually the third trimester), and "other specific types" (due to gestational diabetes or less common secondary conditions such as pancreatic disorders, drug related).

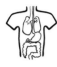

PATHOPHYSIOLOGY

Type 1 DM is typically an autoimmune disease and accounts for approximately 10% of diabetes cases, with a higher incidence among whites, a 10% to 13% incidence among first-degree relatives, a peak incidence at age 12, and more cases reported during autumn and winter. Although it is generally diagnosed before the age of 30, it can develop at any age. Nonautoimmune DM is due to known genetic defects.

Two distinct types of Type 1 have been identified: immune-mediated Type 1 (more common in whites) and nonimmune/idiopathic Type 1 (more common in African Americans and Asian Americans). In immune-mediated Type 1 DM, genetic and environmental factors have been implicated in cell-mediated pancreatic beta cell destruction, with autoantibodies found in 85% to 90% of individuals. Studies indicate a long preclinical period when autoantibodies are detectable before the abrupt onset of clinical manifestations, when 80% to 90% of the beta cells are destroyed, resulting in an insulin deficit. C peptide, which is formed in the process of converting proinsulin to insulin, can be measured in the blood and used as an indicator of the level of functioning beta cells. Type 1 DM is associated with HLA-DR3 and HLA-DR4 antigens, suggesting a genetic susceptibility to environmental factors, such as drugs and chemicals, viruses, and nutritional factors in the etiology. Nonimmune Type 1 DM has no identified etiology.

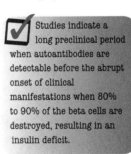

Studies indicate a long preclinical period when autoantibodies are detectable before the abrupt onset of clinical manifestations when 80% to 90% of the beta cells are destroyed, resulting in an insulin deficit.

Carbohydrate, fat, and protein metabolism are affected by the lack of insulin and relative excess of glucagon. As a result, insulin-mediated glucose uptake by hepatic and skeletal muscle cells is disrupted, enabling glucose accumulation in the blood with subsequent overflow of glucose into the urine when the renal threshold is exceeded. Breakdown of fats and protein leads to weight loss and also to high circulating levels of ketones, which causes metabolic acidosis. The metabolic disruption may also cause cardiovascular and neurological problems.

Type 2 DM accounts for 90% of all reported cases, with the highest percentage reported among African Americans, Hispanics, and Native Americans. Type 2 is characterized by insulin resistance and elevated fasting glucose levels. It mainly affects individuals over age 40 and those who are obese. The etiology of Type 2 DM is unknown. Genetic factors interact with environmental factors to affect both insulin action and secretion. Abdominal obesity and high intake of calories and fats are the strongest risk factors and are associated with insulin resistance. It appears that there are two genetic loci involved: one for obesity and one for insulin resistance. The mechanism for insulin resistance is related to defects in insulin receptors, glucose transport mechanisms, and enzymes involved in postreceptor activities in skeletal muscle and hepatic and adipose tissue. The sequence of progression of the disorder begins with the inability of the skeletal muscle cells to take up glucose, especially after meals, resulting in mainly postprandial hyperglycemia. The pancreas may secrete more insulin to counteract the hyperglycemia, causing **hyperinsulinemia.** The hyperglycemia appears to have a toxic affect on the pancreatic beta cells, which then results in a decrease secretion of insulin as the disease progresses.

Abnormal secretion of glucagon has also been demonstrated. Insulin no longer suppresses hepatic gluconeogenesis and glycogenolysis, thus, in addition to postprandial hyperglycemia, fasting blood glucose, HgbA1c, triglycerides, and possibly ketones rise later in the disease.

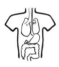

MANIFESTATIONS

DM is diagnosed based on random and fasting blood glucose levels and symptoms. Four clinical stages of glucose tolerance have been identified: normoglycemic, impaired glucose tolerance, impaired fasting glucose, and diabetes (refer to p. 189). Patients may be diagnosed while asymptomatic, with early symptoms, with chronic complications established, or at the time of an acute, life-threatening complication.

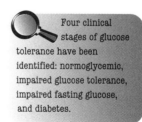

Four clinical stages of glucose tolerance have been identified: normoglycemic, impaired glucose tolerance, impaired fasting glucose, and diabetes.

The hypertonicity of the blood that results from the hyperglycemia causes symptoms such as **polyuria, polydipsia,** temporary blurred vision, and dehydration, and later, acute complications such as hypovolemia, shock, and **hyperglycemic hypertonic nonketotic syndrome.** Hyperglycemia and ketogenesis can be aggravated by counterregulatory hormones such as catecholamines, cortisol, growth hormone, and glucagon (which may be released in situations of stress, infection, or trauma), resulting in another acute complication, diabetic ketoacidosis. Whereas diabetic ketoacidosis is more prevalent in Type 1 DM because of the absolute insulin deficit and relative excess glucagon, hyperglycemic hypertonic nonketotic syndrome is more prevalent in Type 2 DM because of the profound hyperglycemia that can result (see above).

In addition to the acute problems, chronic problems such as neuropathies and macrovascular and microvascular disorders can result and are commonly present for years before diagnosis. Neuropathies are the most common chronic complications of DM and are relevant in both types of DM. These result from a combination of metabolic, genetic, and environmental factors and result in problems with motor (Charcot's joints, foot drop), sensory (painful paresthesias, silent myocardial infarction), and autonomic dysfunction (orthostatic hypotension, gastroparesis, diabetic diarrhea, bladder atony, impotence). Macrovascular problems result from premature atherosclerosis. Hyperglycemia, dyslipidemias (high triglycerides, oxidized low-density lipoproteins, and low high-density lipoproteins), and glycation end products damage vascular endothelium, stimulate smooth muscle proliferation, and increase lipid deposits in plaque. Macrovascular problems lead to hypertension, coronary artery disease (most common cause of death in Type 2 diabetics, also common in Type 1), stroke, and peripheral vascular disease.

Neuropathies are the most common chronic complications of DM and are relevant in both types of DM.

Microvascular disorders result from a thickening of the basement membrane of the capillaries, resulting in ischemia and hypoxia of tissues. Two areas often affected are the eyes and kidneys. Retinopathy develops more readily in Type 2 DM and can lead to retinal detachment and progressive loss of vision. Diabetic nephropathy develops in 30% of Type 1 diabetics and 5% to 10% in Type 2 diabetics and is the leading cause of end-stage renal disease. The exact mechanism that results in **glomerulosclerosis (Kimmelstiel-Wilson disease)** is unknown. Proteinuria is a reliable sign of renal damage.

The neurological and vascular problems contribute to increased risk of infection throughout the body (skin, bladder, and gingiva). Neurological deficits prevent awareness of skin breaks; vascular deficits prevent delivery of defensive cells and oxygen; diminished protein synthesis reduces healing; elevated glucose provides a source of nutrition for pathogens; and white blood cells are abnormal in DM.

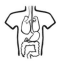

TREATMENT

The main goals of diabetic treatment focus on normalization of blood sugar and prevention of acute and chronic complications. Controlling hypertension and dyslipidemias are essential aspects of a treatment plan. Therapeutic life-style changes that include dietary measures, exercise, and weight management are part of all treatment regimens.

Endogenous insulin is required to sustain life in Type 1 diabetics. Type 2 diabetics may be managed with diet and exercise alone, oral hypoglycemic agents, and/or insulin. Oral hypoglycemic agents may act by diminishing intestinal absorption of glucose, increasing insulin sensitivity, decreasing insulin resistance, or increasing pancreatic insulin. Areas of research include genetic engineering, stem cell research, and beta cell/islet cell transplantation.

Two new classes of drugs for treatment of Type 2 DM, called D-PPIV inhibitors and incretin mimetics, were introduced in 2006 and are showing promising results in control of DM. Inhaled insulin also debuted on the market in 2007 after many years of speculation and intensive research.

PART V · QUESTIONS

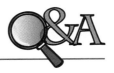

1. The sensitivity of a target cell to a circulating hormone is a result of what?
   a. The number of receptors for that hormone
   b. The amount of hormone in the blood
   c. The amount of bound hormone in the blood
   d. The percentage of body fat

2. Which of the following is an example of an iatrogenic endocrine disorder?
   a. Graves' disease
   b. Cushingoid syndrome from exogenous glucocorticoids
   c. Ectopic hormone production by a malignant tumor
   d. Addison's disease

3. If thyroxine levels are too high, the anterior pituitary produces less TSH. What is this an example of?
   a. Positive feedback
   b. Negative feedback
   c. Facilitated diffusion
   d. Pituitary dysfunction

4. Aging affects endocrine physiology. With aging, there may be
   a. Increased sensitivity of target organs
   b. Increased receptor binding
   c. Glandular structural changes
   d. Decreased amount of connective tissue

5. Increases in parathyroid hormone levels result in which of the following?
   a. Bone catabolism
   b. Bone deposition
   c. Renal excretion of calcium
   d. Renal reabsorption of phosphorus

6. Hyperparathyroidism puts one at risk for what?
   a. Hypothyroidism
   b. Hypertension
   c. Fractures
   d. Gingivitis

7. Which hormone from the parathyroid gland controls calcium homeostasis?
   a. Parathyroid hormone
   b. Calcitonin
   c. Thyroid hormone
   d. Parathyroid-releasing hormone

8. What is the most common cause of hyperparathyroidism?
   a. Graves' disease
   b. Adenoma of the parathyroid
   c. Hashimoto disease
   d. Surgical excision of the parathyroids

9. What measure has been taken in the United States to help prevent dietary deficiencies that lead to thyroid dysfunction?
   a. Adding vitamin B to flour
   b. Adding calcium to orange juice
   c. Adding iodine to salt
   d. Adding vitamin D to milk

10. Because of the thyroid's role in metabolic function, which of the following manifestations would you expect in someone with hyperthyroidism?
    a. Lethargy
    b. Decreased appetite
    c. Weight gain
    d. Heat intolerance

11. The thyroid gland produces all of the following *except*
    a. T_3
    b. T_4
    c. Calcitonin
    d. TSH

12. All of the following are normal changes in the thyroid gland with aging *except*
    a. Atrophy
    b. An increased risk of malignant changes
    c. Fibrosis
    d. An increase in inflammatory infiltrates

13. When does cortisol secretion peak?
    a. In the morning
    b. In the late afternoon
    c. In the evening
    d. During the night

14. Your patient is on long-term glucocorticoid treatments. All of the following are important for her to learn. Which is the *most* important?
    a. Do not stop taking the drug abruptly.
    b. Take the medication with food.
    c. Monitor cuts for healing.
    d. Contact her primary care provider if she has signs of infection.

15. Which of the following is the correct sequence of events in glucocorticoid (cortisol) production?
    a. ACTH-CRH-cortisol
    b. CRH-cortisol-ACTH
    c. CRH-ACTH-cortisol
    d. Cortisol-CRH-ACTH

16. What is an uncommon but potentially life-threatening disorder of the adrenal medulla?
    a. Addison's disease
    b. Pheochromocytoma
    c. Cushing's disease
    d. Hyperaldosteronism

17. Which of the following insulin functions is lost in diabetes mellitus?
    a. Insulin-facilitated breakdown of protein
    b. Insulin-facilitated uptake of glucose by the hepatic and skeletal muscle cells
    c. Insulin-facilitated breakdown of adipose tissue
    d. Insulin-facilitated excretion of glucose by the kidneys

18. Which of the following characteristics more commonly applies to Type 1 diabetes, differentiating it from Type 2?
    a. Stronger genetic component
    b. More common in obese individuals
    c. Greater tendency for ketosis
    d. More common in older individuals

19. Which of the following individuals would be diagnosed with diabetes mellitus?
    a. Individual 1 with a fasting plasma glucose of 126 mg/dL
    b. Individual 2 with a random plasma glucose above 200 mg/dL and symptoms of diabetes
    c. Individual 3 with a random plasma glucose less than 140 mg/dL
    d. Individual 4 with a fasting plasma glucose between 110 mg/dL and 125 mg/dL

20. Which of the following is a complication of diabetes related to autonomic neurological dysfunction?
    a. Orthostatic hypotension
    b. Coronary artery disease
    c. Painful paresthesias of the lower extremities
    d. Renal failure/nephropathy

21. Appropriate therapy for a newly diagnosed Type 2 diabetic includes
    a. Diet and exercise
    b. Oral hypoglycemic agents
    c. Insulin
    d. A combination of A and B

22. Glucocorticoids increase blood glucose levels by
    a. Increasing cellular uptake of glucose
    b. Promoting protein synthesis
    c. Promoting glucogenesis in the liver
    d. Decreasing protein catabolism

23. A decrease in serum calcium levels
    a. Stimulates PTH
    b. Inhibits PTH
    c. Produces renal calculi
    d. Causes insulin resistance

24. The most common cause of Hashimoto thyroiditis is due to
    a. Antibodies that destroy thyroid tissue
    b. Underproduction of TSH
    c. Hypersecretion of T_4
    d. Decreased levels of T_3

25. Which of the following hormones is not affected by iodide?
    a. T_3
    b. T_4
    c. TSH
    d. Thyroglobulin

PART V · ANSWERS

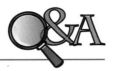

1. **The correct answer is a.** Receptors are necessary for hormones to produce their effects on the target tissue. Choices b, c, and d all play a role in the action and effects of hormones but not in the sensitivity of the target cell.

2. **The correct answer is b.** Iatrogenic disorders are those caused by medical care. The other choices are all diseases.

3. **The correct answer is b.** Negative feedback is a process by which a substance secreted centrally (TSH) is reversed or decreased based on feedback received from the periphery (thyroxine levels). Choices a, c, and d represent different processes/problems.

4. **The correct answer is c.** This is the only change associated with aging among the options given.

5. **The correct answer is a.** The main function of the parathyroid hormone is to maintain serum calcium levels by releasing stored calcium from the bone. Choices b, c, and d are related to bone metabolism in some way but are not directly related to increases in parathyroid hormone.

6. **The correct answer is c.** Hyperparathyroidism causes the release of calcium from bone into the blood, resulting in demineralization that puts one at risk for fractures. The other choices are not related to hyperparathyroidism.

7. **The correct answer is a.** The other choices regulate other processes.

8. **The correct answer is b.** This is the most common cause. Choices a and c are related to the thyroid. Choice d results in hypoparathyroidism.

9. **The correct answer is c.** Iodine is necessary for the formation of thyroxine. The other nutritional additives do not relate to the thyroid.

10. **The correct answer is d.** Heat intolerance is one of many manifestations of a hypermetabolic state. The others can be anticipated with hypothyroidism.

11. **The correct answer is d.** TSH is produced by the anterior pituitary.

12. **The correct answer is b.** Malignant changes are more likely in a younger population.

13. **The correct answer is d.** Diurnal variation is an important consideration in understanding the pathophysiology of certain diseases and administration of selected medications. Choices a, b, and c are incorrect.

14. **The correct answer is a.** Abrupt cessation of exogenous glucocorticoids can cause adrenal insufficiency due to iatrogenic adrenal atrophy that can be reversed by tapering the dose before discontinuing the drug. The other options are important but have less immediate life-threatening consequences.

15. **The correct answer is c.** Corticotropin-releasing hormone from the hypothalamus stimulates adrenocorticotropic hormone from the pituitary, which stimulates cortisol secretion from the adrenal cortex. The other options are not in the correct sequence.

16. **The correct answer is b.** This is the best choice because it is most immediately life threatening. Choices a, c, and d are chronic diseases and can usually be managed effectively.

17. **The correct answer is b.** In diabetes, the relative or total lack of insulin prevents uptake of glucose by hepatic and skeletal muscle cells, thus leading to hyperglycemia (i.e., the accumulation of glucose in the blood). Without glucose for energy production, fats may be broken down, creating ketone bodies, leading to acidosis. Insulin facilitates the synthesis, not breakdown, of protein, thus leading to problems of skin breakdown and poor tissue healing. Insulin facilitates the storage of fats in adipose tissue, not the breakdown. It is lack of insulin that leads to the breakdown of adipose tissue, leading to serum lipid problems.

18. **The correct answer is c.** Because of the absolute lack of insulin in Type 1 diabetes, glucose cannot enter hepatic and skeletal muscle cells; therefore fats are broken down for energy, leading to the creation of ketone bodies, causing ketosis/metabolic acidosis. The other answers apply to Type 2 diabetes.

19. **The correct answer is b.** A random plasma glucose of 200 mg/dL or above with symptoms of diabetes meets the criteria for a diagnosis of diabetes. Other criteria for the diagnosis of diabetes are a fasting plasma glucose of 126 mg/dL or above on two occasions or a plasma glucose value equal to or above 200 mg/dL in the 2-hour sample on a glucose tolerance test. A random plasma glucose of 140 mg/dL or less is normoglycemic. A fasting plasma glucose of 110 mg/dL to 125 mg/dL is considered impaired fasting

plasma glucose (IPFG) and represents an increased risk for diabetes and a need for life-style changes to prevent the onset of diabetes.

20. **The correct answer is a.** Disruption of function of the sympathetic nerves in the lower extremities may lead to orthostatic hypotension. Other manifestations of autonomic dysfunction include gastroparesis, diabetic diarrhea, bladder atony, and impotence. Coronary artery disease is related to the macrovascular problems. Painful paresthesias are related to dysfunction of sensory nerves. Renal failure is due to microvascular problems.

21. **The correct answer is a.** Diet and exercise is recommended for Type 2 diabetics who are newly diagnosed. Medications are added if there is not adequate blood sugar control with diet and exercise alone.

22. **The correct answer is c.** The metabolic effect of glucocorticoids increases blood glucose levels by promoting synthesis of glucose from the liver.

23. **The correct answer is a.** Parathyroid hormone is the most important regulator of serum calcium levels.

24. **The correct answer is a.** Hashimoto thyroiditis or autoimmune thyroiditis is caused by antibodies that destroy thyroid tissue.

25. **The correct answer is d.** Thyroglobulin is not affected by iodide.

Part VI

Respiratory System

Bernadette Madara, BC, APRN

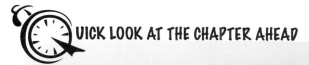
The functions of the respiratory system are to provide oxygen to cells during inhalation; to remove carbon dioxide, which is a byproduct of cell metabolism, during exhalation; and to help regulate serum pH. Oxygen is needed to produce **adenosine triphosphate (ATP)**, which is a nucleic acid that powers cellular activity. Cellular activity produces carbon dioxide that must be removed to prevent a buildup of **carbonic acid** (carbon dioxide + water = carbonic acid) in the bloodstream, which would lower blood pH to life-threatening levels. Although the term respiration is frequently used to denote respiratory activity, ventilation and respiration are more precise descriptors. **Ventilation** means the movement of air and thus denotes inhalation and exhalation, whereas **respiration** denotes the exchange of oxygen and carbon dioxide between cells, the alveoli, and the environment.

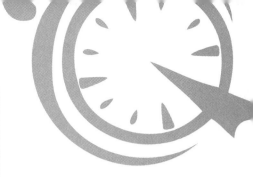

24

Anatomy and Physiology of the Respiratory System

TERMS
- [ ] accessory muscles
- [ ] adenosine triphosphate
- [ ] carbonic acid
- [ ] carbonic anhydrase
- [ ] parietal pleura
- [ ] pleural effusion
- [ ] respiration
- [ ] surfactant
- [ ] ventilation
- [ ] visceral pleura

Figure 24-1 Laboratory tests.

Test	Rationale
Arterial blood gases	Evaluates acid-base balance. **Respiratory acidosis:** Caused by respiratory depression or pulmonary disease—retention of carbon dioxide decreases pH below 7.35. Kidneys compensate by increasing the production and retention of bicarbonate. **Respiratory alkalosis:** Caused by hyperventilation—carbon dioxide rapidly exhaled, leading to a pH increase above 7.45. Kidneys compensate by excreting bicarbonate. **Metabolic acidosis:** Caused by increased production or retention of hydrogen ions as in shock, ketoacidosis, renal failure; pH decreases, bicarbonate decreases. Lungs compensate by increasing ventilation rate. **Metabolic alkalosis:** Caused by loss of hydrogen ions or ingestion of bicarbonate as in prolonged vomiting or bicarbonate overdose; pH increases, bicarbonate increases. Lungs compensate by slow ventilation in order to retain carbon dioxide.
Bronchoscopy	Allows for visualization of the larynx, trachea, and bronchi. Local or general anesthesia or conscious sedation may be used. Biopsies are collected to test for infection or cancer. Aspirated foreign objects, such as peanuts, are removed. Requires nothing by mouth (NPO) status until gag reflex returns.
Pulmonary function tests	Measures the amount of air inhaled and exhaled during a normal breath (tidal volume: about 500 mL) and after maximum inspiration and/or expiration. Abnormal readings signal pulmonary disease. Effectiveness of bronchodilators is evaluated by comparing results before and after their use.
Ventilation-perfusion scan	Perfusion of the pulmonary vessels is determined by injecting radiotagged albumin IV. Pulmonary blood flow distributes the albumin. Ventilation scan detects areas of poor ventilation. Radiotagged gas is inhaled and lungs are scanned for gas distribution. If all lung areas are ventilated and perfused equally, a pulmonary embolus is ruled out. If the lungs are equally ventilated but not perfused, a pulmonary embolus is suspected.

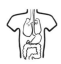

FUNCTIONAL ANATOMY

The pulmonary system consists of the airways (nasal passages, mouth, nasopharynx, larynx, trachea), lungs (two lobes on the left, three on the right), diaphragm, and pulmonary blood vessels. Turbinates are tissue protrusions in each nostril that create air turbulence. Large pollutants, such as dust, are trapped by nasal hairs, whereas the tiny capillaries of the nares warm and humidify the air. Stimulation of nasal irritant receptors by triggers such as pollen activates the sneeze reflex and clears the nares. Insensible water loss of approximately 1 pint per day occurs as we provide humidity to the air we breathe. The frontal, maxillary, and ethmoid sinuses are air-filled spaces that provide resonance to the voice. The larynx contains the vocal cords. Aspiration is prevented by the epiglottis, a tissue flap that closes over the tracheal opening during swallowing.

> The functions of the respiratory system are to provide oxygen to cells during inhalation; to remove carbon dioxide, which is a byproduct of cell metabolism, during exhalation; and to help regulate serum pH.

The trachea branches into the right and left bronchus and then further divides 16 times, finally ending in terminal bronchioles. Mucus and cilia, which line the airway, trap and remove inspired foreign particles by an escalator motion. When the mucus reaches the pharynx, it is either swallowed or expectorated. If tracheal or large airway irritant sensors are triggered, the cough reflex is activated and the lower airways are cleared. The ability to clean and humidify the airway and prevent an environment in which bacteria can flourish is impaired by anything that damages the mucociliary system, such as dehydration, smoking, dry air, or by mouth breathing or a tracheostomy, which bypasses the nares.

> The ability to clean and humidify the airway and prevent an environment in which bacteria can flourish is impaired by anything that damages the mucociliary system.

There is a double-layered membrane that lines the inside of the thoracic cavity (**parietal pleura**) and the outside of the lungs (**visceral pleura**) so that the lungs slide up and down easily during inhalation and exhalation. A thin layer of serous fluid lubricates the pleura and reduces friction associated with ventilation. Accumulation of excess pleural fluid is called **pleural effusion** and results in lung tissue compression and inadequate ventilation.

 Accumulation of excess pleural fluid is called pleural effusion and results in lung tissue compression and inadequate ventilation.

VENTILATION

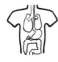

The medulla oblongata in the lower brainstem contains "pacemaker" cells that stimulate autonomous ventilation. The phrenic nerve, which innervates the diaphragm and internal intercostal muscles, transmits neural impulses that trigger inhalation. Stimulation of the apneustic center in the pons triggers gasping ventilation when the higher respiratory center is damaged by trauma.

Chemoreceptors located in the carotid and aortic bodies, the brainstem, stretch and irritant receptors in the airways, and motion receptors in the joints and muscles also help regulate the rate and depth of ventilation. If we require additional oxygen, such as occurs during exercise, the ventilatory rate and volume increases. Although ventilation is mainly an involuntary process controlled by the brainstem, the rate and depth of breathing can be consciously altered up to a point.

When peripheral chemoreceptors in the carotid and aortic bodies sense a rise in the level of arterial carbon dioxide or a decrease in arterial oxygen or serum pH, the respiratory center is stimulated to increase the ventilatory rate and depth. When the central chemoreceptors located near the respiratory center sense a drop in cerebrospinal fluid pH, which closely mirrors serum pH, the respiratory center is again stimulated, resulting in a deeper and faster rate of ventilation to blow off carbon dioxide and lower carbonic acid production.

> When peripheral chemoreceptors in the carotid and aortic bodies sense a rise in the level of arterial carbon dioxide or a decrease in arterial oxygen or serum pH, the respiratory center is stimulated to increase the ventilatory rate and depth.

The diaphragm and external intercostal muscles contract during inhalation, causing an enlarged chest wall and decreased pressure in the lungs, enabling air to enter. Approximately 500 cc of air is inhaled and exhaled with a normal, relaxed breath. **Accessory muscles** are used during dyspnea to assist in ventilation; these include the sternocleidomastoid and scalenus muscles in the neck and possibly facial muscles.

Airway diameter plays an important role in successful ventilation. Bronchodilation occurs because of sympathetic nerve stimulation in an attempt to increase the body's oxygen supply during times of stress. Irritant receptors in the pharynx, trachea, and bronchus, when stimulated by cold air, secretions, or pollutants such as pollen, dust, and tobacco smoke, cause bronchoconstriction and/or coughing and sneezing. If bronchoconstriction continues, the ventilatory effort increases, resulting in dyspnea.

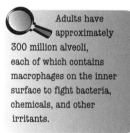

Bronchodilation occurs because of sympathetic nerve stimulation in an attempt to increase the body's oxygen supply during times of stress.

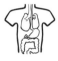

OXYGEN AND CARBON DIOXIDE

Adults have approximately 300 million alveoli, each of which contains macrophages on the inner surface to fight bacteria, chemicals, and other irritants. A fluid, called **surfactant,** coats the inner surface of each alveoli and allows it to remain partially opened during exhalation.

Adults have approximately 300 million alveoli, each of which contains macrophages on the inner surface to fight bacteria, chemicals, and other irritants.

The pulmonary artery, which receives deoxygenated blood from the right ventricle, divides into arterioles and finally pulmonary capillaries, which are composed of capillary endothelium and a basement membrane. These pulmonary capillaries surround the alveoli. Each surfactant-coated alveolar wall

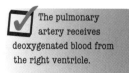

The pulmonary artery receives deoxygenated blood from the right ventricle.

consists of epithelial cells and a basement membrane. A very thin layer of interstitial fluid separates the pulmonary capillary basement membrane from the alveolar basement membrane. Oxygen and carbon dioxide diffuse across this alveolocapillary respiratory membrane. A thick or damaged respiratory membrane impairs this diffusion process.

Hemoglobin, a protein contained in red blood cells, is responsible for transporting 99% of dissolved oxygen to the cells, with 1% transported in plasma. Oxygen and hemoglobin combine in the lungs to form oxyhemoglobin. At the cellular level the oxygen is released in a process called *hemoglobin desaturation.* Acidosis, hypercapnia, high altitude, heart failure, and anemia cause the oxygen–hemoglobin bond to weaken, thereby easily releasing oxygen to the cells. In contrast, alkalosis or a subnormal body temperature makes the oxygen–hemoglobin bond stronger.

Hemoglobin is responsible for transporting 99% of dissolved oxygen to the cells.

An enzyme in red blood cells, called **carbonic anhydrase,** causes 60% of the carbon dioxide produced by cell metabolism to rapidly combine with water and create carbonic acid. The carbonic acid, in turn, rapidly ionizes in the red blood cells to form bicarbonate and hydrogen ions. Hemoglobin acts as a buffer by combining with the hydrogen ions while the bicarbonate diffuses into the plasma. Some carbon dioxide (30%) also forms a weak bond with hemoglobin (carbaminohemoglobin), which transports it to the alveoli. The remaining 10% of carbon dioxide produced is dissolved in the plasma.

Acidosis, hypercapnia, high altitude, heart failure, and anemia cause the oxygen–hemoglobin bond to weaken, thereby easily releasing oxygen to the cells. In contrast, alkalosis or a subnormal body temperature makes the oxygen–hemoglobin bond stronger.

Table 24-1 Common Signs and Symptoms of Lung Disease

Sign/Symptom	Significance
Dyspnea Pathophysiological processes • Airflow obstruction (asthma) • Decreased pulmonary compliance (congestive heart failure, fibrosis) • Change in chest wall compliance (obesity) • Respiratory muscle weakness (chronic respiratory failure) • Hyperinflation (asthma, emphysema) Acute hypercapnia → stimulus Stimulation of airway irritant receptors → stimulus Determine if activity tolerance has decreased	• Subjective phenomena • Sensory input from multiple sites integrated in the cerebral cortex to produce "feeling" of air hunger • Weak correlation between feeling of dyspnea and actual quantitative measure of airflow or exercise intolerance • If patients on a ventilator have an inadequate inspiratory flow rate; they may experience dyspnea which may be manifested as agitation • Use a rating scale similar to the pain rating scale to assess dyspnea • Opioids may mask dyspnea
Cough	Acute episode: less than 3 weeks duration • Viral/bacteria upper respiratory tract infection—25% of people who develop a cough related to a common cold continue to cough for 2–8 weeks • Asthma • Aspiration • Pneumonia • Pulmonary embolism • Pulmonary edema Subacute episode: 3–8 weeks duration Chronic episode: over 8 weeks duration • Chronic bronchitis • Postnasal drip • Gastroesophageal reflux disease (cough may be present without heartburn) • Asthma • Angiotensin-converting enzyme (ACE) inhibitors • Chronic sinusitis

(continued)

Table 24-1 *Continued.*

Hemoptysis (expectoration of blood → bleeding begins below the vocal cords) → usually a sign of serious disease
Anatomical location of bleeding:
• Airways
  • Chronic bronchitis
  • Bronchiectasis
  • Bronchogenic carcinoma
• Pulmonary vasculature
  • Left ventricular failure
  • Mitral stenosis
  • Pulmonary emboli
  • Arteriovenous malformation
• Pulmonary parenchyma
  • Pneumonia
  • Inhalation of crack cocaine
  • Some autoimmune diseases
    (i.e., Goodpasture's disease)
• Iatrogenic
  • After biopsy
  • Anticoagulant therapy
  • Pulmonary artery rupture related to placement of a balloon-tipped catheter
	• Massive → more than 200–600 mL/24 hours or any amount that produces hemodynamic instability or ventilatory difficulty

Table 24-2 Types of Dyspnea

	Common Causes
Acute dyspnea	Asthma Pneumothorax Pulmonary edema Metabolic acidosis Lung infection Panic attack Acute respiratory distress syndrome (ARDS)
Orthopnea (dyspnea when lying down)	Asthma Gastroesophageal reflux disease (GERD) Left ventricular dysfunction Obstructive sleep apnea
Platypnea (dyspnea when sitting upright)	Rare: may signify arteriovenous malformation at lung bases or hepatopulmonary syndrome
Chronic dyspnea	Progressive Symptoms first with exertion—people learn to limit activity Dyspnea then progresses to occur at rest Episodic → asthma, congestive heart failure, acute/chronic bronchitis, recurrent pulmonary emboli Constant → chronic obstructive pulmonary disease (COPD), pulmonary fibrosis, pulmonary vascular disease, severe asthma

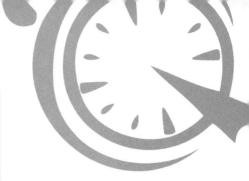

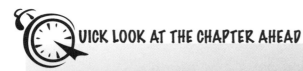

Chronic airflow limitation consists of three common respiratory diseases: asthma, chronic bronchitis, and emphysema. Asthma is the only one of the three chronic disease entities that produces intermittent, reversible airway obstruction. **Asthma,** which is characterized by acute airway inflammation, bronchoconstriction, bronchospasm, edema of the bronchioles, and increased production of mucus, is the most common chronic illness in children. Of the 15 million people in the United States with asthma, approximately 5% of adults and 8% of children are diagnosed.

25
Asthma

TERMS
- [ ] asthma
- [ ] chronic airflow limitation
- [ ] extrinsic asthma
- [ ] intrinsic asthma
- [ ] status asthmaticus

Figure 25-1 Asthma.

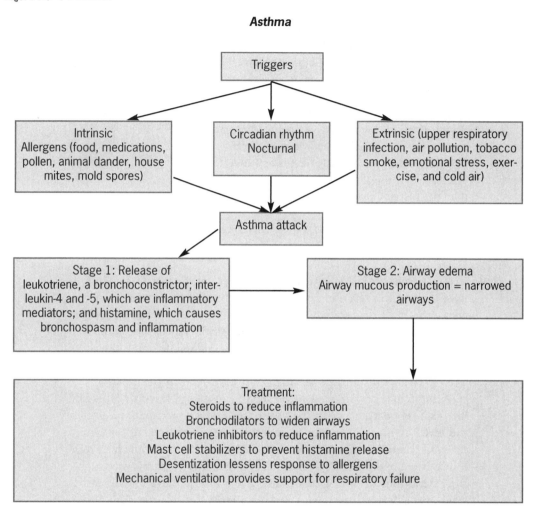

Asthma

Triggers

Intrinsic
Allergens (food, medications, pollen, animal dander, house mites, mold spores)

Circadian rhythm
Nocturnal

Extrinsic (upper respiratory infection, air pollution, tobacco smoke, emotional stress, exercise, and cold air)

Asthma attack

Stage 1: Release of leukotriene, a bronchoconstrictor; interleukin-4 and -5, which are inflammatory mediators; and histamine, which causes bronchospasm and inflammation

Stage 2: Airway edema
Airway mucous production = narrowed airways

Treatment:
Steroids to reduce inflammation
Bronchodilators to widen airways
Leukotriene inhibitors to reduce inflammation
Mast cell stabilizers to prevent histamine release
Desentization lessens response to allergens
Mechanical ventilation provides support for respiratory failure

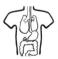

PATHOPHYSIOLOGY

Approximately 470,000 people are admitted to the hospital each year because of asthma, and approximately 5,000 people die each year because of the disease. Children and African Americans have the highest hospital admission

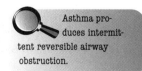

Asthma produces intermittent reversible airway obstruction.

rates for asthma; African-American teens and young adults (aged 15–24 years) have the highest death rates. The number of people diagnosed with asthma, the number of hospitalizations, and the number of deaths have all increased in the past 20 years. Characteristic signs and symptoms of asthma are chest tightness, cough, tachypnea, wheezing, anxiety, and dyspnea caused by airway narrowing. Unless treated promptly, asthma can lead to ineffective gas exchange and death. **Status asthmaticus** is a severe, prolonged asthma attack that does not respond to usual treatment and is life threatening.

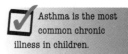 Asthma is the most common chronic illness in children.

 Children and blacks have the highest hospital admission rates for asthma; African-American teens and young adults (ages 15–24) have the highest death rates.

 Status asthmaticus does not respond to usual treatment.

Wearing a face mask, which warms the air and retains airway humidity, is helpful in preventing exercise-induced asthma. Asthma caused by allergens can be managed by removing as much of the offending allergen as possible from the person's environment. Air filters, absence of tobacco smoke, hardwood floors rather than carpets, and dusting daily are some of the measures used to control dust mites and other allergens. Desensitization treatments are also useful in controlling extrinsic asthma.

Asthma may be classified according to cause (e.g., extrinsic [allergic], intrinsic [idiopathic], nocturnal, exercise-induced, occupational, drug-induced) or more precisely by severity (e.g., mild intermittent, mild persistent, moderate persistent, and severe persistent). People with mild intermittent asthma have symptoms less than twice a week with night-time symptoms occurring less than twice a month, have few exacerbations of the disease, and have a peak expiratory flow greater than 80% of the predicted rate. Those with mild persistent asthma have symptoms more than twice a week but less than once a day, nighttime symptoms more than twice a month, and also have a peak expiratory flow greater than 80% of the predicted rate. Once the asthma symptoms occur daily, nighttime symptoms occur more than once a week, and the peak expiratory flow is more than 60% but less than 80%

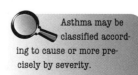 Asthma may be classified according to cause or more precisely by severity.

Table 25-1 Histopathology of Asthma Leading to Symptoms

Denudation (erosion) of airway epithelium	Collagen deposits under the basement membrane
Airway edema	Activation of mast cells
Inflammatory cell infiltration (neutrophils, eosinophils, T lymphocytes)	Hypertrophy of bronchial smooth muscle
Hypertrophy of mucous glands	Airway hyperresponsiveness
Airflow limitation	

of the expected rate, the person is said to have moderate persistent asthma. A person with severe persistent asthma has daily symptoms, must limit physical activity, has frequent nighttime symptoms, and has a peak expiratory flow less than 60% of the predicted rate.

Extrinsic asthma is a result of increased IgE synthesis and hypersensitivity of the airways, resulting in mast cell destruction and release of inflammatory mediators. When stimulated by allergens such as house mites, food additives, pollen, animal dander, drugs (e.g., aspirin [acetylsalicylic acid, or ASA], nonsteroidal antiinflammatory drugs [NSAIDs], nonselective beta-blockers), or mold spores, mast cells in the bronchial tissue release leukotrienes, which cause bronchoconstriction; histamine, which causes increased vascular permeability; and prostaglandins, which cause increased mucus production. The onset of extrinsic asthma generally occurs in childhood or adolescence and is more common in males than in females.

> ✓ The onset of extrinsic asthma generally occurs in childhood or adolescence and is more common in males than in females.

In contrast to extrinsic asthma, **intrinsic asthma** (nonallergic) commonly occurs after age 35. Triggers for intrinsic asthma are an upper respiratory infection, air pollution, tobacco smoke, emotional stress, exercise, and exposure to cold air. Exercise-induced asthma is fairly common, affecting approximately 70% of the people who have asthma. In this type of asthma, the attack usually begins 3 minutes after the activity ends, peaks within 10–15 minutes, and lasts approximately 60 minutes. Hypotheses related to exercise-induced asthma focus on increased airway cooling and drying of the mucosa. It is thought that exercise-induced asthma is a response to the body's attempt to warm and humidify the increased volume of expired air during exercise. Wheezing that occurs in uncompensated congestive heart failure is called cardiac asthma.

In exercise-induced asthma, the attack usually begins 3 minutes after the activity ends.

Occupational asthma is caused by a reaction to substances, such as fumes from plastic, formaldehyde, or cedar dust. Each exposure to the offending substance produces increasingly severe asthma attacks. Time away from work, such as during the weekend, results in clearing of symptoms. It may take years for occupational asthma to develop.

A common cause of drug-induced asthma is ASA, and it may be fatal. ASA intolerance usually develops in patients who have nasal polyps, sinusitis, and asthma. Delayed reactions may occur 12 hours after the ingestion of ASA or may occur shortly after taking the drug. There appears to be a cross-sensitivity to NSAIDs in the person with ASA-induced asthma. Both ASA and NSAIDs prevent the conversion of arachidonic acid to prostaglandins, thereby stimulating leukotriene release, which is a powerful bronchoconstrictor. Food additives, such as yellow dye no. 5 used in pharmaceutical, hair, and food products; monosodium glutamate; and hops, commonly found in beer, have also been indicated in asthma attacks.

Drug-induced asthma may be fatal.

Nocturnal asthma, which generally occurs between 3 AM and 7 AM, is thought to be related to circadian rhythms. At night, natural cortisol and epinephrine levels decrease and plasma histamine levels increase. Epinephrine is a naturally occurring bronchodilator; thus a decrease in epinephrine release produces bronchoconstriction. Nocturnal airway diameter in asthmatics can decrease by as much as 50% during the night. This narrowing, coupled with airway cooling and drying, impaired mucociliary clearance, increased vagal tone, and gastroesophageal reflux disease, causing microaspiration, are thought to be contributing factors to nocturnal asthma. The role of late-phase response

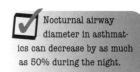
Nocturnal airway diameter in asthmatics can decrease by as much as 50% during the night.

to allergens, which may occur 6 to 12 hours after exposure, is also under investigation.

Regardless of classification, asthma attacks are the body's response to bronchial inflammation. Stage one of an acute asthma attack, generally signaled by coughing, is primarily bronchospastic in nature and reaches a peak within 15 to 30 minutes of the beginning of the attack. Chemical inflammatory mediators responsible for stage one include leukotrienes, interleukin-4 and -5, and histamine.

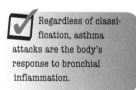

Regardless of classification, asthma attacks are the body's response to bronchial inflammation.

Stage two of an asthma attack peaks within 2 to 6 hours of onset and is a result of airway edema and mucus production. The mucus produced during stage two is generally thick and contains bronchial casts. Air trapping during expiration with resulting alveolar hyperinflation is common. Bronchospasm, smooth muscle contraction, inflammation, and increased mucus production combine to produce a narrowed airway.

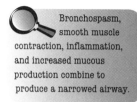

Bronchospasm, smooth muscle contraction, inflammation, and increased mucous production combine to produce a narrowed airway.

Pulmonary function tests, arterial blood gas analysis, complete blood count, challenge testing, and allergy testing are mainstays of asthma diagnosis. Pulmonary function testing in a person with asthma reveals a decreased peak expiratory flow rate, indicating trapped air. Arterial blood gas analysis reveals a decreased carbon dioxide level and respiratory alkalosis related to tachypnea. As respiratory exhaustion takes place, there is an increase in the arterial carbon dioxide level and a decrease in the oxygen level. The person may experience dehydration, general exhaustion, and respiratory failure. Eosinophilia, as reflected in a complete blood count, indicates the body's response to an allergen. Allergy testing is used to pinpoint the offending allergen(s).

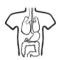

MANAGEMENT

Inhaled steroids, nebulizer treatments, inhaled bronchodilators, and leukotriene modifiers are some of the pharmaceutical agents used to control and/or prevent asthma attacks. Beta agonists are useful in preventing exercised-induced asthma, as is cromolyn sodium, which is a mast cell stabilizer. Ipratropium bromide, an inhaled anticholinergic, is used to relax bronchial smooth muscle. During status asthmaticus, intravenous steroids, intravenous bronchodilators, and mechanical ventilation may be necessary.

Prevention of nocturnal asthma is vital because most asthma-related fatalities occur during the early morning hours. The treatment for nocturnal asthma includes longer acting beta agonists and histamine blockers to control gastroesophageal reflux disease (GERD). Left untreated, long-term asthma may result in bronchial tissue damage and scarring, which in turn leads to increased hyperreactivity of the airways.

Prevention of nocturnal asthma is vital because most asthma-related fatalities occur during the early morning hours.

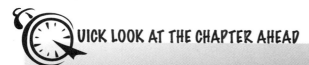

This section provides an explanation of the pathophysiology related to acute respiratory distress syndrome and pulmonary emboli. Both of these conditions are life threatening.

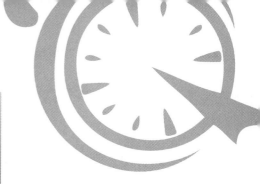

26

Acute Respiratory Distress Syndrome and Pulmonary Emboli

TERMS
- ☐ acute respiratory distress syndrome (ARDS)
- ☐ Greenfield filter
- ☐ polycythemia
- ☐ pulmonary capillary wedge pressure
- ☐ pulmonary embolism (PE)
- ☐ Virchow's triad
- ☐ ventilation-perfusion scan

Figure 26-1 Acute respiratory distress syndrome.

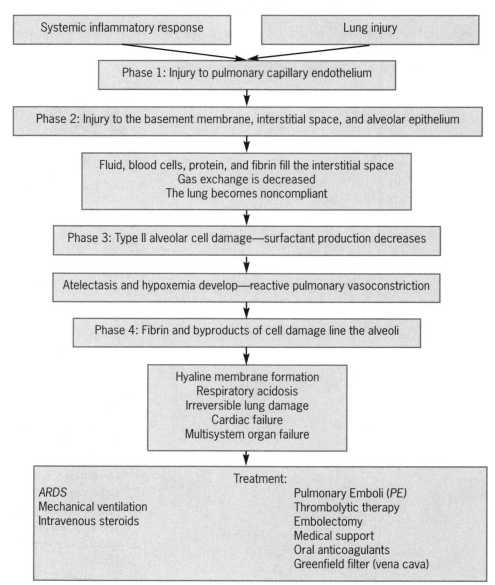

Acute Respiratory Distress Syndrome (ARDS)

| Systemic inflammatory response | Lung injury |

Phase 1: Injury to pulmonary capillary endothelium

Phase 2: Injury to the basement membrane, interstitial space, and alveolar epithelium

Fluid, blood cells, protein, and fibrin fill the interstitial space
Gas exchange is decreased
The lung becomes noncompliant

Phase 3: Type II alveolar cell damage—surfactant production decreases

Atelectasis and hypoxemia develop—reactive pulmonary vasoconstriction

Phase 4: Fibrin and byproducts of cell damage line the alveoli

Hyaline membrane formation
Respiratory acidosis
Irreversible lung damage
Cardiac failure
Multisystem organ failure

Treatment:

ARDS
Mechanical ventilation
Intravenous steroids

Pulmonary Emboli (*PE*)
Thrombolytic therapy
Embolectomy
Medical support
Oral anticoagulants
Greenfield filter (vena cava)

Acute respiratory distress syndrome (ARDS), also known as shock lung, wet lung, Vietnam lung, noncardiogenic pulmonary edema, and adult hyaline membrane disease, was first identified in 1967 as a cause of pulmonary edema resulting from alveolocapillary membrane injury. ARDS is an acute hypoxemia as the result of a systemic or pulmonary event that is not cardiac in origin. The patient with ARDS has widespread pulmonary infiltrates but a normal **pulmonary capillary wedge pressure** (below 18 mm Hg). This type of pulmonary edema affects approximately 150,000 patients per year and has a mortality rate of 30–40% and as high as 90% if the patient also is septic. Patients who survive ARDS may have permanent lung damage, and most have a persistent cough, dyspnea, and sputum production.

Risk factors for developing this noncardiogenic pulmonary edema include aspiration of gastric contents, all types of shock, oxygen toxicity, fat embolism, major trauma, smoke inhalation, multiple blood transfusions, viral pneumonia, and burns. Approximately 3 in

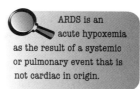

ARDS is an acute hypoxemia as the result of a systemic or pulmonary event that is not cardiac in origin.

10 patients who develop ARDS have had sepsis. Prevention of ARDS relies on avoidance of the occurrences that cause the syndrome.

 This type of pulmonary edema has a mortality rate of 30–40% and as high as 90% if the patient also is septic.

Any bolus of bloodborne material such as air from an intravenous line, fat from a long bone fracture or trauma, amniotic fluid that enters the circulation during childbirth, tumor tissue, or a thrombus that blocks a pulmonary artery is termed a **pulmonary embolism (PE)**, the third most common cardiovascular disease process in the United States. Approximately 64% of autopsies reveal a PE regardless of the cause of death. PE causes a sudden obstruction of blood flow to lung tissue and may cause death, especially within the first 1 to 2 hours after the initial insult. The most common sources of blood clots include the right ventricle, as a consequence of atrial fibrillation, and deep vein thrombosis arising in the pelvis or calf muscles. Deep vein thrombosis is the most common cause of PE, accounting for approximately 5 million cases in the United States each year. Annually, PE is

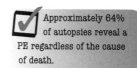

Approximately 64% of autopsies reveal a PE regardless of the cause of death.

responsible for approximately 200,000 deaths and is the third leading cause of death among hospitalized patients. Over half of patients with proximal deep vein thrombosis develop PE, many of which are asymptomatic.

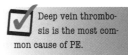
Deep vein thrombosis is the most common cause of PE.

 PE causes a sudden obstruction of blood flow to lung tissue and may cause death, especially within the first 1 to 2 hours after the initial insult.

Over half of patients with proximal deep vein thrombosis develop PE, many of which are asymptomatic.

Prevention of PE lies in removing or reducing risk factors that create clots. Risk factors that create **Virchow's triad** (venous stasis, vessel wall injury, hypercoagulability) such as bed rest, **polycythemia,** and pregnancy, may lead to a PE. Low-dose subcutaneous heparin every 12 hours helps to reduce the likelihood of deep vein thrombosis after surgery or during periods of immobility. Some of the measures used to reduce the risk of PE are encouraging movement and using sequential compression devices (Venodyne boots) in postoperative or bed-ridden patents, avoiding oral contraceptives in women who smoke, using anticoagulant medication for patients with atrial fibrillation, and using an inferior vena cava filter **(Greenfield filter)** to stop clots from traveling to the heart.

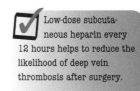
Low-dose subcutaneous heparin every 12 hours helps to reduce the likelihood of deep vein thrombosis after surgery.

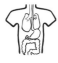

ACUTE RESPIRATORY DISTRESS SYNDROME

Pathophysiology

ARDS develops rapidly, often within 90 minutes of a systemic inflammatory response and within 24 to 48 hours of an initial lung injury. There are four phases of the ARDS process, during which there is progressive respiratory distress caused by atelectasis resulting from reduced surfactant production, reactive pulmonary vasoconstriction caused by hypoxemia,

Table 26-1 Disorders Associated with ARDS Development

Systemic Causes of ARDS	Pulmonary Causes of ARDS
Trauma	Free-base cocaine smoking
Pancreatitis	Lung contusion
Drugs and drug overdose	Toxic gas inhalation
• Opioids	• Ammonia
• Aspirin	• Smoke
• Amiodarone	• Chlorine
• Chemotherapeutic drugs	• Nitrogen dioxide
• Nitrofurantoin	• Sulfur dioxide

and cardiac failure caused by an increase in right ventricular afterload. The pulmonary capillary endothelium is injured during phase 1. Phase 2 follows with injury to the basement membrane, interstitial space, and alveolar epithelium. The damaged capillaries and alveolar walls become permeable during phase 2, allowing fluid, blood cells, protein, and fibrin to fill the space around the alveoli, decreasing gas exchange, creating a noncompliant lung, and increasing the work of breathing. The protein-rich fluid filling the alveoli causes damage to type II alveolar cells that produce surfactant in phase 3, ultimately leading to atelectasis and hypoxemia. Fibrin and byproducts of cell damage line the inside of the alveoli in phase 4, leading to hyaline membrane formation, respiratory acidosis, irreversible lung damage, and possibly multisystem organ failure.

ARDS develops rapidly, often within 90 minutes of a systemic inflammatory response and within 24 to 48 hours of an initial lung injury.

Assessment of a patient who has ARDS reveals tachypnea, dyspnea, crackles related to pulmonary edema, hypoxemia not relieved by oxygen therapy, respiratory acidosis, restlessness, anxiety, and right-sided heart failure. Stress ulcers frequently occur. Clinical and x-ray examinations cannot differentiate between pulmonary edema that has a cardiogenic cause and one that has a noncardiogenic cause. Pulmonary capillary

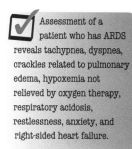

Assessment of a patient who has ARDS reveals tachypnea, dyspnea, crackles related to pulmonary edema, hypoxemia not relieved by oxygen therapy, respiratory acidosis, restlessness, anxiety, and right-sided heart failure.

wedge pressure (PCWP), reflecting left ventricular filling pressure, enables a definitive diagnosis to be made. Pulmonary capillary wedge pressure is elevated in pulmonary edema caused by congestive heart failure but is normal (6–18 mm Hg) in pulmonary edema caused by ARDS because the edema is created by damage to the alveolar-capillary membrane, not a deficient heart muscle.

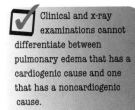

Clinical and x-ray examinations cannot differentiate between pulmonary edema that has a cardiogenic cause and one that has a noncardiogenic cause.

Management

The treatment goals for a patient with ARDS include supplying oxygen to vital organs by supporting the respiratory system with mechanical ventilation until the process has reversed itself, as well as prevention of bronchopulmonary dysplasia. Although the lowest concentrations of oxygen, tidal volume, and airway pressure are used to accomplish these goals, high concentrations of oxygen may be necessary to maintain the PO_2 around 90%. Intravenous steroid therapy is used to halt the progression of late-stage fibrin deposits, enabling the lungs to function at an optimal level.

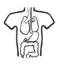

PULMONARY EMBOLI

Pathophysiology

As clots pass through the right atrium to the right ventricle of the heart, they are broken into smaller units that can subsequently block peripheral branches of the pulmonary artery. This blockage results in decreased perfusion and ventilation ability. Respiratory distress may be slight if only a few small capillaries are blocked or major if larger vessels are blocked. If one or more large clots block a large pulmonary vessel, the right ventricle pumps harder in a futile attempt to bypass the blockage. As blood builds up in the right ventricle (right ventricular afterload), the intraventricular septum shifts to the left, making the left ventricle smaller. As a result, the left ventricle is able to pump far less blood to the circula-

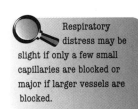

Respiratory distress may be slight if only a few small capillaries are blocked or major if larger vessels are blocked.

tion, leading to decreased coronary perfusion, myocardial ischemia, and cardiogenic shock.

Assessment of a patient who has a small PE may reveal no signs or symptoms of hypoxia. Large PEs cause abrupt onset of signs and symptoms of respiratory distress, such as dyspnea, pain on inspiration, chest pain, anxiety, cough, tachypnea, and crackles. Massive clots cause cyanosis, syncope, and sudden death.

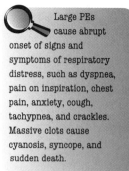

Large PEs cause abrupt onset of signs and symptoms of respiratory distress, such as dyspnea, pain on inspiration, chest pain, anxiety, cough, tachypnea, and crackles. Massive clots cause cyanosis, syncope, and sudden death.

In contrast to emboli caused by clots, fat emboli occur as fat droplets and enter the circulation after orthopedic surgery, bone fracture, or surgery on an obese patient. As the pulmonary fat emboli are hydrolyzed, free fatty acids are released, resulting in increased capillary permeability. Sections of alveolar collapse occur, resulting in dyspnea and rapid heart and ventilatory rates. Confusion, delirium, and petechiae on the chest and arms are also signs of fat emboli.

Confusion, delirium, and petechiae on the chest and arms are signs of fat emboli.

Most diagnostic tests are not conclusive and only suggest a diagnosis of PE. Blood gas analysis reveals a PO_2 of less than 80 mm Hg, chest x-ray that may show pulmonary infiltration, and a lung scan (**ventilation-perfusion scan**) may demonstrate ventilation but lack of perfusion. A definitive test for PE is the pulmonary angiogram. During this test, a contrast medium is injected into the pulmonary arteries and the vessels are visualized.

Most diagnostic tests are not conclusive and only suggest a diagnosis of PE.

Management

Treatment for a PE includes thrombolytic therapy directly into the pulmonary artery to dissolve clots if the patient has immediate access to medical care or possible surgical embolectomy and medical support of cardiac and respiratory functions. Intravenous heparin administered as a continuous infusion for approximately 5 days followed by oral

Table 26-2 Laboratory Tests

Test	Significance + Procedure
Electrocardiogram	• Abnormal in 70% of patients with a PE • Sinus tachycardia, nonspecific T-wave changes (40% of patients)
Arterial blood gas analysis	• Suggestive but not diagnostic • Acute respiratory alkalosis (hyperventilation) • Profound hypoxia
D-dimer (fragment D-dimer, fibrin degradation fragment)	• Elevated (300–500 ng/mL) • Below 500 ng/mL, highly likely that PE not present • Positive test indicates high level of fibrin degradation products in plasma • Signals significant clot formation and breakdown • Recent surgery, trauma, infection, liver disease, pregnancy, eclampsia, heart disease, and some cancers also cause elevated levels
Chest radiography	• Used to rule out other lung diseases and causes of hypoxia
Lung scan (ventilation-perfusion scan)	• The ventilation portion involves inhaling a radioactive gas into the lungs. This part of the scan shows areas of the lungs that are not receiving adequate inhaled air. The perfusion portion involves scanning a radioactive substance injected into an arm vein. This part of the scan shows areas of the lungs that are not receiving enough blood because of a blockage in the pulmonary vasculature.
Computed tomography (helical computed tomographic arteriography)	• False negative in approximately 20% of PE cases • Intravenous radiocontrast dye allows visualization of pulmonary vasculature

Venous thrombosis studies
• Venous ultrasonography
  • Test of choice for proximal deep vein thrombosis
• Impedance plethysmography
  • Noninvasive medical test
  • Measures changes in electrical resistance of a specific area of the body, reflecting blood volume changes
• Contrast venography
	• 70% of patients with a PE also have a DVT
	• 50% of patients with a deep vein thrombosis have a PE detected by angiography
	• Invasive test
	• Allergic reaction to contrast and discomfort accessing dorsal foot veins limit use of test

Pulmonary arteriography	• Research indicates a high level of reliability as a diagnostic tool for PE • Invasive • Contrast media injected into blood vessels
Magnetic resonance imaging	• Used primarily as a research tool • Noninvasive • No contrast dye used • Expensive

Figure 26-2 Pulmonary emboli.

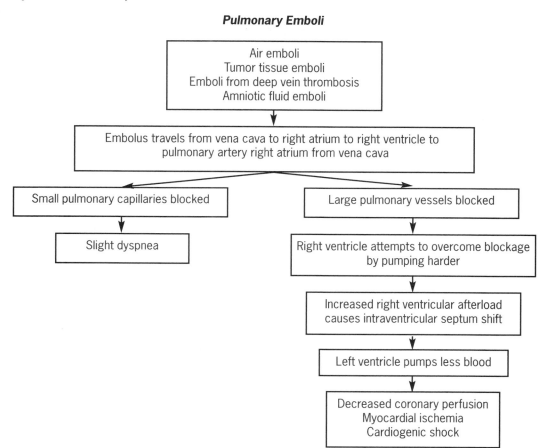

anticoagulant therapy for several months are used if a diagnosis of PE has been made and the patient survives. Treatment for fat emboli includes respiratory support via oxygen and/or mechanical ventilation and systemic steroids to reduce the inflammatory response.

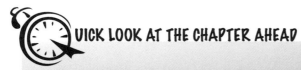

QUICK LOOK AT THE CHAPTER AHEAD

Chronic obstructive pulmonary disease (COPD) occurs when there is chronic, often progressive, airflow limitation related to **chronic bronchitis** or **emphysema.** It has been estimated that 28 million people have COPD, although only 50% have been diagnosed. The death rate from COPD is increasing, with elderly men the most affected.

27

Chronic Bronchitis and Emphysema

TERMS
- [ ] α_1-antitrypsin (AAT) enzyme
- [ ] blebs
- [ ] bullae
- [ ] centrilobular emphysema
- [ ] chronic bronchitis
- [ ] chronic obstructive pulmonary disease (COPD)
- [ ] cor pulmonale
- [ ] emphysema
- [ ] hypercapnia
- [ ] panlobular emphysema
- [ ] pulmonary hypertension

Figure 27-1 Chronic obstructive pulmonary disease.

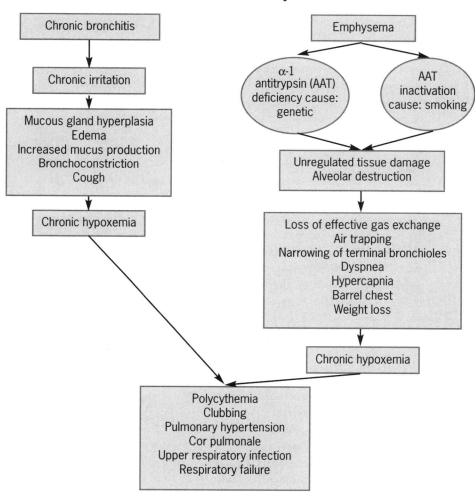

Chronic Obstructive Pulmonary Disease

Chronic bronchitis

Chronic irritation

Mucous gland hyperplasia
Edema
Increased mucus production
Bronchoconstriction
Cough

Chronic hypoxemia

Emphysema

α-1 antitrypsin (AAT) deficiency cause: genetic

AAT inactivation cause: smoking

Unregulated tissue damage
Alveolar destruction

Loss of effective gas exchange
Air trapping
Narrowing of terminal bronchioles
Dyspnea
Hypercapnia
Barrel chest
Weight loss

Chronic hypoxemia

Polycythemia
Clubbing
Pulmonary hypertension
Cor pulmonale
Upper respiratory infection
Respiratory failure

Treatment:
Smoking cessation
Antibiotics for infection
Percussion and postural drainage
Bronchodilators
Inhaled or systemic steroids

Replacement of ATT enzyme if deficiency exists
Surgical removal of lung segments
Low flow oxygen for maintenance
Lung transplant
Mechanical ventilation during respiratory failure

Approximately one in four adults in the United States has chronic bronchitis, which is defined as inflammation of the bronchi, a productive cough, and increased mucus production for at least 3 months of the year for 2 consecutive years. Current or former smokers are at greatest risk for developing this disease, as are people exposed to inhaled irritants such as second-hand cigarette smoke and air pollution.

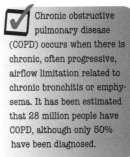

Chronic obstructive pulmonary disease (COPD) occurs when there is chronic, often progressive, airflow limitation related to chronic bronchitis or emphysema. It has been estimated that 28 million people have COPD, although only 50% have been diagnosed.

 Current or former smokers are at greatest risk for developing chronic bronchitis.

Emphysema, which affects 2.5 million Americans, is an anatomical term that denotes loss of lung elasticity as a result of the breakdown of connective tissue support of the lower airways, abnormal dilatation of air spaces distal to the terminal bronchioles, and abnormal enlargement and eventual destruction of the alveoli. Risk factors for developing emphysema include chronic bronchitis, smoking, and air pollution.

PATHOPHYSIOLOGY

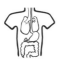

Chronic Bronchitis

As a defense against airborne irritants, the upper and mid-airways set up an inflammatory response that result in mucus gland hyperplasia, edema, increased thick mucus production, bronchoconstriction, and cough. Airway resistance affects both inspiration and expiration, resulting in hypoventilation, hypoxemia, cyanosis, **hypercapnia,** increased red blood cell production (i.e., polycythemia), clubbing of the fingers, and eventually, shortness of breath even at rest.

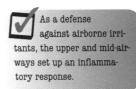

As a defense against airborne irritants, the upper and mid-airways set up an inflammatory response.

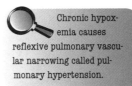

Chronic hypoxemia causes reflexive pulmonary vascular narrowing called pulmonary hypertension.

Chronic hypoxemia causes reflexive pulmonary vascular narrowing called **pulmonary hypertension.** As the right ventricle hypertrophies in an attempt to overcome increased pulmonary artery resistance, **cor pulmonale** (i.e., right-sided heart failure) develops.

Patients with chronic bronchitis are, for unknown reasons, unable to increase their ventilatory effort to effectively overcome airway resistance, and they eventually develop cyanosis ("blue bloaters"). Impaired pulmonary defenses, including cilia damage and decreased phagocytic activity, result in frequent respiratory infections and, in some cases, respiratory failure requiring mechanical ventilation.

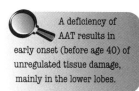 As the right ventricle hypertrophies in an attempt to overcome increased pulmonary artery resistance, cor pulmonale (i.e., right-sided heart failure) develops.

 Impaired pulmonary defenses, including cilia damage and decreased phagocytic activity, result in frequent respiratory infections.

Emphysema

Approximately 2% of emphysema cases are caused by a genetic deficiency of the α_1-**antitrypsin (AAT) enzyme.** Lung tissue normally undergoes a process of remodeling during periods of growth and repair related to lung infections and inflammation. Proteolytic enzymes involved in this process, such as trypsin, are normally inactivated by AAT so that tissue damage is controlled. A deficiency of AAT results in early onset (before age 40) of unregulated tissue damage, mainly in the lower lobes. Smoking, which causes an inflammation of lung tissue, also results in the release of proteolytic enzymes and the inactivation of AAT, resulting in upper lobe structural changes.

A deficiency of AAT results in early onset (before age 40) of unregulated tissue damage, mainly in the lower lobes.

Smoking, which causes an inflammation of lung tissue, also results in the release of proteolytic enzymes and the inactivation of AAT, resulting in upper lobe structural changes.

Two major patterns of emphysema are centrilobular (centriacinar) and panlobular (panacinar). **Centrilobular emphysema** is associated with both smoking and chronic bronchitis, primarily affecting the respiratory bronchioles, whereas **panlobular emphysema** is associated with AAT deficiency and senile emphysema, which affects the terminal and respiratory bronchioles and alveoli. Senile emphysema is a normally occurring degenerative change and does not usually cause symptoms.

Alveolar destruction causes a loss of surface and pulmonary capillary bed area, which reduces effective gas exchange, decreases surfactant production, and produces large, ineffective air spaces called **bullae**

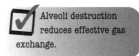

Alveoli destruction reduces effective gas exchange.

or **blebs.** The loss of elastic recoil of lung tissue results in air trapping during expiration, and hyperinflation of the alveoli causes a narrowing of the terminal bronchioles. Inspiration is not affected, and cough is not a usual symptom. Assessment reveals diminished breath sounds and a rapid, shallow respiratory pattern ("pink puffers").

A person with emphysema initially presents with dyspnea upon exertion. In later stages of the disease, weight loss is marked due to severe dyspnea and tachypnea, even at rest. The work of breathing is so difficult that most calories taken in are expended in maintaining respiration and normal pH blood gas levels. Hypercapnia (i.e., elevated carbon dioxide level) because of CO_2 trapping is evident, as is the use of accessory muscles, leading to the development of a barrel chest as the lungs maintain a hyperinflated state. Normally, the diaphragm does 65% of the work of respiration and the accessory muscles do 35% of the work. In emphysema, lost lung elasticity and hyperinflation of the airways causes the accessory muscles to work more and the diaphragm to work less.

The work of breathing is so difficult that most calories taken in are expended in maintaining respiration and normal pH blood gas levels.

Pursed-lip breathing, either instinctive or learned, and assuming a tripod position ease the work of breathing. Pursed-lip breathing increases the resistance to the expiratory phase of respiration and produces airway back pressure, which helps to prevent alveolar and airway collapse. The tripod position is assumed when the person sits up and leans forward, thus supporting the ribcage and allowing for fuller chest expansion.

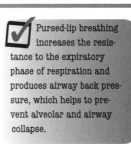

Pursed-lip breathing increases the resistance to the expiratory phase of respiration and produces airway back pressure, which helps to prevent alveolar and airway collapse.

A patient with COPD has an abnormal pulmonary function test, most notably a reduction of the forced expiratory volume, forced vital capacity, increased residual vol-

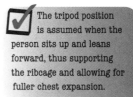

The tripod position is assumed when the person sits up and leans forward, thus supporting the ribcage and allowing for fuller chest expansion.

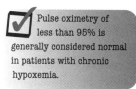

ume, and increased airway resistance. Decreased elastic recoil results in an increased residual volume and an increased total lung capacity. Arterial blood gases may reflect hypercapnia, hypoxemia, and respiratory acidosis, especially in patients with airway obstruction due to chronic bronchitis. Pulse oximetry of less than 95% is generally considered normal in patients with chronic hypoxemia. Because of tachypnea, some patients have mild respiratory alkalosis. Chest x-rays show increased anterior-posterior diameter, low flat diaphragm, and possibly bullae and blebs.

Pulse oximetry of less than 95% is generally considered normal in patients with chronic hypoxemia.

COPD produces an increased hemoglobin and hematocrit count as the body attempts to overcome hypoxemia by supplying more red blood cells to carry oxygen. If infection is present, the white blood cell count is increased with a shift to the left, indicating release of immature white blood cells. Long-term severe COPD may eventually result in cor pulmonale, which can be diagnosed by a noninvasive Doppler echocardiogram.

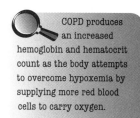

COPD produces an increased hemoglobin and hematocrit count as the body attempts to overcome hypoxemia by supplying more red blood cells to carry oxygen.

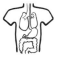

MANAGEMENT

Prevention of chronic bronchitis and emphysema focuses on smoking avoidance or cessation, yearly flu vaccines and a pneumococcal vaccine to prevent pneumonia, and support of clean air legislation. Antibiotic therapy for bacterial respiratory infections, mucolytics, increased fluid intake to thin secretions, bronchodilators, inhaled or systemic steroids, oxygen, and mechanical ventilation during periods of respiratory failure are treatment options.

Percussion and postural drainage may be required to assist in mobilizing thick secretions and prevent mucous plug formation. Pulmonary rehabilitation programs are aimed at increasing respiratory function through participation in regular exercise programs. Education and psychosocial support are achieved through the use of support groups. To prevent weight loss, small, frequent feedings and supplemental vitamins are encouraged.

Continuous low-flow (1 to 2 L/min) oxygen therapy has been shown to reduce mortality in persons with severe COPD and PO_2 levels below

55 mm Hg. Episodes of hypoxemia during sleep are common because of shallow breathing. Oxygen therapy is titrated to maintain PO_2 around 60 mm Hg. In COPD, the drive to breathe is controlled by the amount of oxygen in the blood, not by the amount of carbon dioxide. Flooding the person with oxygen therefore decreases the respiratory drive.

If emphysema is caused by an ATT deficiency, enzyme replacement is a treatment option; however, this treatment is expensive and its efficacy is uncertain. Screening should be done for people with a family history of this genetic defect.

The most recent advance in treatment for severe emphysema is surgical lung volume reduction, which removes bullous lung segments. This procedure seems to restore support to the distal airways, improving expiration. Lung transplantation has also been used for patients with severe COPD and has a 75% 2-year survival rate.

Table 27-1 Comparison of Emphysema and Chronic Bronchitis

	Emphysema	Chronic Bronchitis
History and physical	Severe dyspnea Usually no cough Thin appearance Use of accessory muscles No adventitious sounds No peripheral edema	Mild dyspnea Chronic cough Overweight Cyanosis Peripheral edema Wheezing, rhonchi
Laboratory values	Normal hemoglobin PaO_2 slightly reduced Chest x-ray → hyperinflation	Elevated hemoglobin PaO_2 elevated Chest x-ray → interstitial markings
Pulmonary function tests	Total lung capacity increased Airflow obstruction	Total lung capacity normal Airflow obstruction
Nocturnal ventilation	Mild to moderate oxygen desaturation during sleep	Severe oxygen desaturation Frequently associated with sleep apnea

Lung cancer is a neoplasm that arises out of lung tissue. In addition to primary tumors occuring in the lungs, cancer arising from other sites, such as the breast, frequently metastasize to lung tissue. It is currently the leading cause of cancer deaths among both men (32%) and women (25%), with more African Americans than whites developing the disease. Mortality rates for lung cancer approach 90%, with a 5-year survival rate after diagnosis approaching only 15%.

28

Lung Cancer

TERMS
- [ ] adenocarcinoma
- [ ] asbestos
- [ ] hemoptysis
- [ ] hila
- [ ] oncogenes
- [ ] paraneoplastic characteristics
- [ ] squamous cell carcinoma
- [ ] superior vena cava syndrome

Figure 28-1 Lung cancer.

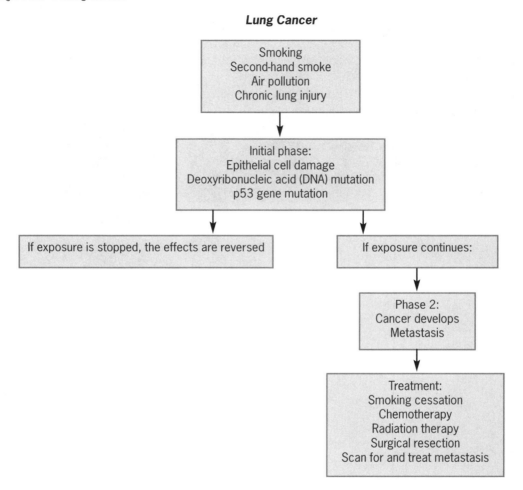

Lung Cancer

Smoking
Second-hand smoke
Air pollution
Chronic lung injury

↓

Initial phase:
Epithelial cell damage
Deoxyribonucleic acid (DNA) mutation
p53 gene mutation

If exposure is stopped, the effects are reversed

If exposure continues:

↓

Phase 2:
Cancer develops
Metastasis

↓

Treatment:
Smoking cessation
Chemotherapy
Radiation therapy
Surgical resection
Scan for and treat metastasis

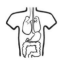

INTRODUCTION

Each year approximately 180,000 new cases of lung cancer are diagnosed, and the vast majority of these cases (80–90%) are directly linked
to smoking. Cigarette smoke contains 4,000 chemicals, 43 of which are
known carcinogens, including tar, which paralyzes cilia. Other causes of
lung cancer include second-hand smoke inhalation, which causes

between 500 and 5,000 deaths per year; inhaled carcinogens such as **asbestos;** and chronic lung disease such as chronic obstructive pulmonary disease in which mucociliary action is diminished, resulting in poor removal of airborne carcinogens.

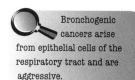 Lung cancer is currently the leading cause of cancer deaths among both men (32%) and women (25%), with more African Americans than whites developing the disease.

There is a direct correlation between the age a person began smoking, how much and how long he or she smoked, and the likelihood of developing lung cancer. People who began smoking in their teenage years, inhale deeply, and smoke at least one-half pack per day have the highest risk of developing the disease. Someone who stops smoking experiences a gradual decline in lung cancer risk. Recently, attention has focused on the risk of developing lung cancer for those exposed to second-hand smoke, such as someone living with a smoker and restaurant/bar workers. Research has indicated that second-hand smoke may contain more carcinogens than inhaled smoke. It takes between 10 and 30 years after exposure to the carcinogens in cigarettes for lung cancers to develop. This accounts for the incidence of lung cancers in people who develop the disease years after they stop smoking. Smokers who are also exposed to other environmental carcinogens, such as air pollution, are at a very high risk for developing lung cancer.

Someone who stops smoking experiences a gradual decline in lung cancer risk.

 It takes between 10 and 30 years after exposure to the carcinogens in cigarettes for lung cancers to develop.

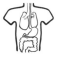

PATHOPHYSIOLOGY

Bronchogenic cancers arise from epithelial cells of the respiratory tract and are aggressive. The first phase of lung cancer development involves irreversible cell deoxyribonucleic acid (DNA) mutation of **oncogenes** and tumor suppressor genes because of exposure to carcinogenic substances. The *p53* gene, a tumor suppressor gene responsible for controlling cell replication, is one of those genes

Bronchogenic cancers arise from epithelial cells of the respiratory tract and are aggressive.

mutated. Over time, exposure to carcinogenic environmental agents alters the growth and reproduction of the affected cells. If exposure to the carcinogens is stopped, the effects are reversible. If the exposure to carcinogens continues, cancer develops.

 If exposure to the carcinogens is stopped, the effects are reversible. If the exposure to carcinogens continues, cancer develops.

Histologic types of bronchogenic cancer, which account for approxmately 90% of all cases of primary lung cancer, include squamous cell carcinoma, which arises from bronchial epithelium; adenocarcinoma, which arises from mucous glands; and bronchioloalveolar carcinoma, which arises from epithelial cells within or distal to the terminal bronchioles. The terms *small cell lung can*cer (SCLC) and *non-small cell lung cancer* (NSCLC) are used for staging and treatment purposes of bronchogenic cancers. Small cell cancers generally occur in the central part of the lungs and are also called oat cell cancers. They tend to be more aggressive than large cell cancers, invade local tissue, and metastasize readily by way of the lymphatic system. Small cell cancers make up approximately 25% of all lung cancers, are the most strongly associated with smoking, and have a poor prognosis. These tumors grow aggressively, metastasize readily, and some have **paraneoplastic characteristics,** meaning that the tumors can produce indirect effects such as the secretion of inappropriate

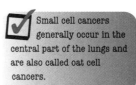
Small cell cancers generally occur in the central part of the lungs and are also called oat cell cancers.

antidiuretic hormone or hyperparathyroidism, producing hypercalcemia. Other paraneoplastic syndromes associated with lung cancer include Cushing's syndrome, myasthenia-like syndrome, peripheral neuropathy, endocarditis, and anemia. Paraneoplastic syndrome does not indicate metastasis.

Non-small cell cancers account for 75% of all lung cancers. Included in this group are **adenocarcinomas,** squamous cell carcinomas, and undifferentiated large cell carcinomas. **Squamous cell carcinoma,** which arises from epithelial cells, is generally located in the **hila** (i.e., the areas where the bronchus splits into the right and left bronchi), tends to be slow growing, is strongly associated with smoking and air pollution, and may take 4 years to become large enough to cause symptoms. Ninety percent of squamous cell cancers occur in men, cause bronchial obstruction, and account for approximately 30% to 40% of lung cancers. Half of the patients diagnosed with squamous cell lung cancer survive 5 years.

Adenocarcinomas arise primarily at sites of previous pulmonary damage, such as fibrotic areas, and are the most common lung tumors in nonsmokers and women. This cancer arises from the bronchial glandular epithelium, including the alveoli and terminal bronchioles. Although this type of lung cancer is slow growing, it also has a tendency to metastasize. The 5-year survival rate for adenocarcinoma is poor.

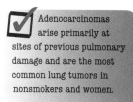

Adenocarcinomas arise primarily at sites of previous pulmonary damage and are the most common lung tumors in nonsmokers and women.

Undifferentiated large cell cancers carry a poor prognosis because of early metastasis. Metastasis to the brain, bone, liver, central nervous system, and adrenal glands is common with this type of lung cancer, and it tends to invade surrounding structures such as the heart, major blood vessels, esophagus, and trachea.

The patient is asymptomatic early in the course of lung cancer. Later signs and symptoms include a chronic cough similar to "smoker's cough" as irritant receptors are stimulated, wheezing as airway obstruction increases, fatigue, and aching joints. Upper respiratory infections may develop because airway defense mechanisms are hampered. **Hemoptysis** is a late sign. **Superior vena cava syndrome** may occur as the tumor compresses that vessel and impairs blood return to the right atrium. Signs of superior vena cava syndrome include headache, upper extremity edema, and facial flushing.

The patient is asymptomatic early in the course of lung cancer.

By the time most lung tumors are detectable by x-ray, they are already 1 cm large and the likelihood of metastasis is great. Fiberoptic bronchoscopy, which enables bronchial washings and the recovery of bronchial cells, can detect lung cancer early in the disease process; however, the prognosis is generally poor because of the tendency of lung cancer to metastasize.

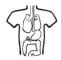

MANAGEMENT

The most efficient method to prevent lung cancer is to eliminate cigarette smoking and exposure to occupational carcinogens. Smoking has been a common activity since ancient times when it was thought to have medicinal properties. Today, smoking is recognized as the primary cause of chronic bronchitis, emphysema, and lung cancer and is associated

Table 28-1 Signs and Symptoms of Lung Cancer

Anorexia, weight loss (55–90%)	Hemoptysis (25–40%)
Nonspecific chest pain	New cough or change in a chronic cough (6–31%)
Pleural effusion (12–33%)	Change in voice (laryngeal nerve compression)
Superior vena cava syndrome	Horner's syndrome—abnormal findings all occurring on the same side of the body (ipsilateral), ptosis (drooping eyelid), sinking in of one eyeball, miosis (constriction of the pupil), anhidrosis (lack of sweating), and flushing of the affected side of the face. The syndrome is caused by paralysis of nerves.
Asthenia	Brain metastasis (headache, nausea, vomiting, seizures, altered mental status)

with the development of pancreatic and bladder cancer. Although cigarette smoking is declining in the United States, due to aggressive marketing techniques, its use is increasing in underdeveloped countries. Because the nicotine in cigarettes is a highly addictive, psychoactive substance, most people find it difficult to stop smoking. The use of nicotine patches, which replace inhaled nicotine with a gradually declining amount of transdermally absorbed nicotine, has enabled some people to stop smoking without suffering from nicotine withdrawal. Smoking cessation support groups, psychotherapy, and hypnosis have

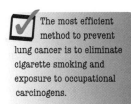

The most efficient method to prevent lung cancer is to eliminate cigarette smoking and exposure to occupational carcinogens.

also been successful. As with any addiction, the key to the success of any smoking cessation program lies with the commitment the person has to give up the addiction.

The nicotine in cigarettes is a highly addictive, psychoactive substance.

Table 28-2 Mesothelioma

Overview	• Primary tumor arising from the surface of the pleura (80% and, of those, 60–80% have had asbestos exposure) or the peritoneum (20%) • Most pleura tumors are diffuse • More men than women are affected • Exposure to asbestos is associated with malignant pleural mesothelioma—20- to 40-year lag time • Asbestos exposure may occur thorough exposure to construction/demolition work, brake linings, insulation, mining, etc.
Signs and symptoms	• Shortness of breath • Nonpleuritic chest pain • Weight loss • Digital clubbing • Percussion dullness • Diminished breath sounds
Complications	• Pleural tumors spread to pericardium, mediastinum, and contralateral pleura • Progressive pain and dyspnea • Superior vena cava syndrome, Horner's syndrome • Dysphagia • Paraneoplastic syndrome (hemolytic anemia, disseminated intravascular coagulation)
Treatment	• Surgery • Radiotherapy • Chemotherapy (treatment is not usually successful)
Prognosis	• Median survival time from onset of symptoms is generally 4–16 months • Five-year survival rate is less than 5%

Treatment for large cell cancers includes pneumonectomy, which is removal of the entire lung, or lobectomy, which is removal of the affected lung segment if distant metastasis has not occurred. Chemotherapy and radiation therapy are also treatment options if local lymph node involvement is detected. Because of their bronchial location small cell cancers are treated with palliative measures such as chemotherapy and radiation therapy but not surgery.

QUICK LOOK AT THE CHAPTER AHEAD

This chapter discusses the pathophysiology associated with two common causes of impaired gas exchange, pneumonia and atelectasis. Pneumonia is an inflammatory process that may be caused by numerous infectious agents. It is the sixth leading cause of death in the United States and the leading cause of death from infection. Atelectasis, or incomplete alveolar expansion or collapse, occurs when the walls of the alveoli stick together.

29

Pneumonia and Atelectasis

TERMS
- [ ] atelectasis
- [ ] bronchopneumonia
- [ ] community-acquired pneumonia
- [ ] lobar pneumonia
- [ ] nosocomial pneumonia
- [ ] pneumonia

Figure 29-1 Atelectasis and pneumonia.

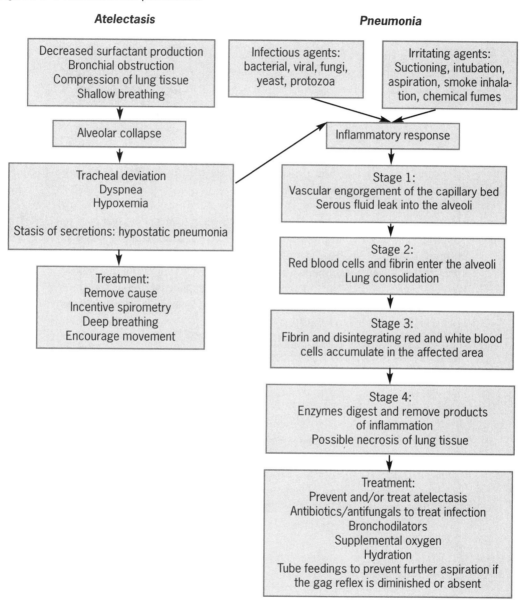

PNEUMONIA

Pneumonia, the sixth leading cause of death in the United States and the leading cause of death from infection, is an inflammatory process that may be caused by numerous infectious agents, such as bacteria, viruses, fungi, yeast, or protozoa. *Streptococcus pneumoniae,* a bacterium, is responsible for up to 75% of all cases of pneumonia. In contrast to bacterial pneumonia, viral pneumonia is usually mild and heals without intervention; however, it can lead to a more virulent bacterial pneumonia.

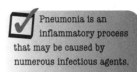
Pneumonia is an inflammatory process that may be caused by numerous infectious agents.

Irritating agents or events, such as suctioning, intubation, aspiration of gastric juice, inhalation of smoke, or chemical fumes, can also lead to pneumonia. Aspiration pneumonia may occur because the gag reflex is impaired as the result of a brain attack or because a nasogastric tube prevents the lower esophageal sphincter from closing, allowing gastric juice or tube-feeding formula to enter the lungs. Gastric secretions and tube-feeding formulas are irritating to lung tissue and set up an inflammatory response when aspirated.

Irritating agents or events, such as suctioning, intubation, aspiration of gastric juice, inhalation of smoke, or chemical fumes, can also lead to pneumonia.

Other common causes of pneumonia are stasis of respiratory secretions and thickened secretions. Stasis of secretions in immobile patients can lead to pneumonia because bacteria can grow in the static secretions. When respiratory secretions become thick, as in a patient with fluid volume deficit, ciliary action cannot remove the bacteria-laden mucus, and pneumonia may result.

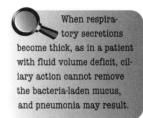
When respiratory secretions become thick, as in a patient with fluid volume deficit, ciliary action cannot remove the bacteria-laden mucus, and pneumonia may result.

Pathophysiology

Pneumonia may be classified by the agent that causes it or by its location in the lung. **Lobar pneumonia** is confined to a single lobe of the lung, whereas **bronchopneumonia,** the most common type, is described as patchy pneumonia in several lobes. Atypical pneumonia, usually caused by viruses (e.g., type A or B influenza) or bacteria (e.g., *Legionella*), is also patchy but does not involve the alveoli. Pneumonia may also be classified according to where it was acquired. **Nosocomial pneumonia** is pneumonia that develops more than 48 hours after admission to the hospital, and **community-acquired pneumonia** is pneumonia acquired outside of a hospital/health care setting. Two to 3 million cases of community-acquired pneumonia, the most deadly infectious disease in the United States, occur each year. There is a 14% mortality rate for patients hospitalized with this type of pneumonia.

When the cough/gag reflex, mucociliary system, or immune system is compromised, bacteria and other pneumonia-causing agents enter the normally sterile lung fields. Bacteria can enter the lungs by inhalation or via the bloodstream. The inflammatory process is responsible for the four stages of pneumonia. The first stage is the *24-hour congestion stage,* during which time there is vascular engorgement of the capillary bed and serous fluid leaks into the alveoli. During this time, the patient may complain of fever, chills, aching chest, malaise, dyspnea, and watery phlegm, and the white blood cells begin to rise. Auscultation reveals fine crackles over the affected area.

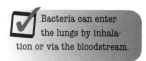

Bacteria can enter the lungs by inhalation or via the bloodstream.

The second stage is called the *red hepatization stage* as red blood cells and fibrin enter the alveoli, creating a red, firm lung appearance. Lung sounds in the consolidated area are absent. The patient may complain of dyspnea (a subjective symptom) and tachypnea.

The third stage, the *gray hepatization stage,* begins as fibrin and disintegrating red/white blood cells accumulate in the affected area. The cough may become blood-tinged or purulent. If the pneumonia has not been treated with antibiotics, the *resolution stage* begins in approximately 8 to 10 days. This is the "cleanup" stage during which time enzymes digest and remove the products of inflammation. The exudate is either coughed up or removed by white blood cells. Necrosis of lung tissue may occur.

Diagnostic tests for pneumonia include a chest x-ray, which shows areas of consolidation; culture and sensitivity of collected sputum; complete blood count; arterial blood gases to determine oxygenation needs, including intubation and ventilation support; and possibly a bronchoscopy to collect samples and/or remove secretions.

Management

Careful and consistent hand washing helps to prevent nosocomial infections. Patients who are in a high-risk group for community-acquired pneumonia benefit from influenza and pneumococcus vaccines. Postoperative patients should be turned every 2 hours, encouraged to deep breathe, and cough, and taught to use incentive spirometry. All three acts assist in preventing atelectasis, a frequent cause of pneumonia in this population. The elderly and immunocompromised patients are most at risk for developing pneumonia.

 The elderly and immunocompromised patients are most at risk for developing pneumonia.

Once pneumonia develops, treatment focuses on eradicating the infection and/or correcting the underlying cause of the inflammation. Bacterial and fungal infectious agents are treated with antibiotic therapy. Few antiviral agents are available at this time. Bronchodilators may be prescribed to reduce or prevent bronchospasm.

Supportive measures include careful monitoring of respiratory and oxygenation status, hydration to thin secretions so they can be expectorated, supplemental oxygen, rest to promote healing, and, in some cases, chest physiotherapy. If aspiration pneumonia occurs, treatment is aimed at eliminating the cause of the aspiration and includes having the patient take nothing by mouth until swallowing studies have been completed and evaluated and possibly placing a permanent feeding tube.

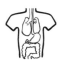

ATELECTASIS

Atelectasis, or incomplete alveolar expansion or collapse, occurs when the walls of the alveoli stick together, producing impaired gas exchange. Atelectasis is caused by a decrease of surfactant, a lipoprotein that coats the inside of the alveoli and allows them to remain open at the end of expiration; by obstruction of a bronchus; or by compression of lung tissue as a result of a tumor, pleural effusion, or pneumothorax. To prevent atelectasis, postoperative patients and those on bed rest should be encouraged to deep breathe, and cough

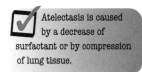

Atelectasis is caused by a decrease of surfactant or by compression of lung tissue.

every 1 to 2 hours. Effective pain management and incisional splinting postoperatively allow the patient to deep breathe and cough.

Pathophysiology

Small areas of atelectasis may produce few, if any, symptoms, whereas larger areas of involvement result in inadequate ventilation and hypoxemia, producing signs such as diminished breath sounds, dyspnea, and restlessness. Tracheal deviation to the affected side occurs if the area of alveolar collapse is large. Atelectasis is diagnosed by chest x-ray, and if left untreated it may lead to pneumonia and/or respiratory failure.

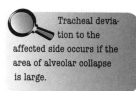

Tracheal deviation to the affected side occurs if the area of alveolar collapse is large.

 Small areas of atelectasis may produce few, if any, symptoms, whereas larger areas of involvement result in inadequate ventilation and hypoxemia.

Management

Treatment focuses on removing the cause (e.g., using bronchoscopy to remove a mucous plug or antibiotic therapy to combat infection). Incentive spirometry is effective because it encourages the patient to take and hold a deep breath, increasing the likelihood of keeping the alveoli open.

QUICK LOOK AT THE CHAPTER AHEAD

Tuberculosis (TB) is a chronic recurrent infection involving the lung and less commonly other tissues, specifically the meninges, liver, kidney, brain, and bone marrow. **Mycobacterium tuberculosis**, an aerobic bacillus that has been around since ancient times, is responsible for causing the infection. It is estimated that 20–43% of the world's population has been infected with this bacillus, and it remains a major health problem in developing countries.

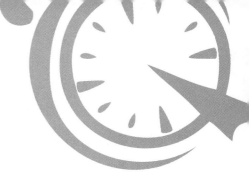

30
Tuberculosis

TERMS
- ☐ bacille Calmette-Guérin vaccine
- ☐ caseous necrosis
- ☐ empyema
- ☐ granulomatous lesions or Ghon's focus
- ☐ Mantoux test
- ☐ purified protein derivative (PPD)
- ☐ tine test
- ☐ tuberculosis (TB)

Figure 30-1 Tuberculosis.

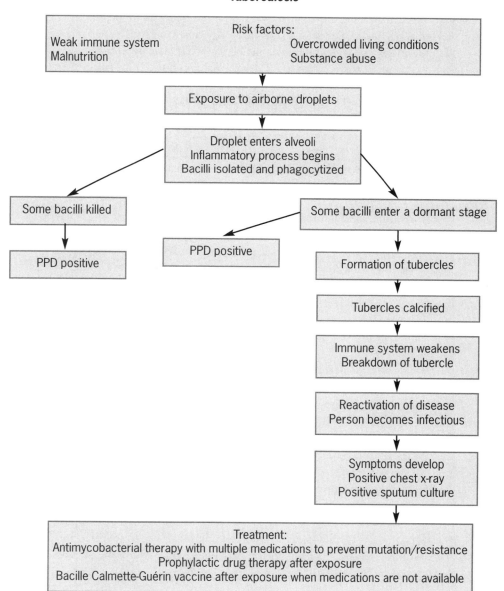

Tuberculosis

Risk factors:
Weak immune system   Overcrowded living conditions
Malnutrition   Substance abuse

Exposure to airborne droplets

Droplet enters alveoli
Inflammatory process begins
Bacilli isolated and phagocytized

Some bacilli killed

PPD positive

PPD positive

Some bacilli enter a dormant stage

Formation of tubercles

Tubercles calcified

Immune system weakens
Breakdown of tubercle

Reactivation of disease
Person becomes infectious

Symptoms develop
Positive chest x-ray
Positive sputum culture

Treatment:
Antimycobacterial therapy with multiple medications to prevent mutation/resistance
Prophylactic drug therapy after exposure
Bacille Calmette-Guérin vaccine after exposure when medications are not available

Approximately 20 million people worldwide have tuberculosis (TB), and it is responsible for 3 million deaths worldwide annually. In the United States, approximately 15 million people are infected with *M. tuberculosis,* with more men infected than women. The incidence is highest among Asians and Pacific Islanders, followed by African Americans, Hispanics, Native Americans, and whites. The incidence of TB is rising in the United States because of the emergence of drug-resistant strains. Fifteen percent of people infected with TB in the United States have a drug-resistant strain. Hospitals and correctional facilities in Florida and New York have reported outbreaks of drug-resistant strains of TB with a mortality rate of 70–90% and a mean survival time of 4–16 weeks.

> The incidence of TB is rising in the United States because of the emergence of drug-resistant strains.

TB is often classified as an opportunistic infection because it is likely to develop in someone with a weakened immune system. People at high risk for contracting TB are those with acquired immunodeficiency syndrome, malnutrition, diabetes, and/or alcoholism. Poverty, overcrowding, homelessness, and drug abuse also place people at risk for the disease.

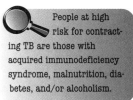

People at high risk for contracting TB are those with acquired immunodeficiency syndrome, malnutrition, diabetes, and/or alcoholism.

TB may be classified as primary (i.e., disease occurs 2 years after infection), reactivation (i.e., disease occurs later than 2 years after infection), pulmonary (i.e., disease occurs in the lungs), or extrapulmonary/miliary (i.e., disease occurs in other tissues). Transmission of TB occurs via airborne droplets when a person with active disease, approximately 5% to 15% of those infected, talks, sings, coughs, or sneezes. High concentrations of the bacilli in the air, such as in small, closed, nonventilated areas, and numerous exposures to the bacilli increase the risk for transmission of the infection.

The incidence of TB can be reduced by education aimed at stopping the transmission of the disease and screening measures to identify persons who have been exposed to the bacillus so that additional further testing and medical treatment can begin.

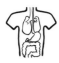

PATHOPHYSIOLOGY

The droplet nuclei that harbor the bacilli are so small that when they are inhaled, they travel directly to the alveoli. Once the bacilli enter the alveoli, usually settling in an upper lobe, an inflammatory response begins. The bacilli are isolated and phagocytized, but not all are destroyed. Some enter a dormant state and can reactivate. From 1 to 3 weeks after the initial infection, tubercles (**granulomatous lesions** or **Ghon's focus**) begin to form. These tubercles are composed of fused, elongated macrophages that have engulfed the bacilli and are surrounded by lymphocytes. In time, the central section of the tubercle becomes necrotic and forms a yellow "cheesy" mass called a **caseous necrosis.** As the immune response continues, scar tissue forms around the tubercle, and it eventually calcifies. The breakdown of a tubercle releases the bacilli and signals an active disease process. If the primary TB progresses, it can erode the bronchus. If the infection spreads to the bloodstream, it can be disseminated to other body areas. Partial immunity develops from infection and offers protection against reinfection.

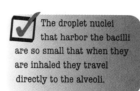
The droplet nuclei that harbor the bacilli are so small that when they are inhaled they travel directly to the alveoli.

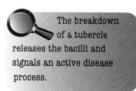
The breakdown of a tubercle releases the bacilli and signals an active disease process.

Secondary, or reactivation, TB occurs if the sealed-off primary lesion breaks apart; this can lead to pleural effusion, **empyema,** and spread of the disease to others. This most likely happens if the person's immune system weakens because of malnutrition, use of systemic steroids, chemotherapy, or acquired immunodeficiency syndrome. Approximately 10% of people who are not given preventative therapy develop active TB. It has been estimated that 50% of people with human immunodeficiency virus develop active TB within 24 months of the primary TB infection.

Reactivation TB most likely happens if the person's immune system weakens.

A person initially infected with TB may be asymptomatic, have non-specific symptoms, or may show signs of pneumonia. Common signs and symptoms of active disease include a low-grade fever, weight loss, weakness, anorexia, night sweats, and malaise. Blood-tinged sputum, chest pain, and chronic cough indicate advanced necrosis. The person appears to be ill and malnourished.

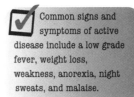

Common signs and symptoms of active disease include a low grade fever, weight loss, weakness, anorexia, night sweats, and malaise.

The tuberculin skin test converts to positive during the granuloma formation stage of the disease. People exposed to the bacilli develop a cellular response within 3 to 10 weeks after exposure, and injecting a small amount of **purified protein derivative (PPD)** of tuberculin activates a local inflammatory response, yielding a positive test result. A positive PPD indicates that the person has been infected and developed a cellular response to the bacillus, not that he or she currently has active disease and is infectious. Intradermal PPD is also called a **Mantoux test,** whereas a multiple-puncture test is called a **tine test.** The tine test is less accurate than the Mantoux test.

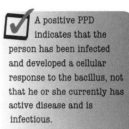

A positive PPD indicates that the person has been infected and developed a cellular response to the bacillus, not that he or she currently has active disease and is infectious.

Active TB is diagnosed by a positive chest x-ray and positive culture. Eighty-five percent of patients with TB have an abnormal chest x-ray involving the apical and posterior segments of the upper lobes, especially in the right lung. Early morning sputum cultures, generally three consecutive specimens, are examined for the acid-fast bacillus. A culture positive for *M. tuberculosis* is definitive for the disease. Ten days is required for the slow-growing bacillus to produce positive culture results.

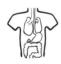

MANAGEMENT

Treatment for TB requires an average of 6 to 9 months of antimycobacterial therapy. The slow-growing bacilli have a high rate of mutation and develop resistance when exposed to monotherapy, so multiple medications are required to treat this disease. Primary drugs used include medications by mouth, such as isoniazid, rifampin, ethambutol, pyrazinamide, and parenteral streptomycin. Because TB is a public health risk, antituberculin medications are provided free of charge by the U.S. Public Health Service. Sputum cultures and chest x-rays are used to evaluate the effectiveness of the treatment regime.

 The slow-growing bacilli have a high rate of mutation and develop resistance when exposed to monotherapy.

In cases in which a person is suspected of having a subclinical case of TB, a year-long treatment with isoniazid is recommended to prevent active disease. Persons who are positive for the human immunodeficiency virus and have a positive PPD or persons who are close contacts of someone with newly diagnosed TB and who have a positive PPD fall into this category.

The **bacille Calmette-Guérin vaccine** is administered when prophylactic isoniazid therapy cannot be used. This vaccine is widely used in developing countries to protect infants and children from becoming infected with TB. In the United States it is recommended for infants, children, and health care workers with a negative PPD who are repeatedly exposed to ineffectively treated or untreated persons with TB. After the vaccine is administered, subsequent PPD tests will be positive.

 After the vaccine is administered, subsequent PPD tests will be positive.

PART VI · QUESTIONS

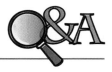

1. The ventilatory rate is controlled by the
   a. Medulla oblongata
   b. Serum bicarbonate level
   c. Pons' apneustic center
   d. Sympathetic nervous system

2. Which of the following statements about carbon dioxide is *true?*
   a. Ninety-nine percent of the carbon dioxide produced by cellular metabolism combines with hemoglobin.
   b. Carbon dioxide combines with water to form carbonic anhydrase.
   c. Serum carbon dioxide levels drive the rate and depth of ventilation in individuals who do not have chronic obstructive pulmonary disease.
   d. A high serum carbon dioxide level results in respiratory alkalosis.

3. Medications that may cause asthma in hypersensitive individuals include
   a. Cardiac glycosides
   b. Beta-blockers
   c. Carbonic anhydrase inhibitors
   d. Serotonin reuptake inhibitors

4. The nurse explains to Karin, a patient newly diagnosed with asthma, that nocturnal asthma is thought to be caused by
   a. Increased cortisol levels
   b. Decreased vagal tone
   c. Decreased epinephrine levels
   d. Increased plasma histamine levels

5. The nurse evaluating Ms. Clayton's ABGs, a patient with ARDS, correctly evaluates the ABGs pH of 7.50 as indicating:
   a. Respiratory acidosis
   b. Respiratory alkalosis
   c. Metabolic acidosis
   d. Metabolic alkalosis

6. Which of the following statements concerning ARDS is true?
   a. One of the causes of ARDS is congestive heart failure.
   b. Pulmonary capillary wedge pressure is elevated in ARDS.
   c. Surfactant production is reduced in ARDS.
   d. ARDS has a low mortality rate.

7. When assessing a client who has fat emboli, the nurse is likely to note which of the following?
   a. Petechiae on the chest
   b. Bradycardia
   c. Bradypnea
   d. Pedal edema

8. What is the major cause of chronic bronchitis?
   a. A deficiency of AAT
   b. Smoking
   c. Aging
   d. Asthma

9. Lung changes that occur in emphysema include
   a. Increased elastic recoil
   b. Increased pulmonary capillary permeability
   c. Increased surfactant production
   d. Narrowing of the terminal bronchioles

10. Which of the following statements about lung cancer is *true*?
    a. Metastasis is rare.
    b. When someone stops smoking, their risk of developing lung cancer declines rapidly.
    c. Second-hand smoke is more likely to cause lung cancer than inhaled smoke.
    d. The 5-year survival rate for adenocarcinoma is high.

11. Signs of superior vena cava syndrome related to lung cancer include
    a. Headache
    b. Pallor
    c. Wheezing
    d. Pedal edema

12. Which of the following statements regarding pneumonia is *true?* (Select all that apply.)
   a. Pneumonia is exclusively caused by bacteria or viruses.
   b. Pneumonia is most commonly caused by a bacterium.
   c. Pneumonia generally produces mild symptoms if the cause is viral.
   d. Pneumonia generally resolves within 3 to 4 days.

13. The nurse auscultating lung sounds in a patient with atelectasis most likely hears
   a. Rhonchi
   b. Rales
   c. Wheezing
   d. Diminished breath sounds

14. Which of the following statements concerning TB is *true?*
   a. A positive PPD indicates active infection.
   b. Bacille Calmette-Guérin vaccine is used prophylactically.
   c. The dormant stage of TB generally lasts a few months.
   d. Developing resistance to antimycobacterial therapy is rare.

15. Classic signs of active pulmonary TB include (select all that apply)
   a. High fever
   b. Weight loss
   c. Night sweats
   d. Wheezing

16. The *most* precise term that denotes the exchange of oxygen and carbon dioxide between cells, the alveoli, and the environment is
   a. Respiration
   b. Ventilation
   c. Inhalation
   d. Exhalation

17. Events that can damage the mucociliary system and allow bacteria to enter the lungs include (select all that apply)
   a. Dehydration
   b. Smoking
   c. Breathing dry air
   d. Mouth breathing

18. When peripheral chemoreceptors in the carotid and aortic bodies sense a rise in the level of arterial carbon dioxide or a decrease in arterial oxygen or serum pH, the respiratory center is stimulated to (select all that apply)
    a. Decrease the ventilatory rate
    b. Increase the ventilatory rate
    c. Decrease the ventilatory depth
    d. Increase the ventilatory depth

19. Which of the following can stimulate irritant receptors in the pharynx, trachea, and bronchus and cause bronchoconstriction? (Select all that apply.)
    a. Warm air
    b. Pollen
    c. Dust
    d. Tobacco smoke

20. The pulmonary artery
    a. Receives oxygenated blood from the left atrium
    b. Returns oxygenated blood to the right atrium
    c. Receives deoxygenated blood from the right ventricle
    d. Returns deoxygenated blood to the left ventricle

21. Events that cause the oxygen–hemoglobin bond to weaken, thereby easily releasing oxygen to cells, include
    a. Alkalosis
    b. Subnormal temperature
    c. Hypocapnia
    d. Anemia

22. The nurse, explaining the term *dyspnea* to a new graduate, correctly states that dyspnea is
    a. An objective sign of pulmonary disease
    b. Directly correlated to airflow measurements
    c. Manifested by agitation in some ventilated patients
    d. Made apparent when sedatives are given to a patient

23. Hemoptysis may be caused by (select all that apply)
    a. Bronchogenic carcinoma
    b. Pulmonary emboli
    c. Smoking marijuana
    d. Daily aspirin use

24. The nurse notes that the term *platypnea* has been used to describe Mr. Dunges' dyspnea. The nurse knows that this term means that his dyspnea occurs
   a. During activity
   b. At night
   c. As a result of gastroesophageal reflux disease
   d. When sitting upright

25. The nurse conducting a community health education program about asthma correctly states that asthma (select all that apply)
   a. Has declined in the past 10 years
   b. Results in approximately 25,000 hospital admissions per year
   c. Has a higher death rate in African Americans
   d. Causes approximately 5,000 deaths per year

26. The pathological changes that occur because of asthma include
   a. Increased mucus production
   b. Drying of the large airways
   c. Infiltration of B cells in the small airways
   d. Deactivation of mast cells

27. The nurse explains to Karen's parents that extrinsic asthma is a result of
   a. An allergic reaction to household pets
   b. A recent upper respiratory infection
   c. Breathing cold air
   d. Exposure to second-hand cigarette smoke

28. The nurse caring for Mr. Irons, a patient with ARDS, can expect that
   a. Oxygen will reduce his dyspnea.
   b. Assessment will reveal pedal edema.
   c. Chest x-ray will differentiate between cardiogenic and noncardiogenic pulmonary edema.
   d. Mechanical ventilation will be required.

29. Which of the following conditions alerts the nurse to the possible development of pulmonary emboli?
   a. Deep vein thrombosis
   b. Smoke inhalation
   c. Aspirin toxicity
   d. Cocaine use

30. The nurse understands that the term *Virchow's triad* indicates (select all that apply)
    a. Venous stasis
    b. Vessel wall injury
    c. Hypocoagulability
    d. Elevated pulmonary capillary wedge pressure

31. The nurse caring for Ms. Temple, a patient with a pulmonary embolus blocking a large pulmonary vessel, recognizes that which of the following pathological changes is taking place?
    a. The intraventricular septum has shifted to the right.
    b. The right ventricle has becomes smaller.
    c. Decreased coronary perfusion has occurred.
    d. Decreased pulse rate is apparent.

32. A fat embolus causes
    a. The release of free fatty acids
    b. Decreased capillary permeability
    c. Cerebral edema
    d. Increased surfactant production

33. The nurse conducting a community health education program about COPD is correct when stating which of the following?
    a. More men in the 45- to 55-year-old age bracket have COPD than men in other age groups.
    b. Approximately 10 million Americans have COPD.
    c. The death rate from COPD has declined in the past 5 years.
    d. Approximately 50% of people with COPD are unaware they have COPD.

34. One of the major causes of pulmonary hypertension is
    a. Asthma
    b. COPD
    c. Congestive heart failure
    d. High salt intake

35. The nurse notes that Ms. Kling has cor pulmonale. This means that Ms. Kling has
    a. Bilateral pulmonary infiltrates
    b. Right-sided congestive heart failure
    c. Left-sided congestive heart failure
    d. Emphysema

36. Mr. Taylor has been diagnosed with emphysema. He asks the nurse what to expect because of this diagnosis. The nurse correctly replies that he will
   a. Have difficulty with expiration
   b. Have difficulty taking a deep breath
   c. Develop a productive cough
   d. May have severe dyspnea

37. The nurse teaches Ms. Gordon, a patient with emphysema, the pursed-lip breathing technique. The purpose of this technique is to
   a. Decrease resistance to expiration
   b. Encourage deep breathing
   c. Prevent alveolar collapse
   d. Give added support to the ribcage and allow for chest expansion

38. The nurse is asked to explain mesothelioma for Mr. Singh, who has just been diagnosed with this condition. The nurse correctly responds that mesothelioma (select all that apply)
   a. Is associated with prolonged exposure to asbestos
   b. Has signs and symptoms that appear 3–5 years after exposure to asbestos
   c. Is associated with occupations such as construction/demolition and brake repair
   d. Has a positive prognosis

39. The nurse conducting a community health education program stresses that community-acquired pneumonia
   a. Infects over 2 million people each year
   b. Rarely results in death
   c. Is a mildly infectious disease
   d. Is primarily caused by a virus

40. The nurse working at a prison system discusses drug-resistant strain TB with administrative personnel and stresses that this type of TB
   a. Is relatively rare
   b. Has a high mortality rate
   c. Has a mean survival rate of 10–15 years
   d. Reverts to a dormant stage quickly

PART VI · ANSWERS

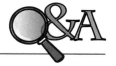

1. **The correct answer is a.** The medulla oblongata contains "pacemaker" cells that control the rate and depth of respiration.

2. **The correct answer is c.** Chemoreceptors in the carotid and aortic bodies react to high serum carbon dioxide levels and trigger ventilation in healthy individuals.

3. **The correct answer is b.** Nonselective beta-blockers block sympathetic nervous system stimulation and cause bronchoconstriction.

4. **The correct answer is c.** Epinephrine is a natural bronchodilator. In the early morning hours, epinephrine levels decrease by as much as 50%.

5. **The correct answer is a.** Alveoli damage results in a decreased ability to exchange carbon dioxide for oxygen, resulting in respiratory acidosis. Carbon dioxide + water = carbonic acid.

6. **The correct answer is c.** Type II alveolar cells are damaged as part of the ARDS cascade, leading to a decrease in surfactant production and alveolar collapse.

7. **The correct answer is a.** Petechiae on the arms and chest are a classic sign of fat emboli.

8. **The correct answer is b.** Smoking and/or inhalation of second-hand smoke are the major causes of chronic bronchitis.

9. **The correct answer is d.** Loss of elastic recoil and alveolar hyperinflation result in narrowing of the terminal bronchioles.

10. **The correct answer is c.** Second-hand smoke contains more carcinogens than inhaled smoke.

11. **The correct answer is a.** Impaired blood return to the right atrium because of vessel compression by a tumor results in a headache as cerebral blood vessels become engorged.

12. **The correct answers are b and c.** *Streptococcus pneumonia* is responsible for causing 75% of all pneumonia cases. Pneumonia may be caused by pathogens or from any activity, such as deep suctioning, which causes an inflammatory response.

13. **The correct answer is d.** Areas of alveolar collapse result in diminished or absent breath sounds.

14. **The correct answer is b**. After exposure to TB, the bacille Calmette-Guérin vaccine may be used as a prophylactic measure if antimycobacterial medications are not available.

15. **The correct answers are b and c**. Night sweats and weight loss are classic signs of active pulmonary TB.

16. **The correct answer is a**. Ventilation means the movement of air and thus denotes inhalation and exhalation.

17. **All answers are correct**.

18. **The correct answers are b and d**.

19. **The correct answers are b, c, and d**. Inhaling cold air causes bronchoconstriction.

20. **The correct answer is c**. Deoxygenated blood enters the right atrium from the inferior and superior vena cava. It then enters the right ventricle. From the right ventricle it is pumped through the pulmonary artery to the pulmonary circulation where it is oxygenated and then returns to the left atrium, left ventricle, and back into the general circulation via the aorta.

21. **The correct answer is d**. Acidosis and hypercapnia also cause the bond to weaken. A subnormal temperature causes the bond to strengthen.

22. **The correct answer is c**. Dyspnea is a subjective symptom of breathlessness. It is not directly correlated to airflow measurements and is masked by sedatives and opioids.

23. **The correct answers are a, b, and d**. Inhalation of crack cocaine may cause hemoptysis.

24. **The correct answer is d**. Dyspnea during activity may be acute (asthma) or chronic, with dyspnea eventually occurring even at rest. Orthopnea describes dyspnea that occurs at night when the person lies down and may be the result of asthma or gastroesophageal reflux disease.

25. **The correct answers are c and d**. Asthma rates have increased for the past 20 years. Approximately 470,000 hospital admissions per year are due to asthma.

26. **The correct answer is a**. Asthma results in activation of mast cells and inflammatory cell infiltration, especially of neutrophils, eosinophils, and T lymphocytes.

27. **The correct answer is a**. Extrinsic (allergic) asthma is caused by increased IgE synthesis. All the other choices reflect causes of intrinsic asthma (nonallergic).

28. **The correct answer is d**. Oxygen does not reduce dyspnea associated with ARDS. Pedal edema is not present. A chest x-ray cannot differentiate between cardiogenic and noncardiogenic pulmonary edema. Mechanical ventilation will most probably be required to support this patient.

29. **The correct answer is a**. Over half of patients with proximal deep vein thrombosis develop pulmonary emboli, many of which are asymptomatic. Smoke inhalation, aspirin toxicity, and cocaine use may lead to ARDS.

30. **The correct answers are a and b**. Elements of Virchow's triad are venous stasis, vessel wall injury, and hypercoagulability.

31. **The correct answer is c**. As blood builds up in the right ventricle (right ventricular afterload), the intraventricular septum shifts to the left, making the left ventricle smaller. As a result, the left ventricle is able to pump far less blood to the circulation, leading to decreased coronary perfusion, myocardial ischemia, and cardiogenic shock.

32. **The correct answer is a**. As the pulmonary fat embolus is hydrolyzed, free fatty acids are released, resulting in increased capillary permeability.

33. **The correct answer is d**. Elderly men have the highest mortality rate from COPD. Approximately 28 million Americans have COPD. The death rate from COPD is rising.

34. **The correct answer is b**.

35. **The correct answer is b**. Cor pulmonale is caused by chronic hypoxia. The pulmonary artery constricts because of hypoxia, increasing the force with which the right ventricle must pump blood into the pulmonary circulation.

36. **The correct answer is a**. People with chronic bronchitis have a cough and severe dyspnea. Emphysema causes the loss of alveolar recoil, trapping air and making expiration difficult.

37. **The correct answer is c**. Tripod positioning gives added support to the ribcage and allows for chest expansion. Pursed-lip breathing is used to help keep the alveoli open during expiration.

38. **The correct answers are a and c**. Signs and symptoms appear 20–40 years after exposure to asbestos, and a poor prognosis is seen, with a median survival of 4–16 months.

39. **The correct answer is a.** Fourteen percent of people admitted to the hospital with community-acquired pneumonia die each year. It is the most virulent infectious disease in the United States and is frequently caused by a bacterium.

40. **The correct answer is b.** Outbreaks of drug-resistant TB are frequent in correctional facilities. The mean survival time is 4–16 weeks.

Part VII

Cardiovascular System

Vanessa Pomarico-Denino, MSN, APRN

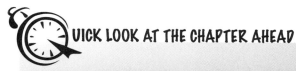

The main function of the heart and blood vessels is to transport oxygen and nutrients to the body tissues. This is needed to remove metabolic waste products such as carbon dioxide, nitrogenous wastes, and acids from tissues to the kidneys for elimination. The heart provides a pumping mechanism, and the blood vessels provide the transport system. The arterial system delivers the blood to the tissues, whereas the venous system returns the blood to the heart. The cardiovascular system works in an integrated fashion and has both intrinsic and extrinsic control mechanisms to accomplish its task.

31

Anatomy and Physiology of the Cardiovascular System: Part I

TERMS
- [ ] diastole
- [ ] endocardium
- [ ] myocardium
- [ ] pericardium
- [ ] systole

Figure 31-1 Phases of the cardiac cycle.

The term *cardiac cycle* is used to describe the rhythmic pumping action of the heart and consists of a sequence of interdependent electrical and mechanical events. Each contraction and relaxation that follows constitutes one cardiac cycle.

Systole

Phase 1—Isovolumetric Contraction
At the beginning of systole, all valves are closed and the myocardial muscle tension begins to rise. When the pressure in the ventricles exceeds the pressure in the aorta and pulmonary artery, the aortic and pulmonic valves open.

Phase 2—Rapid Ventricular Ejection
Pressures in the ventricles exceed diastolic pressures, allowing the semilunar valves to open, and blood flows into the arteries.

Phase 3—Isometric Relaxation phase
Ventricular pressures fall below arterial diastolic pressure, causing semilunar valves to close, creating the second heart sound, the "dub." Pressures continue to fall and rapid ventricular filling begins again.

Diastole

Phase 1—Isovolumetric Relaxation
At the beginning of diastole all valves are closed. The atria are filling. The ventricular muscles begin to relax. As atrial pressures rise and ventricular pressures fall, the tricuspid and mitral valves open, allowing for blood flow from the atria to the ventricles.

Phase 2—Rapid Ventricular Filling
Seventy percent to 80% of the blood flows into the ventricles, increasing ventricular volume and pressure.

Phase 3—Atrial Kick
The atria contract, sending 20–30% more blood into the ventricles, after which ventricular pressure rises above atrial pressure. The mitral valve closes immediately, followed by the tricuspid valve. The closing of the mitral and tricuspid valves causes the first heart sound, the "lub," signifying the beginning of systole. During diastole, blood in the aorta and pulmonary artery flow out to the body and lungs, diminishing the pressure in these two vessels.

The anatomy and physiology of the heart are such that the right side of the heart receives carbon dioxide–laden deoxygenated blood from the body via the venous system and delivers it to the lungs for carbon dioxide removal and oxygenation. Oxygenated blood returns to the left side of the heart for delivery out to the body via the arterial system.

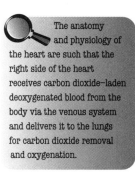

The anatomy and physiology of the heart are such that the right side of the heart receives carbon dioxide–laden deoxygenated blood from the body via the venous system and delivers it to the lungs for carbon dioxide removal and oxygenation.

The heart is a four-chambered muscular organ divided into right and left sides. The two sides of the heart function separately but simultaneously and in a coordinated fashion. The superior and inferior vena cavae deliver deoxygenated blood to the right atrium. The blood then passes through the tricuspid valve into the right ventricle. The blood leaves the right ventricle through the pulmonic valve and the pulmonary artery to the lungs. Blood enters the left atrium via the pulmonary veins and passes through the mitral valve into the left ventricle. It is then ejected through the aortic valve and out the aorta. The two sides of the heart are separated by the septum.

The heart wall comprises three layers. The **endocardium** is the internal lining and is composed of connective tissue and squamous cells. It covers the heart valves and is continuous with the endothelium that lines all the arteries, veins, and capillaries. The **myocardium** is the middle layer, consisting of cardiac muscle. It is the thickest layer, thicker in the left ventricle than the right because of the greater pressures against which the left ventricle must pump. The **pericardium** is a double-walled membranous sac that surrounds the heart and serves as a protective barrier against infection and inflammation. The visceral and parietal pericardia are separated by the pericardial cavity and lubricated by pericardial fluid.

Blood vessels have three layers: the innermost intima, composed of smooth endothelium; the middle tunica media, composed of elastic and smooth muscle fibers; and the outermost adventitia. The endothelium produces substances that promote relaxation (e.g., prostacyclin and nitric oxide) and others that promote constriction (e.g., endothelial derived constricting factor). Prostacyclin also inhibits platelet aggregation. Another substance, thromboxane, is produced and promotes platelet aggregation. Elastic arteries (e.g., aorta and major branches) and pulmonary arteries have many elastic fibers to withstand the pressure of the blood pumped from the heart. Muscular arteries are medium- and small-sized arteries, and arterioles precede capillaries. Capillaries are thin, single layers of endothelial cells that allow for exchange of substances between blood and tissues.

Veins are thinner and have greater distensibility than arteries. This is known as a *capacitance system*. The valves within the veins allow only for one-way blood flow toward the heart.

Stimulation of parasympathetic cholinergic receptors on the heart decreases the rate. Stimulation of sympathetic adrenergic β_1 receptors increases the heart rate, conductivity, and contractility. Stimulation of β_2 receptors causes vasodilation of the coronary arteries as well as the arteries of skeletal muscles and lungs. Stimulation of α_1 receptors on the peripheral arterioles and veins causes vasoconstriction.

Stimulation of β_2 receptors causes vasodilation of the coronary arteries as well as the arteries of skeletal muscles and lungs. Stimulation of α_1 receptors on the peripheral arterioles and veins causes vasoconstriction.

The heart achieves its pumping action by means of the relaxation and contraction of the myocardium and the opening and closing of valves in a cyclic, coordinated fashion. This creates pressure gradients that move the blood forward. Events on the left side of the heart occur at approximately the same time as events on the right. The period of the cardiac cycle during which the ventricles relax and fill is **diastole** and the period of ventricular contraction is **systole** (Figure 31-1). Normally, diastole is longer in duration than systole. It is also the phase during which the coronary arteries are being perfused because their ostia are not covered by the aortic valve cusps as they are in systole. With excessive heart rates, ventricular filling and coronary artery perfusion are diminished.

 With excessive heart rates, ventricular filling and coronary artery perfusion are diminished.

Figure 31-2 Direction of blood flow through the heart.

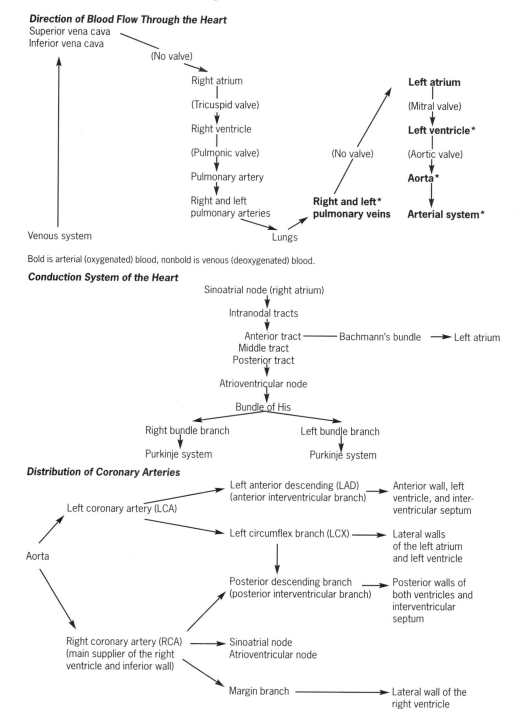

Direction of Blood Flow Through the Heart

Superior vena cava
Inferior vena cava

(No valve)

Right atrium

(Tricuspid valve)

Right ventricle

(Pulmonic valve)

Pulmonary artery

Right and left
pulmonary arteries

Venous system

Lungs

(No valve)

Right and left*
pulmonary veins

Left atrium

(Mitral valve)

Left ventricle*

(Aortic valve)

Aorta*

Arterial system*

Bold is arterial (oxygenated) blood, nonbold is venous (deoxygenated) blood.

Conduction System of the Heart

Sinoatrial node (right atrium)

Intranodal tracts

Anterior tract ———— Bachmann's bundle ——→ Left atrium
Middle tract
Posterior tract

Atrioventricular node

Bundle of His

Right bundle branch   Left bundle branch

Purkinje system   Purkinje system

Distribution of Coronary Arteries

Aorta

Left coronary artery (LCA)

Left anterior descending (LAD)
(anterior interventricular branch)
→ Anterior wall, left
ventricle, and inter-
ventricular septum

Left circumflex branch (LCX) ——→ Lateral walls
of the left atrium
and left ventricle

Posterior descending branch ——→ Posterior walls of
(posterior interventricular branch)   both ventricles and
interventricular
septum

Right coronary artery (RCA)
(main supplier of the right
ventricle and inferior wall)
→ Sinoatrial node
Atrioventricular node

Margin branch ————————————→ Lateral wall of the
right ventricle

The heart is a muscular organ located in the chest, between the lungs and above the diaphragm. Its four chambers are designed to work in a systematic fashion, each relying on the ability to work efficiently. There are several factors that influence the size and weight of the heart, including gender, age, and body weight. Disease states also affect the quality of heart function.

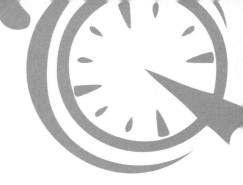

32

Anatomy and Physiology of the Cardiovascular System: Part II

TERMS
- [ ] afterload
- [ ] automaticity
- [ ] conductivity
- [ ] contractility
- [ ] excitability
- [ ] Frank-Starling law of the heart
- [ ] preload
- [ ] refractory period
- [ ] rhythmicity

Figure 32-1 P Wave.

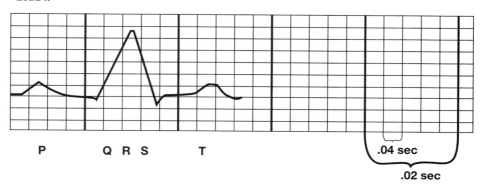

Lead II

P   Q R S   T   .04 sec

.02 sec

P wave

- Begins with firing of the sinoatrial (SA) node and represents depolarization of the atria
- Duration is 0.06 to 0.12 seconds

QRS wave

- Represents depolarization of the atrioventricular (AV) node through the ventricles
- Duration is 0.04 to 0. 12 seconds (The height of the Q wave should be <one third the height of the R wave)

T wave

- Represents repolarization of the ventricle
- Duration is 0.16 seconds

P-R wave

- A measure of time required for the impulse to spread from the SA node through the ventricles
- Duration is 0.12 to 0.20 seconds

QT interval

- Represents the time it takes for depolarization of the ventricles
- Duration varies with the pulse; at a heart rate of 72, it is 0.31 to 0.38 seconds

Regulation and coordination of contractions of the atria and ventricles are essential for effective pumping of the heart. There are both intrinsic and extrinsic mechanisms to accomplish these goals.

Intrinsic mechanisms achieve coordination through precise timing and routing of electrical impulse formation and conduction, which are tied to stimulation of contractility. In the healthy heart, impulses originate in the sinoatrial (SA) node and spread rapidly through the atrial myocardial fibers that respond by contracting. These impulses are further conducted toward the atrioventricular (AV) node, where there is a slight delay before being transmitted to the ventricles. The impulse then continues through the His-Purkinje system and the ventricles and ultimately stimulates ventricular contraction.

Four properties of cardiac tissue enable the initiation and conduction of impulses and myocardial contractility: automaticity, rhythmicity, conductivity, and excitability. **Automaticity** is the ability of specialized tissue cells in the SA node, parts of the atria, and AV node to spontaneously initiate impulses. **Rhythmicity** regulates the generation of impulses. **Conductivity** is the ability to transmit impulses from one fiber to another. **Excitability** is the ability to respond to an impulse and generate an action.

Cardiac cells achieve these tasks by initiating and conducting action potential (AP), which is a self-propagating wave of depolarization followed by repolarization. The APs are generated by sodium ions (Na^+), potassium ions (K^+), and calcium ions (Ca^{++}) moving in and out of cells through channels in the cell membranes. In a resting myocardial cell, negatively charged ions line up inside the cell membrane, whereas positively charged ions line up outside, creating an electrical charge difference, and the cell is said to be polarized. With or without stimulation, channels in the membrane open, allowing positive ions to enter and eliminating the charge differences, and the cell is then said to be depolarized. After depolarization, the positively charged ions are extruded and the cell membrane repolarized.

Cardiac excitation normally begins in the SA node where autorhythmic fibers undergo rapid spontaneous depolarization, initiating APs at a rate of 90 to 100 times per minute, before any spontaneous depolarization in other regions. APs from the SA node spread to other areas of the conduction system, stimulating them before they are able to generate an AP at their own slower rate. Thus the SA node becomes the primary pacemaker for the heart. Hormones or neurotransmitters can slow or speed pacing of the heart. Slow conduction in the small size fibers of the AV node allows time for the atria to contract, moving blood forward into the ventricles before they contract.

If, because of disease or damage, the SA node fails to initiate an impulse, the slower AV node fibers can pick up the pacing chores; however, with AV pacing, the pacing rate is 40 to 50 beats per minute. If activity in the nodes is suppressed, the heartbeat may be maintained by autorhythmic fibers in the ventricles such as the AV bundle, a bundle branch, or conduction myofibrils. These fibers fire AVs very slowly, only about 20 to 40 beats per minute, a rate that is too slow to adequately perfuse the brain. Sometimes a site other than the SA node develops abnormal self-excitability. Such a site is called an *ectopic focus.*

The level of excitability of myocardial cells is determined by the length of time since the previous depolarization. The recovery time is called the **refractory period** and is subdivided into the absolute refractory period, which extends through depolarization and most of repolarization when no other AP can be stimulated, and relative refractory period, which occurs slightly later when excitability is more likely (i.e., approximately on the second half of the T wave on an electrocardiogram [ECG]). The refractory period is normally longer than the period of contraction, giving the ventricles time to fill before another contraction can occur.

The electrical activity of the heart leads to myocardial muscle fiber contraction by initiating the influx of Ca^{++} through calcium channels in the cell membranes, raising its concentration among contractile fibers. Ca^{++} binds to a regulator protein, troponin, which allows actin and myosin fibers to slide past one another, tension mounts, and fibers shorten. The muscle contraction moves the blood out of the heart. The volume expelled with each contraction is called the *stroke volume.* The portion of the end-diastolic volume that is ejected is called the *ejection fraction.*

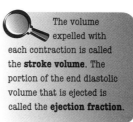
The volume expelled with each contraction is called the **stroke volume.** The portion of the end diastolic volume that is ejected is called the **ejection fraction**.

The electric currents produced by the impulses as they are conducted in the heart can be detected on the body surface by an ECG tracing. The tracing represents the net electrical activity of the atria and ventricle as they depolarize and repolarize. Conventionally, 12 leads are placed on different areas of the chest wall and limbs to evaluate electrical activity from different perspectives. A lead is a pair of electrodes with a positive and a negative pole that can detect electrical current. The electrical currents drive a stylus that can make a tracing of the impulse. An impulse traveling toward the positive pole causes an upward deflection in the ECG tracing, and one traveling away from the positive pole causes a downward deflection. In addition to the direction of the current, the voltage and timing of the electric current can be determined by the vertical and horizontal calibrations of the graphic paper. The deflections or waves on the ECG, which have been arbitrarily designated as P, Q, R, S, and T, represent events during the cardiac cycle (Figure 32-1).

Extrinsic neurohumoral control mechanisms also influence cardiac function. These mechanisms are initiated by changes in the *cardiac output* (CO), which is a function of the stroke volume times the heart rate (CO = SV × R). The stroke volume is influenced by the preload, contractility, and afterload.

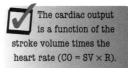
The cardiac output is a function of the stroke volume times the heart rate (CO = SV × R).

Preload is the degree of stretch in muscle length before contraction or at the end of diastole. Venous return is a function of both the blood volume of the body and venous constriction. Stretch determines the amount of tension in the wall and is known as the **Frank-Starling law of the heart,** or the Frank-Starling mechanism. This mechanism results in more ventricular volume during diastole and greater stroke volume with contraction. The renin-angiotensin-aldosterone system, which is activated when decreased CO diminishes renal blood flow, increases the blood volume. Sympathetic nervous system (SNS) stimulation also activates the renin-angiotensin-aldosterone system and increases secretion of antidiuretic hormone (ADH), contributing to the increased blood volume. SNS stimulation causes venous vasoconstriction. All these mechanisms increase venous return. Over-stretching (e.g., excessive fluid volume), however, can diminish contractility. **Contractility** is the ability of the myocardial fibers to shorten. It is a function of the amount and quality of the fibers, the physiological environment such as adequate oxygen and calcium, and sympathetic stimulation. Increased contractility improves the stroke volume.

Preload is the volume of work on the heart before contraction begins and is determined by the stretch of muscle fibers and the subsequent return of venous blood to the heart.

Afterload is the amount of pressure or tension on the heart that moves blood into the aorta and occurs after contraction. It is most commonly a factor of blood pressure. SNS stimulates arteriole constriction and increases the blood pressure and afterload.* Increased afterload decreases stroke volume.

> Afterload is the amount of pressure or tension on the heart that moves blood into the aorta and occurs after contraction.

The factors that determine CO (i.e., stroke volume [preload, contractility, and afterload] and the heart rate) are all influenced by the nervous system. Nervous system control of the heart stems from the cardiovascular center in the medulla oblongata, which receives sensory input from receptors in blood vessels. The SNS is the first mechanism to be activated when CO falls. Changes in CO alter pressure in blood vessels, which is sensed by baroreceptors located in the aortic arch, carotid arteries, and other arteries and veins. The baroreceptors have connections to the cardiovascular center in the brainstem, which then provides output to the heart and blood vessels via the autonomic nervous system. Other influences on the cardiovascular center are higher brain centers, such as the limbic system and cerebral cortex; chemoreceptors that monitor chemical changes in blood, such as oxygen changes; and proprioceptors that are stimulated during exercise.

Sympathetic stimulation increases heart rate, conduction, and contractility, all of which increase CO. SNS stimulation of β receptors in the kidneys increases the production of renin and ultimately the preload. α_2 Receptors in the smooth muscle walls of arterioles and veins are also stimulated by norepinephrine. The venous constriction increases the preload. Decreased pressure sensed by baroreceptors also increases ADH secretion, thus also contributing to preload.

> Sympathetic stimulation increases heart rate, conduction, and contractility, all of which increase CO.

The activation of the renin-angiotensin-aldosterone system and ADH secretion are later compensatory responses to decreased CO than is the SNS. CO is one of the factors that influences systemic arterial blood pressure. Blood pressure is a function of the CO times the systemic vascular resistance (blood pressure = CO × SVR). Systemic vascular resistance is a factor of the caliber of the arterioles that is influenced by the SNS. Thus the neuroendocrine mechanisms that influence heart function and CO are the same mechanisms that regulate blood pressure.

Decreased blood pressure increases firing of the baroreceptor, which activates SNS, thus increasing heart rate, contractility, arteriole and venous constriction, ADH secretion, and renin production, all of which serve to increase blood pressure. With an elevation of blood pressure, these mechanisms are not initiated and the blood pressure falls. A substance produced in the atria known as *atrial natriuretic hormone* promotes excretion of fluids, causing a reduction in blood pressure.

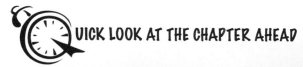

Dyslipidemia, also called hyperlipidemia, is an increased level of plasma lipid concentration made up of cholesterol and/or triglycerides. These lipid levels have been well documented in their relationship to the development of atherosclerotic vascular disease, especially coronary artery disease (CAD), cerebrovascular disease, and peripheral vascular disease. Alterations in the lipid profile are associated with the increased risk of CAD.

It is estimated that approximately 50% of Americans have dyslipidemia, with a higher incidence among diabetics, those with hypertension, and African Americans. Familial or inherited forms of hypercholesterolemia occur in approximately 1 in 500 persons. More than 100 million Americans have borderline high levels of cholesterol.

Atherosclerosis is a chronic disease characterized by thickening and hardening of the arterial wall. Lesions/plaques containing lipids develop and calcify, causing vessel obstruction, platelet aggregation, and abnormal vasoconstriction.

Atherosclerotic heart disease is the leading cause of death in the United States, although there has been a gradual decline in those deaths possibly due to earlier intervention and improved medical therapies. Atherosclerotic cerebrovascular disease is the leading cause of stroke, accounting for more than 40% of deaths in the United States. Peripheral vascular disease and its increased incidence of complications is common among those persons with diabetes mellitus and atherosclerosis.

33

Dyslipidemia and Atherosclerosis

TERMS
- [ ] atherosclerosis
- [ ] chylomicrons
- [ ] dyslipidemia
- [ ] high-density lipoprotein (HDL)
- [ ] low-density lipoprotein (LDL)
- [ ] triglycerides

Figure 33-1 NCEP ATP III classification of LDL, total, and HDL cholesterol (mg/dL).

LDL Cholesterol

<100	Optimal
100–129	Near optimal/above optimal
130–159	Borderline high
160–189	High
≥190	Very high

Total Cholesterol

<200	Desirable
200–239	Borderline high
≥240	High

HDL Cholesterol

<40	Low
≥60	High

Reprinted courtesy of ATP III Guidelines, National Cholesterol Education Program. Third Report of Expert Panel on Detection, Evaluation and Treatment of High Blood Cholesterol in Adults (Adult Treatment Panel III). National Heart, Lung, and Blood Institute/National Institute of Health. NIH Publication no. 02-5215. September 2002.

Table 33-1 Therapeutic Life-Style Changes

Diet
    Saturated fat < 7% of calories
    Cholesterol < 200 mg/d
    Increase soluble fiber 10–25 g/d
    Increase plant stanols/sterols 2 g/d
Weight management
Increased physical activity
    Thirty to 40 minutes of aerobic activity minimum three times a week

Reprinted courtesy of Third Report of Expert Panel on Detection, Evaluation and Treatment of High Blood Cholesterol in Adults (Adult Treatment Panel III). National Heart, Lung, and Blood Institute/National Institute of Health. NIH Publication no. 02-5215. September 2002.

The risk factors for atherosclerotic vascular disease include dyslipidemia, cigarette smoking, hypertension, male or postmenopausal female, age > 50, diabetes/insulin resistance, increased serum fibrinogen, and hyperhomocystinemia. Other contributory factors include a diet high in saturated fat, obesity, sedentary life-style, and family history of atherosclerosis.

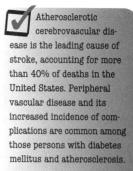

Atherosclerotic cerebrovascular disease is the leading cause of stroke, accounting for more than 40% of deaths in the United States. Peripheral vascular disease and its increased incidence of complications are common among those persons with diabetes mellitus and atherosclerosis.

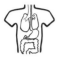

PATHOPHYSIOLOGY

The two main lipids in the blood are **triglycerides** (TGs) and cholesterol. Saturated fats in the diet are the source of serum TGs. Some cholesterol is absorbed from food, but most is synthesized by the liver from breakdown products of saturated fats.

Because lipids are insoluble, they combine with carrier proteins called *apoproteins* that are carried in the blood. These lipoproteins are classified on the basis of their density. This is determined by the amount of TG, which has less density, and protein, which has greater density. The main classes of lipoproteins are chylomicrons, very-low-density lipoproteins (VLDLs), **low-density lipoproteins (LDLs)** or "bad cholesterol," and **high-density lipoproteins (HDLs),** or "good cholesterol."

Chylomicrons are large lipoproteins that serve as a transport system of exogenous or dietary lipids to the liver, adipose, cardiac, and skeletal tissue. They are composed mainly of TGs and some cholesterol. TGs, a highly concentrated energy source, are found in fats and oils that are absorbed from the diet. Stored TGs are then broken down by lipolysis into fatty acids to form adenosine triphosphate. If there is no need to use TGs this way, a limited amount is stored in the liver, and the rest is stored in adipose tissue. The capacity to store TGs in the adipose tissue is unlimited. Excess dietary carbohydrates, proteins, fats, and oils are all stored in the adipose tissues as TGs.

Some cholesterol is absorbed from the diet, but most is endogenously produced in the liver at night. Increases in dietary cholesterol produce only a slight elevation of blood cholesterol because ingestion reduces endogenous hepatic production. An increase in dietary saturated fats, however, produces a substantial increase in blood cholesterol because they serve as a substrate for endogenous cholesterol production.

From its fat and carbohydrate stores, the liver synthesizes VLDL particles, which are composed mainly of TGs and some cholesterol. The VLDL particles transport the TGs to cells to meet their needs. After losing enough TGs, the VLDL particles become LDL particles. These LDL particles contain the highest concentration of cholesterol and are the major transporter of cholesterol. HDL particles, which contain the largest proportion of apoprotein with some cholesterol, participate in reverse cholesterol transport by transporting cholesterol back to the liver and clearing the blood. HDL is reduced by smoking and is increased by exercise.

Plaque found in the arterial walls of individuals with atherosclerosis contains large amounts of cholesterol. Epidemiological studies have established that the higher the level of serum LDL cholesterol, the higher the risk of atherosclerotic heart disease; conversely, the higher the level of HDL, the lower the risk. Because most serum cholesterol is LDL cholesterol, high total cholesterol levels are also associated with increased risk. The relationship of VLDL and TGs in atherogenesis is less certain. The levels of VLDL and HDL are inversely related; thus, individuals with high TGs and VLDL are likely to have low HDLs, and for this reason alone, are likely to have a higher risk of atherosclerosis. High blood levels of apoprotein A have been identified as a risk factor.

 Plaque found in the arterial walls of individuals with atherosclerosis contains large amounts of cholesterol.

The initiating event in atherogenesis is *endothelial injury.* Dyslipidemia, hypertension, cigarette smoking, diabetes/insulin resistance, elevated homocysteine levels, autoimmune processes, and possibly some bacterial infections have been implicated as causes of injury. The injured cells become more permeable, have increased levels of oxygen radicals, and become inflamed. Once inflamed, these cells recruit leukocytes and macrophages that produce more oxygen radicals, thereby increasing the injury. They also release cytokines and mitogens that stimulate smooth muscle cell proliferation and inhibit the endothelial cells from secreting endogenous vasodilators, such as nitric oxide.

> The initiating event in atherogenesis is endothelial injury. Dyslipidemia, hypertension, cigarette smoking, diabetes/insulin resistance, elevated homocysteine levels, autoimmune processes, and possibly some bacterial infections have been implicated as causes of injury.

Serum LDLs are oxidized and phagocytosed by histiocytes that become foam cells, which penetrate into the intima. This creates further inflammation and injury, forming a lesion called a *fatty streak*. Fibrous tissue and smooth muscle cells migrate and cover the foam cells, forming a cap. Protrusion into the lumen causes narrowing and diminished blood flow or ischemia. This lesion is called a *fibrous plaque*. This is a relatively stable plaque and most likely represents the stage of chronic angina in CAD.

Necrosis and calcification occur below the cap, and as the plaque progresses, it can ulcerate and rupture. This is called a *complicated plaque*. Platelets then aggregate, adhering to the surface of the plaque. Coagulation results, with thrombus formation that may completely obliterate the lumen, possibly resulting in death of tissue or infarction. This can result in unstable angina or infarction of CAD.

The result of the pathological process is a narrowed artery vulnerable to abnormal constriction and thrombosis. If the process occurs slowly, collateral circulation may bypass the lesion and maintain perfusion.

MANIFESTATIONS

Dyslipidemia and atherosclerosis are often asymptomatic for a long period of time, often until the degree of arterial obstruction, approximately 50% to 70% blockage in CAD, is sufficient to compromise blood supply to a target organ. The individual may then complain of symptoms of CAD, such as dyspnea, fatigue, or chest pain. Symptoms of cerebral vascular disease such as transient or permanent neurological deficits or arterial insufficiency (intermittent claudication, hair loss, or skin ulcers) may also occur as a result of impaired blood flow. Physical examination may reveal evidence of plaque or findings related to damage to the organs supplied. Evidence of lipid abnormalities or plaque might include xanthomas and xanthelasma, arcus senilis, abdominal bruits, peripheral thrills, and diminished pulses. Cholesterol screening and lipid profile identify specific lipid abnormalities.

Angiography, ultrasound, or nuclear scanning may be used to specifically locate an atherosclerotic lesion.

Evidence of lipid abnormalities or plaque might include xanthomas and xanthelasma, arcus senilis, abdominal bruits, peripheral thrills, bruits, and diminished pulses.

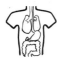

TREATMENT

The goals of treatment for dyslipidemia and atherosclerosis are to normalize lipids, prevent plaque progression, and restore blood supply. Therapeutic life-style changes that reduce the risk of CAD are critical components of the therapeutic regimen.

Pharmacological interventions include lipid-lowering agents, antiplatelet/antiinflammatory agents (e.g., aspirin), thrombolytics, angiotensin-converting enzyme inhibitors (to reduce smooth muscle hypertrophy and increase vasodilation), estrogen, and antioxidants. Diet and drug decisions are based on the level of dyslipidemia and number of other cardiac risk factors (see p. 282). Revascularization procedures that will increase blood flow to areas where it is decreased or compromised, such as coronary artery bypass surgery and percutaneous coronary intervention with stenting, may be used.

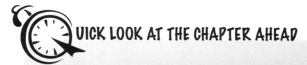
Coronary artery disease (CAD) is caused by diminished blood flow in the coronary arteries with subsequent reduced oxygenation to the myocardium, resulting in transient ischemia or **angina.** It may also cause permanent damage to the myocardial cells or infarction. Atherosclerosis and vasospasm are the most prevalent causes, with atherosclerosis being the most common. The left ventricle is most susceptible. The imbalance in supply and demand of oxygen can also be caused by cardiomyopathy and thrombus formation.

34

Coronary Artery Disease

TERMS
- [ ] angina
- [ ] Dressler's syndrome
- [ ] Prinzmetal's or variant angina
- [ ] remodeling

Figure 34-1 Cross-section of the arteries.

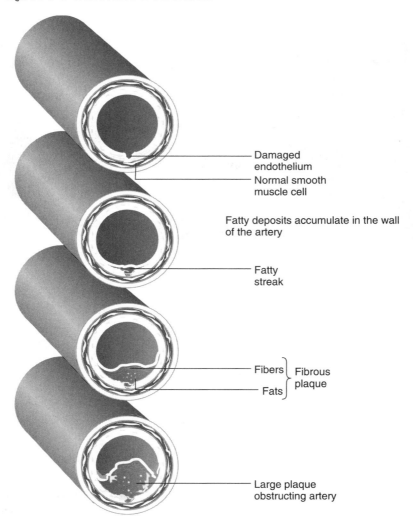

Damaged
endothelium

Normal smooth
muscle cell

Fatty deposits accumulate in the wall
of the artery

Fatty
streak

Fibers ⎱ Fibrous
Fats ⎰ plaque

Large plaque
obstructing artery

Coronary atherosclerosis remains the leading cause of death in the industrialized world and is the leading cause of death in women over age 50 years. CAD is the most common cause of heart attacks. Over 1 million Americans have myocardial infarctions

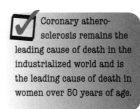

Coronary atherosclerosis remains the leading cause of death in the industrialized world and is the leading cause of death in women over 50 years of age.

Table 34-1 Risk Factors for Coronary Heart Disease

Nonmodifiable	Modifiable	Negative Risk Factor
Age: men ≥ 45 y; women ≥ 55 y or premature menopause	Tobacco use, obesity, physical inactivity	High HDL cholesterol
Gender	Diabetes mellitus	
Family history: history of premature coronary heart disease in first-degree male relative < 55 y or first-degree female relative < 65 y	Hyperlipidemia Hypertension	

(MIs) each year, and it is estimated that there are 2 million Americans with silent ischemia.

Nonmodifiable risk factors for CAD include age, gender, race, and family history. Men are more often affected than women by an overall ratio of 4:1, although after age 70 the ratio is 1:1. The incidence greatly increases among postmenopausal women and is higher among postmenopausal women who smoke. With increasing longevity, the incidence of CAD is expected to rise. White men have a higher incidence than African-American men, but the incidence of CAD among African-American women is higher than among white women. African-Americans have an earlier onset with more severe disease. The nature of the relationship to CAD is unclear and may be related to the higher incidence of other risk factors in African-Americans. The risk of CAD increases if a biological parent manifested CAD before the age of 55.

The incidence greatly increases among postmenopausal women and is higher among postmenopausal women who smoke.

Modifiable risk factors that are most predictive of the development of CAD are dyslipidemia (high total cholesterol, high LDL, and low HDL), hypertension, diabetes, and cigarette smoking. Increased levels of homocysteine are also emerging as an important risk factor. Other, more controversial, risk factors are obesity, sedentary life-style, heavy alcohol consumption, estrogen deficiency, and a personality characterized by hostility. Research also suggests a genetic predisposition to CAD in positive family history. Additional research implicates infection and inflammation.

Figure 34-2 Location of coronary artery blockage and manifestations.

Right Coronary Artery (RCA)

- Main supplier of right ventricle, the inferior wall of the heart, sinoatrial (SA) node, and the atrioventricular (AV) node
- ECG changes appear in leads II, IIIA, and a VF
- Occlusion leads to inferior (also called posterior) myocardial infarction (MI)

Left Coronary Artery (LCA)

- Main supplier of the anterior wall of the left ventricle, interventricular septum, and lateral walls of the left atrium and ventricle
- ECG changes appear in leads V_3, V_4, V_5, V_6, L_1, and a VL
- Occlusion leads to massive anterolateral MI
- Creates major disruption in cardiac output, largest incidence of residual cardiac failure
- High mortality rate

Left Anterior Descending Artery (LAD)

- Main supplier of anterior wall of left ventricle, interventricular septum
- ECG changes in leads V_1, V_2, and V_3
- Occlusion leads to anteroseptal MI
- High incidence of residual cardiac failure

Left Circumflex Artery

- Main suppler of lateral walls of left atrium and ventricle
- ECG changes appear in leads VL, I, V_5, and V_6
- Occlusion leads to lateral MI

Transmural MIs—Penetrate the complete myocardium and are large enough to create a Q wave, thus they are called Q wave MIs

Subendocardial MIs—Do not penetrate the entire myocardial wall, thus they do not create a Q wave and are called non-Q wave MIs

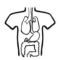

PATHOPHYSIOLOGY

The coronary arteries (Figure 34-2) normally provide oxygen to meet the metabolic demands of the myocardium to perform its work of impulse conduction and contraction. In CAD, if plaque narrows the lumen by more than 75%, blood flow is impaired sufficiently to hamper metabolism when oxygen demand increases with exertion, resulting in ischemia. Byproducts of anaerobic metabolism or lactic acid accumulate, causing substernal pain. This can also cross-stimulate other nerves, causing radiation of pain. During ischemic episodes, conduction disturbances may lead to changes in the electrocardiogram (ECG). Reduction of oxygen demand reverses the ischemia. Predictable ischemia brought on by increased oxygen demand and relieved with reduction of demand is called *stable angina pectoris*.

> In CAD, if plaque narrows the lumen by more than 75%, blood flow is impaired sufficiently to hamper metabolism when oxygen demand increases with exertion, resulting in ischemia. Byproducts of anaerobic metabolism or lactic acid accumulate, causing substernal pain.

If a complicated plaque ulcerates, inflammation occurs, platelets aggregate, and thrombi form, further diminishing the blood supply. Platelets release thromboxane A_1, a potent vasoconstrictor, causing spasms of the arteries. This leads to more platelet aggregation, more spasm, and a recurring cycle. Eventually, transient thrombotic occlusions of the coronary vessels occur unpredictably, often at rest, and with increased frequency, causing unstable angina, which is a preinfarction situation.

If an acute thrombus occludes the vessel completely, MI, or death of cells, occurs. Generally, there is a sequence of ischemia, injury, and infarction with a centrally infarcted area surrounded by an area of injury followed by ischemia. The most common site for an MI is the left ventricle, but it can occur in any region of the heart wall (inferior, lateral, posterior, or septal) depending on the artery involved and can penetrate the myocardium to different depths. Subendocardial infarctions are limited to the inner half of the myocardium, partially penetrating wall thickness. Transmural infarctions involve the full thickness of the wall. Infarcted cells release intracellular substances into the blood, which may cause conduction disturbances.

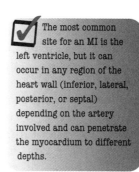

The most common site for an MI is the left ventricle, but it can occur in any region of the heart wall (inferior, lateral, posterior, or septal) depending on the artery involved and can penetrate the myocardium to different depths.

Within 24 hours, cardiac enzymes are released and inflammatory cells infiltrate the necrotic area. By the third week, scar tissue forms. Over time, the necrotic tissue is replaced by fibrotic tissue, which thickens the area of injury. Healing is completed by 6 weeks. Loss of functional tissue can lead to ventricular failure and cardiogenic shock, ventricular wall inertia with stasis of blood and mural thrombi, ventricular aneurysm, papillary muscle dysfunction and mitral regurgitation, dysrhythmias, and pericarditis. **Dressler's syndrome,** pericarditis, fever, and effusion may develop 1 to 4 weeks post-MI.

Myocardial cells in the vicinity of the infarcted area may lose their conductive and contractile functions for a period of time, or they may undergo **remodeling,** a process mediated by the renin-angiotensin-aldosterone system that results in hypertrophy and abnormal contractile function, both leading to ventricular failure. Silent ischemia or infarction may occur in a significant number of individuals, especially diabetics, the elderly, and postcardiac surgery patients because of autonomic dysfunction. **Prinzmetal's** or **variant angina** is a form of angina caused by coronary artery spasm, with or without atherosclerotic plaque, that occurs unpredictably and almost exclusively at rest.

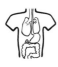

MANIFESTATIONS

Typically, angina is experienced as substernal chest discomfort, ranging from a sensation of pressure or heaviness to moderately severe pain. The discomfort may radiate to the neck or the jaw, left shoulder down the inner aspect of the left arm, or occasionally the back or right arm. It is commonly mistaken for indigestion. The discomfort is precipitated by exertion or exercise, emotional stress, eating a heavy meal, extremes of temperature, sexual activity, and stimulants such as tobacco or cocaine. Other factors that may contribute are dysrhythmias, blood pressure extremes, left ventricular dysfunction, valvular problems, anemia, thyroid toxicosis, stimulant drugs, and lung disease. The discomfort is transient and is relieved within minutes by rest or the use of nitroglycerin. Discomfort lasting longer than 30 minutes suggests unstable angina or infarction. Pallor, diaphoresis, and dyspnea may occur. The blood pressure and pulse are frequently elevated, though hypotension may be present. Dysrhythmias may occur with the presence of S_3 with ventricular dysfunction. On ECG, transient ST segment depression and T wave inversion are signs of subendocardial ischemia and ST segment elevation with transmural ischemia. The ECG lead where the changes occur indicates the location of the ischemia.

Figure 34-3 Cardiac marker changes after myocardial infarction.

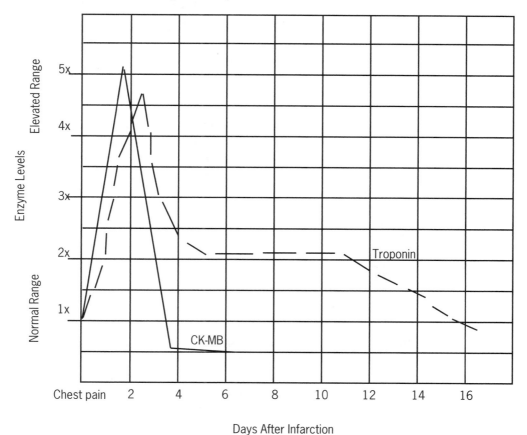

Typically, angina is experienced as substernal chest discomfort, ranging from a sensation of pressure or heaviness to moderately severe pain.

The first symptom of an MI is sudden, prolonged (>30 minutes), severe chest pain often described as heavy and crushing accompanied by dyspnea and diaphoresis. Radiation is similar to angina. It often causes a feeling of "gas" or unrelenting indigestion. Nausea and vomiting may occur. Initially, blood pressure drops, but it may rise along with the pulse because of sympathetic stimulation. Inflammation may cause fever, elevation of white blood cells and erythrocyte sedimentation rate, friction rubs, or murmurs. Serum glucose rises with stress.

ECG changes indicative of infarction are an initial peaked T wave. A depressed ST segment and T wave inversion indicates subendocardial ischemia, and ST segment elevation occurs with transmural ischemia or injury. A Q wave develops with transmural infarction. There is no Q wave with a subendocardial infarction. Gradually, ST segments and T waves return to normal, but Q waves persist.

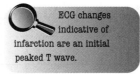

ECG changes indicative of infarction are an initial peaked T wave.

Important cardiac markers released into the blood from necrotic cells are creatine kinase-MB band (>3%, rises in 4 to 8 hours, peaks in 12–24 hours, and is normal in 3–4 days) and troponin I (>3.1 ng/mL, rises in 3 hours, and persists for 7–10 days).

Additional diagnostic tests used to localize areas of obstruction, ischemia, and infarction include stress testing, nuclear imaging with thallium (cold spots) or technetium (hot spots), and coronary angiography.

TREATMENT

Preserving functional cardiac tissue by increasing oxygen supply and decreasing demand is the goal of treatment. Measures to increase perfusion are antihyperlipidemic medications; hemolytic, antiplatelet, and anticoagulating agents; and revascularization procedures. Vasodilators are generally ineffective because of nondistensible vessels. Medications that decrease oxygen demand are nitrates, beta-blockers, calcium channel blockers, angiotensin-converting enzyme inhibitors, and angiotensin blockers. Life-style interventions include diet, exercise, smoking cessation, and stress management. Current research is addressing methods of stimulating myocardial cell repair after infarction such as stem cell stimulation.

Hypertension is the most common primary diagnosis in the United States, accounting for 35 million office visits annually. It is a leading risk factor for cardiovascular disease and is the leading cause of death in the United States. Of these deaths, 83% are caused by myocardial infarction and 17% from stroke, although there has been a steady decline in those statistics because of the lowering of blood pressure in the general population.

35
Hypertension

TERMS
- [ ] hypertensive emergency
- [ ] primary or essential hypertension
- [ ] secondary hypertension
- [ ] systemic vascular resistance (SVR)

Table 35-1 Major Cardiovascular Disease Risk Factors

Hypertension	Physical inactivity
Obesity (body mass index ≥ 30 kg/m²)	Microalbuminuria, estimated glomerular filtration rate <60 mL/min
Dyslipidemia	Age (>55 for men, >65 for women)
Diabetes mellitus	Family history of premature
Cigarette smoking	cardiovascular disease (men age < 55, women age < 65)

Reprinted courtesy of the U.S. Dept. of Health and Human Services, NIH Seventh Report of the Joint National Committee on Prevention, Detection, Evaluation, and Treatment of High Blood Pressure (JNC 7), NIH Publication No. 03-5231, May 2003.

Hypertension is defined as a consistently elevated systolic blood pressure and/or diastolic blood pressure on two or more occasions. Approximately 50 million people have hypertension. Variation exists in the prevalence and consequences of hypertension among different age, gender, and racial and ethnic groups. There is an increasing incidence of hypertension with increasing age.

Hypertension tends to occur at an earlier age in African Americans. The incidence is higher in men than in women until the age of 55, and then the risk is about equal until age 74, after which point women have a higher incidence than men. African Americans have a much higher prevalence, more severe hypertension, and diagnosis at a later stage than whites. The greater severity is accompanied by a much higher rate of stroke mortality, heart disease, and hypertension-related end-stage renal disease. Hispanics have the same or lower prevalence of hypertension despite a high prevalence of obesity and diabetes.

 There is an increasing incidence of hypertension with increasing age.

Hypertension-related consequences of cardiovascular disease, stroke, and end-stage renal disease make hypertension a major public health concern. Cardiac disease and stroke are the first and third leading causes of death in the United States, respectively. Cardiac complications are the major causes of morbidity and mortality in essential

 Cardiac complications are the major causes of morbidity and mortality in essential hypertension. Hypertension is the major predisposing cause of stroke and is the second most common antecedent of end-stage renal disease.

hypertension. Hypertension is the major predisposing cause of stroke and is the second most common antecedent of end-stage renal disease.

Various methods of classification for hypertension based on pathology, severity, and associated risk factors are used to give direction to interventions. It is estimated that 95–99% of people with hypertension have no identifiable cause for it. This is known as **primary** or **essential hypertension.** Primary hypertension may be controlled, but the predisposition remains. **Secondary hypertension** results from a known cause such as renal disease or primary aldosteronism and constitutes 5% to 8% of all hypertensive individuals. It is caused by altered hemodynamics associated with a primary disease or condition that, when removed, results in cure of the hypertension if it has not been prolonged. Isolated systolic hypertension, an elevation of systolic pressure with a normal diastolic pressure, is common in the elderly and appears to be a significant cardiovascular risk factor.

> Isolated systolic hypertension, an elevation of systolic pressure with a normal diastolic pressure, is common in the elderly and appears to be a significant cardiovascular risk factor.

A commonly recognized classification of hypertension according to level of blood pressure elevation is shown in Figure 35-2. Because risk for cardiovascular disease in individuals with hypertension is determined not only by the level of blood pressure elevation but also by other risk factors and end-organ damage, a cardiovascular risk stratification classification for hypertension has been developed to guide treatment and is shown in Figure 35-1.

Figure 35-1 Diagnostic workup of hypertension.

- Assess risk factors and comorbidities.
- Reveal identifiable causes of hypertension.
- Assess presence of target organ damage.
- Conduct history and physical examination.
- Obtain laboratory tests: urinalysis, blood glucose, hematocrit and lipid panel, serum potassium, creatinine, and calcium. Optional: urinary albumin-to-creatinine ratio.
- Obtain electrocardiogram.

Reprinted courtesy of the U.S. Department of Health and Human Services, NIH Seventh Report of the Joint National Committee on Prevention, Detection, Evaluation and Treatment of High Blood Pressure (JNC 7), NIH Publication No. 03-5231,May 2003.

Table 35-2 JNC 7 Classification of Blood Pressure (BP)

Category	Systolic Blood Pressure (mm Hg)	Diastolic Blood Pressure (mm Hg)
Normal	<120 and	<80
Prehypertension	120–139 or	80–89
Hypertension, stage 1	140–159 or	90–99
Hypertension, stage 2	≥160 or	≥100

When systolic and diastolic blood pressures fall into different categories, the higher category should be selected to classify the individual's blood pressure status.

Reprinted courtesy of the U.S. Department of Health and Human Services, NIH Seventh Report of the Joint National Committee on Prevention, Detection, Evaluation and Treatment of High Blood Pressure (JNC 7), NIH Publication No. 03-5231, May 2003.

Hypertensive emergency is a severe level of hypertension with evidence of end-organ damage that needs to be treated within 1 hour. Hypertensive urgency is a severe level of hypertension without end-organ damage. It needs to be treated within a few hours.

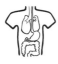

PATHOPHYSIOLOGY

Understanding the pathological mechanism involved in blood pressure elevation is necessary for understanding prevention and implementation of intervention strategies. Blood pressure is a function of the cardiac output (CO) times the **systemic vascular resistance (SVR)** (BP = CO × SVR). Elevation of blood pressure may be caused by increased CO, increased peripheral resistance, or both.

CO is increased by any condition that increases the heart rate or stroke volume (CO = Rate × SV). The heart rate is influenced by the autonomic nervous system. The stroke volume is determined by preload and contractility. Preload is influenced by blood volume and sympathetic stimulation of the veins. Myocardial contractility is influenced by preload, sympathetic activation, condition of myocardial fibers, and the inotropic environment. SVR is the decreased or resistive blood flow by the systemic arteries and determines diastolic blood pressure. SVR is affected by increased blood viscosity, as determined by the hematocrit, or reduced arteriolar diameter, which is determined by vascular compliance, the sympathetic nervous system, and local autoregulation.

CO is increased by any condition that increases the heart rate or stroke volume.

Genetic and environmental causes may also contribute to the development of primary hypertension. The genetic predisposition is thought to be polygenic with multiple defects. Hypotheses suggested in explaining causation of primary hypertension and exploited in interventions include sympathetic nervous system hyperactivity; increased renin-angiotensin-aldosterone, resulting in increased vascular tone and fluid retention, thus increasing preload; a defect in sodium excretion; and defect in vascular smooth muscle cell transport, resulting in an intracellular accumulation of calcium, which increases vascular reactivity.

In addition to family history, gender, and advancing age, environmental risk factors found to precipitate or aggravate hypertension are obesity; cigarette smoking; heavy alcohol intake (more than three drinks a day); high dietary sodium intake; low potassium, calcium, and magnesium consumption; and glucose intolerance.

Secondary hypertension is caused by primary diseases or conditions that increase CO or peripheral resistance, such as catecholamine-secreting adrenal medullary tumors; excessive aldosterone secretion by the adrenal cortex in some disease states; renovascular disease with increased renin-angiotensin production; and iatrogenic causes such as medications (e.g., corticosteroids and estrogen).

High pressures within the arteries and arterioles stimulate hypertrophy and hyperplasia of smooth muscle cells and eventual fibromuscular thickening and endothelial injury. Inflammatory mediators increase permeability of the endothelium, allowing fluids and calcium to enter the wall and increasing reactivity and constriction. Endothelial injury caused by hypertension may also cause or aggravate atherosclerosis further, diminishing lumen patency and vessel distensibility. Eventually, structure and function of the end organs, such as the heart, aorta, kidneys, eyes, brain, and lower extremities, are compromised, with resulting ischemia, edema, and even hemorrhage. Elevation of hydrostatic pressure within arteries can cause tissue edema.

Cardiac complications include left ventricular hypertrophy, coronary artery disease, angina pectoris/ischemia, left ventricular failure, myocardial infarction, and sudden death. Vascular complications include aneurysm formation and arterial insufficiency. Renal complications include parenchymal damage, nephrosclerosis, and renal artery sclerosis, insufficiency, and failure. Retinal complications include retinopathy, papilledema, retinal vascular sclerosis, exudation, and hemorrhage. Cerebral vascular complications include transient ischemic attacks, stroke/brain attack, aneurysm, and hypertensive encephalopathy.

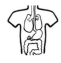

MANIFESTATIONS

Initially, elevated blood pressure is usually asymptomatic. An early symptom might include early morning headache as a result of nighttime cerebral edema that diminishes during the day. Manifestations tend to be related to end-organ damage, including retinopathy, visual disturbance, papilledema, carotid bruits, distended neck veins, left ventricular hypertrophy, angina, heart failure, myocardial infarction, abnormalities of heart rhythm, murmurs, third and fourth heart sounds, lung crackles and bronchospasm, pulmonary edema, abdominal bruits, pulsations, diminished peripheral pulses, proteinuria, hematuria, abnormal creatine clearance, and hypertensive encephalopathy (headache, irritability, confusion, and altered mental status due to cerebral vasospasm).

 An early symptom might include early morning headache as a result of night time cerebral edema that diminishes during the day.

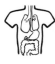

TREATMENT

Life-style modifications to prevent hypertension or to lower blood pressure include weight reduction; alcohol limitation; aerobic exercise; limitation of sodium intake; maintenance of calcium, potassium, and magnesium intake; and stress management. If these measures fail to control blood pressure, pharmacological measures are implemented. Pharmacological measures are aimed at decreasing the fluid volume, decreasing the CO, and vasodilation.

Figure 35-2 Algorithm for treatment of hypertension.

Algorithm for Treatment of Hypertension*

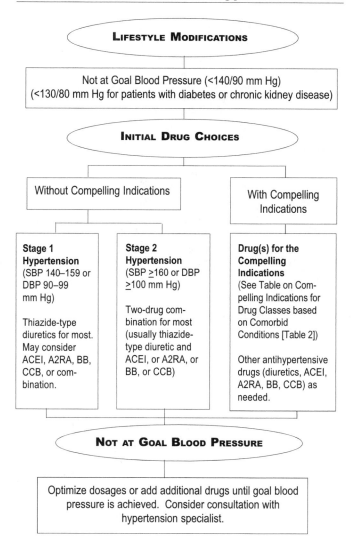

DBP, diastolic blood pressure; SBP, systolic blood pressure.
Drug abbreviations: ACEI, ACE inhibitor; A2RA, angiotensin II receptor antagonist; BB, β-blocker; CCB, calcium channel blocker.

* Source: National Heart, Lung, and Blood Institute National High Blood Pressure Education Program. The seventh report of the Joint National Committee on Prevention, Detection, Evaluation, and Treatment of High Blood Pressure (JNC VII) Express. Bethesda, MD: May 14 2003. From NIH website. (http://www.nhlbi.nih.gov/guidelines/hypertension/jncintro.htm). (Also published in JAMA. 2003; 289.)

Table 35-3 Life-Style Modification Recommendations

Modification	Recommendation	Average Systolic Blood Pressure Reduction Range
Weight reduction	Maintain normal body weight (body mass index 18.5–24.9 kg/m²)	5–20 mm Hg/10 kg
DASH (Dietary Approaches to Stop Hypertension) eating plan	Adopt a diet rich in fruits, vegetables, and low-fat dairy products with reduced content of saturated and total fat	8–14 mm Hg
Dietary sodium intake	Reduce sodium intake to <2.4 g sodium or 6 g sodium chloride	2–8 mm Hg
Aerobic physical activity	Regular aerobic physical activity (e.g., brisk walking) at least 30 minutes per day, most days of the week	4–9 mm Hg
Moderation of alcohol consumption	Men: limit to <2 drinks* per day	2–4 mm Hg
	Women and lighter weight persons: limit to <1 drink* per day	

*One drink = 1/2 oz or 15 mL ethanol (e.g., 12 oz beer, 5 oz wine, 1.5 oz 80-proof whiskey).
Reprinted courtesy of the National Institutes of Health.

Table 35-4 Identifiable Causes of Hypertension

Sleep apnea	Cushing's syndrome or steroid therapy
Drug induced/related	Pheochromocytoma
Chronic kidney disease	Coarctation of aorta
Primary aldosteronism	Thyroid/parathyroid disease
Renovascular disease	

Reprinted courtesy of the National Institutes of Health.

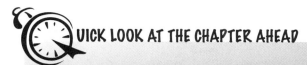
Congestive heart failure (CHF) is a pathophysiological syndrome in which the heart is unable to pump an adequate amount of blood to meet metabolic demands. In addition to inadequate cardiac output (CO), there is an elevation of pressure in the left ventricle caused by **left ventricular dysfunction.** Pressures are reflected backward through the pulmonary veins, causing increased pulmonary pressure and congestion.

36

Congestive Heart Failure

TERMS
- [ ] **afterload**
- [ ] **diastolic dysfunction**
- [ ] **left ventricular dysfunction**
- [ ] **preload**
- [ ] **systolic dysfunction**

Congestive heart failure (CHF) refers primarily to left ventricular failure (LVF). However, the increased pulmonary pressure resulting from LVF increases pressure against which the right ventricle must pump, eventually resulting in right ventricular failure (RVF). The right ventricle is unable to compensate for this increased workload and becomes hypertrophic, leading to failure. Pressures in the systemic venous circulation rise, leading to peripheral edema and hepatosplenomegaly. LVF is the most common cause of RVF. Pulmonary disease, such as chronic obstructive pulmonary disease, cystic fibrosis, or adult respiratory distress syndrome, may also contribute to RVF.

 LVF is the most common cause of RVF. Pulmonary disease, such as chronic obstructive pulmonary disease, cystic fibrosis, or adult respiratory distress syndrome, may also contribute to RVF.

CHF is associated with numerous types of cardiovascular disease, especially hypertension and coronary artery disease. More than half of the deaths from heart disease are due to end-stage CHF. One and a half percent to 2% of the American population is afflicted with CHF. There is a 65% 6-year mortality rate for women and an 80% mortality rate for men. CHF results in 700,000 hospital admissions each year and is the most common admitting diagnosis after age 65. It is associated with extended hospital stays, and the resulting costs for these stays are estimated to be $102 billion a year. Research has demonstrated that better control of CHF can substantially reduce health care expenditures. The prevalence of CHF is expected to continue to rise due to the aging population and because of declines in mortality from other cardiovascular disease. Age is the most common risk factor for CHF.

The causes of CHF may be divided into two subgroups: (1) underlying cardiac diseases and (2) causes that precipitate the onset of CHF in those with underlying cardiac problems. In addition to aging, coronary artery disease, a more common cause in whites, and hypertension, a more common cause in African Americans, are other risk factors. Additional risk factors include cardiomyopathy, diabetes, valvular heart disease, and renal failure. Twenty percent of survivors of myocardial infarction, a common cause of CHF, will be incapacitated by CHF within 6 years. Precipitating causes of decompensation in CHF include anemia, infection, hyperthyroidism, hypothyroidism,

 The causes of CHF may be divided into two subgroups: (1) underlying cardiac diseases and (2) causes that precipitate the onset of CHF in those with underlying cardiac problems.

exacerbation of hypertension, dysrhythmias, endocarditis, and hypervolemia. Noncompliance with diet or medications can precipitate CHF episodes.

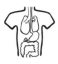

PATHOPHYSIOLOGY

CHF results from complex interaction among factors that affect contractility: **preload,** which is the degree of myocardial stretch just before contraction; **afterload,** the resistance of ejection of blood from the left ventricle; and the subsequent neurohumoral and hemodynamic compensatory responses from decreased CO. Decreased afterload (or lower aortic pressures) allows quicker contractility of the heart. Higher pressures, or increased afterload, reduce contractility, causing higher workload demands upon the heart.

CO is determined by stroke volume multiplied by heart rate. Stroke volume is determined by preload, contractility, and afterload. An increased preload stretches myocardial fibers, increasing the strength of contraction; however, excessive stretch results in decreased contractility. Increased contractility increases stroke volume, but, if excessive, oxygen demand results in decreased contractility. Any increased afterload decreases stroke volume. Heart rate, which is influenced by the autonomic nervous system,

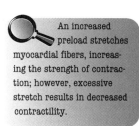

An increased preload stretches myocardial fibers, increasing the strength of contraction; however, excessive stretch results in decreased contractility.

increases the CO until it is excessive (>160 beats/min), in which case the duration of diastole is shortened, reducing ventricular filling and stroke volume.

Several compensatory mechanisms to decrease CO are activated. Initially, the sympathetic nervous system is stimulated, causing increased heart rate, increased contractility, vasoconstriction, and antidiuretic hormone secretion. Venous constriction and antidiuretic hormone increase preload. These mechanisms help restore CO until limits are exceeded, and then excessive myocardial oxygen demand and preload result in decreased contractility and decompensation.

Falling CO with subsequent decreased renal perfusion also activates the renin-angiotensin-aldosterone system, resulting in vasoconstriction and fluid retention. This increases the preload and CO until the preload is excessive and decompensation occurs. Angiotensin II and aldosterone have been implicated as causes of damage to the myocardium.

Ventricular hypertrophy occurs as a compensatory mechanism, but the myocardium eventually outgrows its oxygen supply and increases the oxygen demand, resulting in decreased contractility. Recently, endogenous vasodilators such as atrial natriuretic factor and other peptides have been identified, and their role in compensation of CHF and treatment is being defined.

Ventricular failure can be defined as *systolic dysfunction, diastolic dysfunction,* and *mixed systolic–diastolic dysfunction.*

Systolic dysfunction is characterized by diminished CO (ejection fraction <40%) due to decreased contractility. Activation of the sympathetic nervous system and renin-angiotensin-aldosterone system ultimately excessively increases preload and afterload, further decreasing contractility, thereby causing repeated cycles and further injury to the heart. Increased pressure in the left ventricle causes pulmonary venous congestion. The most common cause of decreased contractility is ischemic heart disease. Cardiac dysrhythmias, dilated cardiomyopathy, chronic alcohol abuse, and myocarditis also decrease contractility.

Diastolic dysfunction has the classic findings of CHF, with abnormal diastolic but normal systolic function and normal ejection fraction. It is characterized by resistance to ventricular filling resulting from abnormal relaxation of the myocardial muscle and increased pressure in the left ventricle at the end of diastole. It is caused by conditions that stiffen the myocardium, such as ischemic heart disease with scarring, hypertrophic and restrictive cardiomyopathies, or pericardial disease. Increases in heart rate decrease filling time, thus exacerbating diastolic dysfunction. The pulmonary congestion that results from LVF may ultimately lead to RVF and systemic congestion.

> It is caused by conditions that stiffen the myocardium, such as ischemic heart disease with scarring, hypertrophic and restrictive cardiomyopathies, or pericardial disease.

A common but acute life-threatening complication of CHF is pulmonary edema, a condition in which there is a redistribution of fluid into the alveoli, making it difficult for lung expansion during respiration. This impairs gas exchange, leading to development of progressive acidosis. Other complications of CHF include cardiogenic shock, pleural effusion, left ventricular thrombus, dysrhythmias, and impaired liver function.

A common but acute life-threatening complication of CHF is pulmonary edema, a condition in which there is a redistribution of fluid into the alveoli, making it difficult for lung expansion during respiration.

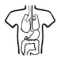

MANIFESTATIONS

The clinical manifestations of CHF reflect both decreased perfusion of body tissues resulting from decreased CO (forward effects) and pulmonary congestion that results from the increased left ventricular pressure (backward effects). The manifestations of right ventricular dysfunction reflect the systemic congestion. Figure 36-1 compares the manifestations of LVF and RVF. Figure 36-2 lists the manifestations of pulmonary edema. A physical examination can often establish the diagnosis of CHF. A chest x-ray may reveal cardiomegaly, pulmonary congestion, edema, and pleural effusion. Arterial blood gases may indicate the alterations in gas exchange that result from CHF. An echocardiogram can estimate the ejection fraction. The New York Heart Association *Functional Classification of Patients With Heart Disease* is one guide used to classify cardiac dysfunction.

TREATMENT

In addition to treating the underlying cause of the CHF and implementing life-style modifications (e.g., reducing dietary salt, exercising), pharmacological therapy involves using angiotensin-converting enzyme inhibitors, diuretics, and inotropic agents for systolic dysfunction. Some calcium blockers are used in diastolic dysfunction, slowing the heart rate; thus, they support diastolic filling. Beta-blockers have an increasing role because of decreased symptoms and decreased mortality. Intravenous inotropics are used in pulmonary edema. An intraaortic balloon pump is sometimes needed for cardiogenic shock.

Figure 36-1 Comparison of the manifestations of left ventricular failure with those of right ventricular failure.

Manifestations of Left Ventricular Failure

Signs
- Increased heart rate
- Pulsus alternans (alternating strong/weak)
- S_3 and S_4 heart sounds
- Displaced or forceful apical impulse
- Left ventricular heave
- Crackles
- Cheyne-Stokes respiration
- Decreased O_2 saturation
- Shortness of breath

Symptoms
- Fatigue
- Dyspnea
- Orthopnea
- Paroxysmal nocturnal dyspnea
- Nocturia
- Dry hacking cough (decreased cardiac output can cause mental status disturbance, activity intolerance, cool, pale extremities with increased capillary refill time, decreased urine output, chest pain possible)

Manifestations of Right Ventricular Failure

Signs
- Right ventricular heave
- Murmurs
- Peripheral edema/tight shoes
- Weight gain
- Dependent edema
- Ascites
- Anasarca
- Increased jugular pressure, hepatojugular reflux
- Hepatomegaly

Symptoms
- Fatigue
- Dependent edema
- Right upper quadrant pain
- Anorexia and bloating
- Nausea

Figure 36-2 Clinical manifestations of CHF.

Dyspnea: shortness of breath

Fluid retention and peripheral edema: occurs as result of impaired pumping ability of the heart

Nocturia: occurs as result of edema returning to circulation when the patient is supine (usually while sleeping), causing increased nocturnal urination

Orthopnea: shortness of breath that occurs with lying down

Paroxysmal nocturnal dyspnea: dyspnea that develops within several hours of going to sleep and awakens the patient

Fatigue and decreased exercise tolerance: occurs as result of decreased left ventricular output

Cyanosis: late sign of heart failure due to decreased oxygenation

Cachexia and malnutrition: caused by congestion of the gastrointestinal system impairing digestion and absorption

Figure 36-3 Precipitating causes of decompensation in heart failure.

- Anemia
- Infection
- Thyrotoxicosis
- Arrhythmias
- Pulmonary disease, pulmonary embolism
- Hypervolemia
- Nutritional deficiency
- Paget's disease (bone disease characterized by thickening and softening of bones; increased vascular bed increases heart workload)
- Myocardial infarction
- Progression of the heart disease
- Noncompliance with prescriptions (e.g., medications, diet)

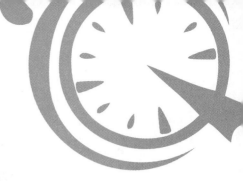

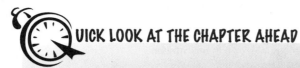
Normal contraction of the heart is achieved by the domination of a single pulse generated by the sinoatrial (SA) node, which is known as the "natural pacemaker" of the heart. This sets off a unique series of impulses throughout the heart. (see Chapter 31 for the conduction system of the heart). The terms **dysrhythmia** or **arrhythmia** are used interchangeably to describe the disturbance of normal cardiac rhythm occurring as a result of alterations within the conduction of electrical impulses. These impulses stimulate and coordinate atrial and ventricular myocardial contractions that provide cardiac output. Dysrhythmias may have serious consequences because coordinated electrical function of the heart is directly related to the coordinated myocardial contraction necessary for normal cardiac output. They can occur intermittently as a "skipped" or rapid beat or may be more serious abnormal conductions leading to heart failure.

37

Dysrhythmias

TERMS
- [ ] **automaticity**
- [ ] **conductivity**
- [ ] **excitability**
- [ ] **reentry**
- [ ] **rhythmicity**

Figure 37-1 Common dysrhythmias.

Common Dysrhythmias

	P Wave	P-R Interval	QRS
Sinus Bradycardia Slow discharge of SA node, R<60/minute, regular rhythm, may cause decreased CO/hypertension Etiology: physical training, sleep, hypothermia hypothyroid, vagal stimulation (suctioning), increased intracranial Sick Sinus Syndrome (SSS) (elderly), certain drugs (beta-blockers)	Normal	Normal	Normal
Sinus Tachycardia Rapid discharge of SA node, >100/minute, regular rhythm may cause decreased CO/hypotension, myocardial ischemia Etiology: hypotension, hypovolemia, fever, anemia, hypoxia, hyperthyroid, heart failure, certain drugs (e.g., Theophyllin [Roxane Laboratories, Inc, Columbus, OH])	Normal	Normal	Normal
Premature Atrial Contraction (PAC) Originate from ectopic atrial foci, usually normal conduction Rate varies, irregular rhythm, impulse conduction through AV node may be delayed or nonconducted May be prelude to supraventricular tachycardia Etiology: stimulants, hyperthyroid, infection, COPD, heart disease	Abnormal	Variable	Normal
Paroxysmal Supraventricular Tachycardia (SVT) Originate from ectopic focus above bundle of His, "re-entry" rate from 100 to 300/minute, regular rhythm If R>180/minute, then decreased CO/hypotension, myocardial ischemia Etiology: exertion, emotion, stimulants, rheumatic heart disease	Abnormal or hidden	Variable	Normal

CO = cardiac output, MI = myocardial infarction, CAD = coronary artery disease, SA = sinoatrial, AV = atrioventricular

(continued)

Figure 37-1 *Continued.*

	P Wave	P-R Interval	QRS

Atrial Flutter
Ectopic atrial focus "re-entry"
Atrial R 250 to 400/minute, usually slow ventricular
    response
AV block, usually fixed 2:1, 3:1
High rate could decrease CO
Etiology: CAD, valve problem, hyperthyroid,
    some drugs
	Saw-tooth
	Shaped
		Variable	Normal

Atrial Fibrillation
Total disorganization, atrial electrical activity
    without effective atrial contraction
Atrial R 300 to 600/minute, irregularly irregular
    ventricular, may be rapid; if rapid, decrease CO,
    mural, thrombi/emboli
Etiology: usually heart disease, also hyperthyroid,
    infection
	Chaotic	Can't be
		measured
			Normal

Junctional/Nodal Arrhythmia
Originates in AV node, may move retrograde,
    producing abnormal P wave before or after QRS
Indicate problem with SA node; if rapid,
    decrease CO			

First-Degree AV Block
AB conduction time is gradually prolonged until an
    atrial impulse is nonconducted and QRS is dropped,
    then repeats
Ventricular rate may be slower
Etiology: CAD, drugs (digoxin, beta blockers),
    rheumatic fever
	Normal	>.20 second	Normal

Second-Degree Block—Type 1
AV conduction time is gradually prolonged until an
    atrial impulse is nonconducted and QRS is
    dropped, then repeats
Ventricular rate may be slower
Etiology: usually myocardial ischemia, drugs
	Normal	Progressive
		lengthening
			Normal width
			one not
			conducted

Figure 37-1 *Continued.*

	P Wave	P-R Interval	QRS

Second Degree—Type 2
Atrial impulses dropped, without antecedent
   lengthening P-R
Certain number of impulses are not conducted
   2:1, 3:1 block
Often progresses to third-degree block; if slow
   pulse, decrease CO
Etiology: CAD, MI, digoxin
	Occurs in
	multiples
		Normal
		or prolonged
			Widened
			Preceded by
			two or more
			P waves

Third Degree—Complete AV Block
No atrial impulses conducted, atrium and ventricle
   contract separately, result is decreased CO
   and heart failure
Etiology: calcification of conduction system, CAD,
   cardiomyopathy
	Normal	Variable	Normal
			or widened

Premature Ventricular Contraction (PVC)
From single or multiple ectopic focus in ventricle
Premature, distorted QRS, R = 60 to 100/minute,
   irregular
Bigeminy, triplets, >3 is ventricular tachycardia
May decrease CO, indicates ventricular irritability
Etiology; ischemia, stimulants, hypokalemia,
   stress, fever
	None	Not
		measurable
			Wide and
			Distorted

Ventricular Tachycardia
Run of three or more PVCs, ventricular focus
   or foci fire repeatedly, take control as
   pacemaker, R = 110 to 250/minute
May cause profound decreased CO, immediate
   intervention
May progress to ventricular fibrillation
	Usually none	Not
		measurable
			Wide and
			distorted

Ventricular Fibrillation
Severe derangement, firing multiple ventricular foci
No effective ventricular contraction, terminal
   if untreated
Etiology: ischemia, infarction, CAD,
   cardiomyopathy
	None	Not
		measurable
			Wide and
			distorted

Four inherent properties make up normal cardiac rhythm: **automaticity** is the ability to generate spontaneous impulses, **rhythmicity** is the regular generation of impulses, **conductivity** allows transmission of impulses, and **excitability** is the response to stimulation. There are two basic types of dysrhythmias: *tachydysrhythmias,* which are the most common, and *bradydysrhythmias.* There are two fundamental causes of dysrhythmias: disorders of impulse formation and disturbances of impulse conduction. In addition to the causes and types, there are two major groups of dysrhythmias: *supraventricular dysrhythmias,* which arise above the ventricles, and *ventricular dysrhythmias,* which arise in the ventricles. Ventricular dysrhythmias are more dangerous because the ventricles are the main pumping chambers.

Causes of dysrhythmia may relate to structural abnormalities of the heart, such as inflammation or scarring after a myocardial infarction, or to an abnormal physiological environment for cardiac cells, such as ischemia or hypoxia, electrolyte imbalance, or the presence of some drugs. Neuroendocrine hormones, such as epinephrine, acetylcholine, and thyroxine, can impact dysrhythmias. Most patients with serious dysrhythmias have underlying cardiac disease, but some have a normal heart. Individuals with underlying cardiac pathology tend to tolerate dysrhythmias less than those without underlying pathology, although a life-threatening dysrhythmia in an individual with a normal heart can result in sudden cardiac death.

Dysrhythmias can range from asymptomatic occasional missed beats to symptomatic and sudden cardiac death. They are dangerous to the extent that they reduce cardiac output, impairing perfusion to the myocardium and brain. Less serious dysrhythmias, if they

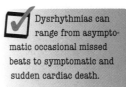

Dysrhythmias can range from asymptomatic occasional missed beats to symptomatic and sudden cardiac death.

compromise the cardiac output, tend to deteriorate into life-threatening dysrhythmias. Thus, prompt recognition and intervention are essential.

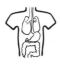

PATHOPHYSIOLOGY

The two fundamental pathophysiological mechanisms underlying dysrhythmias are disordered impulse formation or automaticity and disordered impulse conduction. There are a variety of types of impulse formation problems. Cardiac cells normally capable of automaticity, such as the SA node, atrioventricular (AV) node, and His-Purkinje system, may produce dysrhythmias if their rates of discharge change. The SA node may discharge at a rate slower or faster than normal (60–100 beats/min), producing sinus bradycardia or sinus tachycardia. Pacemakers from the secondary sites may escape the control of the SA node and discharge before the SA node in one of two ways. If the SA node discharges at a rate slower than the rate of the secondary pacemakers, electrical discharges from the secondary sites may automatically discharge at their intrinsic rates (AV node at 40–60 beats/min or the His-Purkinje system at 30–40 beats/min), producing "escape" beats or rhythms. Also, the secondary pacemakers may begin to discharge at a rate faster than the SA node, escaping its control.

Dysrhythmias may be produced if tissues that ordinarily do not express automaticity such as atrial and ventricular muscle develop spontaneous phase 4 depolarization and discharge at a rate faster than the SA node. Then early beats, such as atrial premature beats or ventricular premature beats, may be "triggered" at these ectopic foci and may begin a run of dysrhythmias that replaces normal sinus rhythm. Ectopic beats may originate at a single focus or multiple foci. There are situations in which so many ectopic foci are discharging from many different sites that there is no organized contraction of the heart chamber—only a quivering of the atrial or ventricular muscle, or *fibrillation*.

Disturbances of conduction can occur in the SA node or the AV node, in the intraventricular conduction system, and within the atria and ventricles. They are responsible for SA exit blocks, AV conduction blocks, and establishing reentry circuits (see below). Impulse conduction through the AV node can be impaired to varying degrees. If conduction is slowed but not stopped, it is first-degree block. If some impulses pass through and others do not, it is second-degree block, and if no impulses pass through, it is third-degree block.

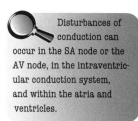

Disturbances of conduction can occur in the SA node or the AV node, in the intraventricular conduction system, and within the atria and ventricles.

Reentry, also called *recirculating activation,* is a generalized mechanism underlying many dysrhythmias, such as premature beats, supraventricular tachycardias, and atrial flutter. Almost all tachyarrhythmias are result of reentry. Reentry establishes localized self-sustaining circuits of repetitive cardiac stimulation. Reentry occurs in areas of slow conduction or in a unidirectional block in one of the branches. Because the block only prevents the impulse from traveling down through the branch, the impulse from the other branch passes up the unidirectionally blocked fiber in a retrograde fashion. It may then pass back down through the unblocked branch, creating a reentrant activation of that branch. The impulse may continue to cycle, creating a circuit that causes repetitive ectopic beats and initiates pathological rhythms or extrasystole.

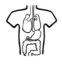

MANIFESTATIONS

Dysrhythmias are detected because they produce symptoms or are detected during some form of cardiac monitoring. Most of the symptoms of dysrhythmias are related to a decreased cardiac output. They can be felt as palpitations, a fluttering sensation, or skipped beats. Both bradycardias and tachycardias, because of the diminished diastolic filling time of the ventricles, can reduce cardiac output. Symptoms of diminished cardiac output include fatigue, lightheadedness, confusion, poor peripheral perfusion, dyspnea, syncope, and sudden cardiac death. Abrupt slowing of the rate can cause convulsions. Dysrhythmias can also precipitate congestive heart failure, angina, and infarction.

They can be felt as palpitations, a fluttering sensation, or skipped beats.

Symptoms of diminished cardiac output include fatigue, lightheadedness, confusion, poor peripheral perfusion, dyspnea, syncope, and sudden cardiac death.

The electrocardiogram is a noninvasive method for detecting dysrhythmias. Twelve leads are placed on different areas of the chest wall and limbs to evaluate electrical activity from different perspectives. An electrocardiogram may be determined at a single point in time or continuously by continuous ambulatory monitoring (Holter monitor) or via telemetry. An invasive method of evaluating dysrhythmias is intracardiac electrophysiological studies, which require cannulation of veins or arteries.

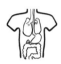

TREATMENT

Medications are a common method of intervention for significant dysrhythmias. Symptomatic bradycardias and AV conduction blocks may also be treated with pacemakers. Carotid massage, cardioversion or controlled defibrillation, and pacemakers may be used to treat supraventricular tachydysrhythmias. Immediate intervention by defibrillation (conventional or implanted) is necessary for life-threatening ventricular dysrhythmias. Radiofrequency catheter ablation uses high-frequency electromagnetic energy to destroy points of origin or pathways necessary for the propagation of some dysrhythmias. Avoidance of stimulants, such as caffeine and tobacco, and stress management are other important measures.

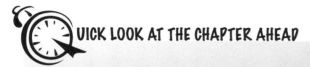

Cardiomyopathy is a term used to describe a diverse group of cardiac diseases that primarily affect the structure and function of the myocardium and its pumping ability. Two major divisions of cardiomyopathy are ischemic and nonischemic. This chapter deals only with nonischemic cardiomyopathy.

Ischemic cardiomyopathy refers to the type of myocardial dysfunction that occurs in coronary artery disease (see Chapter 34). **Nonischemic cardiomyopathies** are classified into three groups—dilated, hypertrophic, and restrictive—based on their pathophysiological effects on the heart. Although some cardiomyopathies may be secondary to specific causes, most are idiopathic.

38

Cardiomyopathies

TERMS
- ☐ dilated cardiomyopathy
- ☐ exertional dyspnea
- ☐ orthopnea
- ☐ paroxysmal nocturnal dyspnea
- ☐ syncope

Figure 38-1 Distinguishing pathophysiologic features of the types of cardiomyopathies.

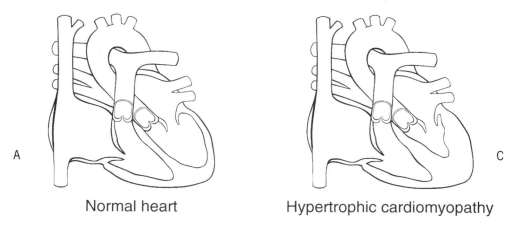

A — Normal heart

C — Hypertrophic cardiomyopathy

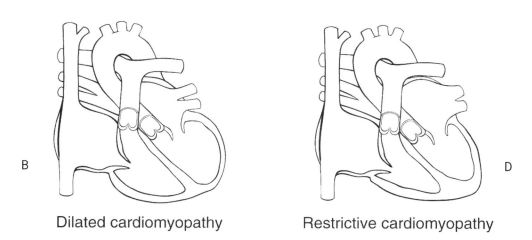

B — Dilated cardiomyopathy

D — Restrictive cardiomyopathy

Diagram showing the major distinguishing pathophysiologic features of the types of cardiomyopathies. (A) The normal heart. (B) In the dilated type of cardiomyopathy, the heart has a globular shape and the largest circumference of the left ventricle is not at its base but midway between the apex and base. (C) In the hypertrophic type, the wall of the left ventricle is greatly thickened and the cavity reduced, but the left atrium may be dilated because of poor diastolic relaxation of the ventricle. (D) In the restrictive type, the left ventricular cavity is of normal size, but again, the left atrium is dilated because of the reduced diastolic compliance of the ventricle.

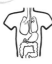

DILATED CARDIOMYOPATHY

Dilated cardiomyopathy accounts for more than 90% of all cardiomyopathies and results in 20,000 deaths per year. It can occur at any age, but its peak incidence occurs in the fourth or fifth decade. African-American men have 2.5 times higher risk than whites and women. Half the cases of dilated cardiomyopathy are idiopathic, and the remainder can be attributable to a known cause. Certain chemotherapeutic agents, particularly doxorubicin and daunorubicin, cause serious myocardial damage.

> ✓ Nonischemic cardiomyopathies are classified into three groups—dilated, hypertrophic, and restrictive—based on their pathophysiological effects on the heart. Although some cardiomyopathies may be secondary to specific causes, most are idiopathic.

A disproportionate number of individuals with dilated cardiomyopathy are alcoholics—approximately 4%—and this is the second leading cause of dilated cardiomyopathy. Damage may be due to direct toxic effects or to nutritional deficiencies. Dilated cardiomyopathy is now seen more frequently in cocaine abusers. Peripartum cardiomyopathy generally develops in the last month of pregnancy and up to 5 months postpartum. Another form of dilated cardiomyopathy may be the consequence of previous viral, bacterial, or parasitic infections. Autoimmune factors, thyrotoxicosis, diabetes, neuromuscular diseases, and hypersensitivity reactions to some medications have also been associated with cardiomyopathy.

Pathophysiology

Dilated cardiomyopathy is characterized by cardiomegaly due to ventricular dilation and by impaired myocardial contractility and mixed systolic and diastolic dysfunction, a condition in which poor systolic function (weakened muscle function) is further compromised by dilated ventricular walls that are unable to relax. A decreased ejection fraction and/or cardiac output, increased end-diastolic pressure with pulmonary congestion, and stasis of blood with mural thrombi are the result. The walls of the ventricle do not become

> 🔍 Dilated cardiomyopathy is characterized by cardiomegaly due to ventricular dilation and by impaired myocardial contractility and mixed systolic and diastolic dysfunction, a condition in which poor systolic function (weakened muscle function) is further compromised by dilated ventricular walls that are unable to relax.

thickened as in congestive heart failure, which is thought to be due to diffuse inflammation and rapid degeneration of myocardial fibers and fibrosis. Deterioration is rapid after the onset of symptoms, and 20% to 50% of patients die within 1 year. Most deaths occur within 5 years.

Manifestations

Clinical manifestations of dilated cardiomyopathy develop insidiously. Patients present with signs and symptoms of congestive heart failure. The most common symptoms are dyspnea and fatigue. A dry cough, orthopnea, and **paroxysmal nocturnal dyspnea** occur. Palpitations are common, and exertional chest pain indistinguishable from angina occurs in some patients. Dizziness may result from dysrhythmias. A decrease in activity tolerance occurs. Signs may include increases or decreases of blood pressure, tachycardia, S_3 and S_4 heart sounds, and murmurs of mitral or tricuspid regurgitation. Pulmonary congestion results in increased respiratory rate, crackles, and abnormal blood gases. There may be peripheral edema, ascites, weak pedal pulses, and cool, pale extremities with poor capillary refill. Hepatomegaly and jugular venous distention may occur. Systemic and pulmonary emboli are common complications. Left heart failure is the cause of death in 75% of the patients. Sudden death from dysrhythmia may occur.

The best diagnostic tool is the echocardiogram, which shows dilated ventricles, global diminished ventricular wall motion, and an ejection fraction of less than 45%.

Treatment

Few causes of dilated cardiomyopathy are reversible; these include nutritional or alcohol-related causes. Treatment is mainly supportive by relief of symptoms of heart failure by decreasing afterload and enhancing contractility through the use of digoxin or other afterload-reducing agents. Patients with terminal end-stage dilated cardiomyopathy may require heart transplantation. Fifty percent of heart transplants are performed due to dilated cardiomyopathy.

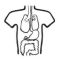

HYPERTROPHIC CARDIOMYOPATHY

Hypertrophic cardiomyopathy, also known as idiopathic hypertrophic subaortic stenosis, is less common than dilated cardiomyopathy. It is more common in men and is often seen in active athletic individuals. It appears to have an autosomal dominant genetic basis. Sudden cardiac death can occur in relation to physical activity in those who are completely asymptomatic.

Pathophysiology

The hallmark of hypertrophic cardiomyopathy is massive ventricular wall thickening with disproportionate thickening of the intraventricular septum. This results in a hyperdynamic state with increased contractility and increased ejection fraction. The loss of ventricular wall compliance and impaired diastolic relaxation or diastolic dysfunction combined with the thickened septum may obstruct left ventricular outflow through the aorta. The decreased ventricular filling and obstruction to outflow may result in decreased cardiac output. Any condition that increases the contractility also increases the obstruction, such as exertion or cardiotonic medications like digoxin.

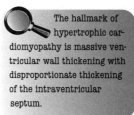

The hallmark of hypertrophic cardiomyopathy is massive ventricular wall thickening with disproportionate thickening of the intraventricular septum.

Manifestations

Major clinical manifestations are **exertional dyspnea,** fatigue, **syncope, orthopnea,** angina, and left heart failure. If the hypertrophied muscle outgrows its blood supply, a myocardial infarction may occur. Palpitations are common and often related to dysrhythmias. Common dysrhythmias are supraventricular tachycardia, atrial fibrillation, ventricular tachycardia, and ventricular fibrillation. Any of these dysrhythmias may lead to loss of consciousness or to sudden cardiac death, which is the most common cause of death. Diagnosis is made by electrocardiogram (ECG) and echocardiogram. Increased voltage (height) and duration (width) of QRS complexes indicate ventricular hypertrophy on ECG. Dysrhythmias are also frequently seen. The primary diagnostic tool is the echocardiogram, which reveals the classical feature—asymmetrical left ventricular hypertrophy. It may also demonstrate abnormal wall motion and diastolic dysfunction.

Treatment

The goals of treatment are to reduce the ventricular stiffness, improve the ventricular filling, and relieve the left ventricular outflow obstruction by decreasing the contractility and cardiac rate with beta-blockers.

Verapamil has also been successful. Surgical resection of the hypertrophied tissue, ventriculomyotomy and myectomy, may relieve symptoms in those who do not respond to medications.

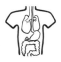

RESTRICTIVE CARDIOMYOPATHY

Restrictive cardiomyopathy is the least common of the cardiomyopathies and is endemic to parts of South and Central America, India, Asia, and Africa. Although the specific etiology is unknown, it is usually associated with an infiltrative disease of the myocardium. The most common cause is due to amyloidosis, but other causes include sarcoidosis, hemochromatosis, glycogen storage disease, myocardial fibrosis, and radiation to the thorax.

Pathophysiology

Myocardial fibrosis, hypertrophy, and infiltration produce stiffness of the ventricular wall, which results in diminished compliance and decreased ventricular diastolic filling with high diastolic filling pressures to maintain cardiac output.

Manifestations

The most common clinical manifestation of restrictive cardiomyopathy is heart failure, particularly right-sided heart failure. The most common symptom is exercise intolerance because the ventricle cannot increase the rate without further compromising the diastolic filling. Angina, fatigue, syncope, paroxysmal nocturnal dyspnea, orthopnea, and dyspnea on exertion are also common. Signs of both right- and left-sided heart failure and peripheral edema, hepatomegaly, ascites, and jugular venous distention may be present. Pulmonary congestion, or crackles, may be evident. The most common dysrhythmia that may be produced is atrial fibrillation. Diagnosis is made by chest x-ray, which may reveal pulmonary congestion, or by ECG, which demonstrates tachycardia or dysrhythmia. An echocardiogram may reveal thickened ventricular walls, small cavities, and enlarged atria. Endomyocardial biopsy and a computed tomography may aid diagnosis. Cardiac catheterization may also be considered.

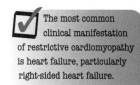

The most common clinical manifestation of restrictive cardiomyopathy is heart failure, particularly right-sided heart failure.

Treatment

There is no specific treatment for restrictive cardiomyopathy other than treating the underlying disease. Interventions may be aimed at improving the diastolic filling by controlling the heart rate and treatment of congestive heart failure. A heart transplant may need to be considered. Prognosis is generally poor, and death occurs due to congestive heart failure.

Table 38-1 Pathophysiological Characteristics of Cardiomyopathies

Type of Cardiomyopathy	Associated Conditions	Anatomic Derangement	Physiologic Derangement	Manifestations
Dilated or congestive	Infection Alcohol Pregnancy Some drugs	Cardiomegaly—ventricular dilation without hypertrophy Chamber volume increased Decreased contractile muscle fibers Diffuse necrosis Mitral valve incompetence	Poor systolic function Diminished contractility Decreased ejection fraction Increased end diastolic (residual) volume Blood stasis Mural thrombi	Fatigue Weakness Dyspnea Palpitations Left ventricular failure Dysrhythmias
Hypertrophic	Autosomal dominant inheritance	Disproportionate thickening of interventricular septum Aortic outflow obstruction in some cases Chamber volume is decreased Mitral valve incompetence	Increased contractility Decreased compliance Poor diastolic function	Dyspnea Angina Syncope Palpitations Dysrhythmias Left ventricular failure Sudden death
Restrictive	Infiltrative diseases (e.g., amyloidosis)	Rigid, noncompliant myocardium Mild cardiomegaly Fibrotic myocardium Atrioventricular valve incompetence	Impeded ventricular filling Diastolic dysfunction Decreased compliance	Right ventricular failure Dysrhythmias

Adapted from Huether, S., & McChance, K. (2000). Understanding pathophysiology (2nd ed.). St. Louis, MO: C. V. Mosby Co.

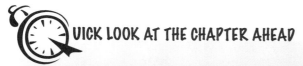

QUICK LOOK AT THE CHAPTER AHEAD

Pericarditis, or inflammation of the pericardium, may be a primary condition or result from secondary disease. It can be caused by viral, bacterial, or fungal infections or by neoplasm or uremia. Males under 50 years old are most commonly affected. Other causes include systemic disease such as autoimmune and connective tissues diseases, such as rheumatoid arthritis, systemic lupus erythematosus, or rheumatic fever, and trauma due to radiation, chest injury, open heart surgery, or pacemaker insertion. It may also be the result of diseases of adjacent structures, myocardial infarction, and pulmonary disease. Pericarditis may spread from or to the **myocardium.**

Infective endocarditis, formerly known as bacterial endocarditis, is an infection of the endocardium, or inner lining of the heart, and most often involves the valves. Before the era of antibiotics, it was a lethal disease. It is now relatively rare, although there are approximately 5,000 to 8,000 new cases in the United States each year. Two forms of endocarditis are described: subacute and acute. The subacute form has a longer course, a more insidious onset, less toxicity, and causative organism of low virulence, commonly **Streptococcus viridans**. It responds well to treatment. The acute form has a shorter course, more rapid onset, more toxicity, and more virulent organism, commonly caused by **Staphylococcus aureus**. It can cause death within days or weeks if untreated.

39

Inflammatory Heart Disease

TERMS
- ☐ myocarditis
- ☐ myocardium
- ☐ pericarditis

Figure 39-1 Clinical manifestations of endocarditis, myocarditis, and pericarditis.

Clinical Manifestations of Endocarditis

History

- Fever
- Anorexia, weight loss
- Back pain
- Night sweats
- Embolization to coronary arteries could cause myocardial infarction
- Preexisting heart defects or murmurs
- Cough, dyspnea, or flank pain

Physical Examination

- New or significantly changed heart murmur
- Petechial lesions of skin, conjunctiva, oral mucosa
- Splinter hemorrhages under nails of fingers and toes

Diagnostic Tests

- Positive blood cultures
- Elevated erythrocyte sedimentation rate
- Electrocardiographic changes: prolonged P-R interval, conduction blocks
- Echocardiogram or transesophageal echocardiogram

Clinical Manifestations of Myocarditis

History

- May be asymptomatic
- Dyspnea, fatigue, syncope
- Palpitations, chest discomfort
- Flu-like symptoms

Physical Examination

- Cardiac enlargement
- Tachycardia
- Faint heart sounds, friction rub, gallop or S_3
- Pericardial effusion, congestive heart failure

Diagnostic Tests

- Electrocardiographic changes: ST-T wave abnormalities, ischemia
- Elevated serum creatinine kinase and troponin T and/or I
- Leukocytosis, atypical lymphocytes, erythrocyte sedimentation rate
- Echocardiogram, myocardial biopsy

Clinical Manifestations of Pericarditis

History

- Chest pain—Pleuritic pain is relieved by sitting; retrosternal and left precordial radiating to neck, shoulders, back, and epigastrium. Pain may be severe, sharp, or aching and worsens with sneezing, coughing, or change of position; relieved with sitting up and leaning forward
- Dyspnea
- Flu-like symptoms as prodrome

Physical Examination

- Pericardial friction rub heard best at apex and lower left sternal border
- Fever

Diagnostic Tests

- Leukocytosis
- Electrocardiogram may show S-T segment elevations without Q waves, PR segment depression
- Chest x-ray may show cardiac enlargement
- Echocardiogram—most effective diagnostic tool. May show pericardial effusion or localization and estimation of quantity of pericardial fluid
- Computed tomography or magnetic resonance imaging detects loculated pericardial effusion and pericardial thickening

Pericardial Effusion

- Pain may or may not be present, dyspnea, cough, friction rub
- Faint heart sounds
- If tamponade, tachycardia, tachypnea, narrow pulse pressure
- Pulsus paradoxus (>10 mmHg fall in systolic pressure with inspiration)
- Increased central venous pressure, edema, ascites
- Diagnostic tests: chest x-ray—may reveal enlarged heart; electrocardiogram, echocardiogram may reveal pericardial fluid; magnetic resonance imaging

Constrictive Pericarditis

- Progressive dyspnea, fatigue, weakness, pedal edema
- Hepatomegaly, ascites (early finding), jugular venous distention
- Atrial fibrillation
- Diagnostic tests: chest x-ray, echocardiogram, computed tomography, magnetic resonance imaging

Infective endocarditis occurs when turbulent blood flow in the heart allows causative organisms to grow on damaged valves or other endothelial surfaces. Conditions predisposing individuals to endocarditis have changed with the decreasing incidence of rheumatic heart disease and recognition

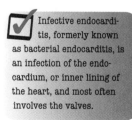

Infective endocarditis, formerly known as bacterial endocarditis, is an infection of the endocardium, or inner lining of the heart, and most often involves the valves.

and treatment of mitral valve prolapse. Risk factors include congenital and degenerative heart diseases that damage valves and endothelial surfaces. Individuals with artificial valve replacement may develop endocarditis. Organisms may gain entry to the bloodstream during intrusive procedures such as dental procedures, gynecological examinations, and placement of urinary catheters. Intravenous drug abusers are at high risk. Organisms other than bacteria can be involved, such as gram-negative bacilli, fungi, and yeast, particularly in the immunocompromised individual.

Myocarditis is a focal or diffuse inflammatory process involving the myocardium and resulting from a variety of etiological agents, including pathological organisms (mainly viruses but also fungi, parasites, and rickettsiae), radiation, toxins, systemic diseases such as systemic lupus erythematosus or rheumatic fever, and immune reactions. It often follows an upper respiratory infection but may also occur from chemotherapy drugs, radiation, or cocaine abuse. It is frequently associated with pericarditis and endocarditis. The most common causative organism is Coxsackievirus A and B. It is also thought to be caused by exposure to chemical or physical agents.

Acute rheumatic fever is an acute, febrile, inflammatory disease caused by a delayed immune response to an untreated pharyngeal infection caused by group A β-hemolytic streptococcus. In its acute form it results in inflammation of the joints, skin, nervous system, and heart. Inflammation in the heart may involve the pericardium, endocardium, and myocardium. If the streptococcal infection is untreated, damage to the heart can result in rheumatic heart disease, a chronic condition characterized by destruction, scarring, and deformity of the heart valves. Antibiotic treatment of streptococcal infections within 9 days usually prevents acute rheumatic fever.

Initial and recurrent episodes of acute rheumatic fever are most common in childhood between the ages of 5 and 15 as a complication of streptococcal pharyngitis. Recurrent attacks may occur. Chronic rheumatic heart disease can appear approximately 10 years after the initial illness. The incidence of acute rheumatic fever has declined in recent years with socioeconomic and medical improvements. However, because overcrowding and poor hygiene are risk factors for acute rheumatic

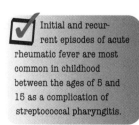
Initial and recurrent episodes of acute rheumatic fever are most common in childhood between the ages of 5 and 15 as a complication of streptococcal pharyngitis.

fever, the disease continues to be a concern in underprivileged populations. It has a tendency to run in families.

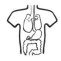

PERICARDITIS

Pathophysiology

In pericarditis, the pericardial membranes become inflamed with formation of proteinaceous exudates on epi- and pericardial surfaces, causing a pericardial effusion, filling the pericardial sac. The fluid may be serous (heart failure), purulent (bacterial infection), serosanguineous (neoplasm, uremia), or hemorrhagic (ruptured aneurysm or trauma). If fluid accumulates slowly, it may not be clinically significant; however, when fluid accumulates rapidly, cardiac tamponade or compression of the heart may occur, impairing venous return, filling the heart, and causing systemic congestion and decreased cardiac output. Cardiac failure, cardiogenic shock, and death can result.

> If fluid accumulates slowly, it may not be clinically significant; however, when fluid accumulates rapidly, cardiac tamponade or compression of the heart may occur, impairing venous return, filling the heart, and causing systemic congestion and decreased cardiac output.

Chronic inflammation can gradually lead to constrictive pericarditis, in which pericardial membranes become thickened and fibrous and adhere, encasing the heart in a hard shell that restricts cardiac filling and causing systemic congestion and reduced cardiac output.

Manifestations

See Figure 39-1 for the clinical manifestations of pericarditis.

Treatment

Treatment is specific to the underlying cause (e.g., antibiotics for infection) and to reduce inflammation and its sequelae. Small effusions are treated with nonsteroidal antiinflammatory drugs and corticosteroids if the inflammation is refractory to the nonsteroidal antiinflammatory drugs. A pericardiocentesis may be needed for large effusions or a pericardial fenestration for continuous drainage. In

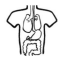

constrictive pericarditis, a pericardectomy, or removal of the pericardium, may be needed.

INFECTIVE ENDOCARDITIS

Pathophysiology

Pathogenesis of infective endocarditis first involves endothelial damage, which attracts platelets and stimulates thrombus formation. This facilitates the adherence of organisms that entered the bloodstream and survived body defenses, allowing their colonization. Some very virulent organisms do not require the initial endothelial damage. This mass of fibrin, leukocytes, platelets, and microorganisms forms a "vegetation." This process commonly involves valves and surrounding endothelium. The valves may become scarred and perforated. Valvular incompetence and invasion of the myocardium may result in heart failure. Emboli may break free from the vegetative growth, travel in the bloodstream to distant organs, and form abscesses.

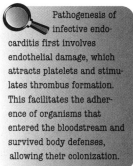

Pathogenesis of infective endocarditis first involves endothelial damage, which attracts platelets and stimulates thrombus formation. This facilitates the adherence of organisms that entered the bloodstream and survived body defenses, allowing their colonization.

Manifestations

See Figure 39-1 for the clinical manifestations of endocarditis.

Treatment

Prophylactic treatment involves administration of antibiotics before invasive procedures such as dental cleanings and procedures and certain gynecological or surgical procedures. With infection of valves, antibiotics are started and continued for 4 to 6 weeks. Deteriorated valves are surgically replaced if necessary.

Prophylactic treatment involves administration of antibiotics before invasive procedures such as dental cleanings and procedures and certain gynecological or surgical procedures.

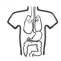

MYOCARDITIS

Pathophysiology

The pathogenesis of myocarditis is poorly understood because there is a period of several weeks (in some forms, a decade) between exposure to the infecting organism and development of manifestations. Infiltration of organisms, blood cells, toxins, and immune substances around coronary arteries and between muscle fibers can result in fiber dysfunction and degeneration that may impede contractility and conduction and may cause dilation of the heart or diminished wall motion. Though commonly benign, it can result in heart failure, dysrhythmias, and mural thrombi. It has been theorized that dilated cardiomyopathy is a manifestation of myocarditis.

Manifestations

See Figure 39-1 for the clinical manifestations of myocarditis.

Treatment

Specific treatment is not yet established. Treatment usually consists of managing any cardiac decompensation. Immunosuppressive agents are used in some cases after the infective stage of the disease to reduce myocardial inflammation and prevent damage. Bed rest and restriction of activity and fluid are also recommended to decrease demand on the heart.

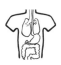

RHEUMATIC HEART DISEASE

Pathophysiology

Rheumatic fever causes carditis or inflammation in all three layers of the heart, but the primary lesions involve the endocardium, which lines the chambers and heart valves. Inflammation causes swelling of the valve leaflet and erosion along the edges. Vegetative growths containing fibrin and platelets are deposited on the eroded tissue, valve elasticity is lost, and leaflets become adherent to one another over time. Valvular dysfunction, most commonly mitral stenosis, develops. Fibrinoid necrotic deposits called *Aschoff's bodies* develop in the myocardium. Pericardial inflammation is characterized by serosanguineous effusion. Cardiomegaly and heart failure may develop with chronic rheumatic heart disease. Conduction disturbances and atrial fibrillation are common.

Treatment

Penicillin or erythromycin is used to treat the rheumatic fever and is used continuously to prevent recurrence. Salicylate, which is used as an antiinflammatory agent; corticosteroids; and bed rest are used with serious inflammation. The valves may need to be surgically repaired or replaced.

There are four heart valves: two atrioventricular valves (mitral and tricuspid) and two semilunar valves (aortic and pulmonic). It is the coordination of the opening and closing of these valves with the pressure gradients created during the phases of the cardiac cycle that determines the forward flow of the blood. During systole, the aortic and pulmonic valves are normally open, and the mitral and tricuspid valves are closed. During diastole, the mitral and tricuspid valves are open, and the aortic and pulmonic valves are closed.

Valvular disease causes disruption of normal blood flow through the valves, damaging the valves and impeding cardiac function to various degrees. The types of valvular disease are defined according to the valve affected and the type of functional alteration or **stenosis** due to a narrowed orifice and **regurgitation** due to incomplete closure. Although any of the valves may be affected, those on the left side of the heart are more commonly affected. Valvular problems may be congenital or acquired. At one time, most acquired valvular disease in the United States was a result of rheumatic fever, but other causes are more common today, such as atherosclerotic heart disease in the elderly.

40
Valvular Problems

TERMS
- ☐ mitral valve regurgitation
- ☐ mitral valve stenosis
- ☐ regurgitation
- ☐ stenosis

Figure 40-1 Valvular stenosis and regurgitation.

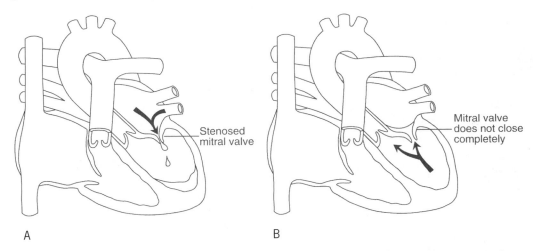

A   B

Valvular stenosis and regurgitation. (A) Hemodynamic effect of mitral stenosis. The stenosed valve is unable to open sufficiently during left atrial systole, inhibiting left ventricular filling. (B) Hemodynamic effect of mitral regurgitation. The mitral valve does not close completely during left ventricular systole, permitting blood to reenter the left atrium.

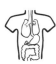

PATHOPHYSIOLOGY

Mitral valve stenosis is a valve in which the leaflets have become thickened and restrict the forward flow of blood, thereby increasing the workload of the chamber behind the diseased valve. As a result, left atrial pressure increases to compensate for the resistance to outflow (increased afterload) and the chamber hypertrophies.

> The types of valvular disease are defined according to the valve affected and the type of functional alteration or stenosis due to a narrowed orifice and regurgitation due to incomplete closure.

    Mitral valve regurgitation (also called *incompetence* or *insufficiency*) occurs when an incompetent valve does not close completely, permitting backward or retrograde flow of blood during ventricular systole into the chamber above the valve. This causes an increased volume of blood, which increases workload and causes hypertrophy of the affected chamber. The mitral and aortic valves are more commonly affected than the tricuspid and pulmonic valves.

The dilation and hypertrophy that occur are compensatory mechanisms to support the pumping ability of the heart. Eventually, contractility and the ejection fraction may diminish, the end-diastolic pressure increases, and the ventricles fail. Abnormal valves also predispose to cardiac infection and thrombus formation. Cardiac dysrhythmias, particularly atrial fibrillation, artial flutter, and atrioventricular blocks, may occur.

> Abnormal valves also predispose to cardiac infection and thrombus formation.

Mitral valve prolapse syndrome is the most common valve disorder in the United States and is more prevalent in young women. It is also associated with other inherited connective tissue disorders. Mitral valve prolapse syndrome is caused by the displacement of the posterior cusp of the mitral valve, causing the valve leaflets to bulge or balloon upward into the left atrium during systole. It has a high incidence, suggesting that it may be a normal variant rather than pathological. It is usually associated with minimal morbidity or mortality, and, although rare, severe sequelae are potentially possible such as mitral regurgitation, ventricular failure, thromboemboli, and sudden death.

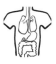

MANIFESTATIONS

Most individuals with mitral valve stenosis have underlying rheumatic heart disease. Initially, it is asymptomatic, with symptoms occurring only when the orifice is reduced by 50%. Symptoms, often precipitated by atrial fibrillation that develops in 80% of the individuals, include those of left heart failure such as dyspnea, orthopnea, paroxysmal nocturnal dyspnea, and dry cough; increased respiratory infection; and hemoptysis. As the stenosis progresses, symptoms of diminished cardiac output appear (fatigue, syncope, chest pain). Eventually, with increasing pulmonary hypertension, manifestations of right-sided heart failure are seen (anorexia, hepatomegaly, ascites, edema, jugular venous distention). The individual may experience palpitations if atrial fibrillation develops. Atrial enlargement may lead to hoarseness. On physical examination, there is a low-pitched, rumbling, mid-diastolic murmur at the apex with an accentuate S_1 and a diastolic snap.

The manifestations of mitral valve regurgitation, related to overfilling of the atrium and increased workload for the left atrium and ventricle, depend on how abruptly it develops. Chronic mitral valve regurgitation may be asymptomatic for years, with slow development of left ventricular failure with exertional dyspnea, fatigue, syncope, palpitations, and atypical chest pain. Patients with acute mitral valve regurgitation develop sudden onset of symptoms after a myocardial infarction or infective endocarditis. Physical examination reveals a loud, high-pitched, blowing, pansystolic murmur radiating to the axilla. A midsystolic click and S_3 may be present. Atrial fibrillation is common. The left atrium and ventricle are dilated and hypertrophied. Acute mitral valve regurgitation may have a fulminant course of pulmonary edema and shock. Surgery to replace the defective valve is indicated for those with severe disease.

> Chronic mitral valve regurgitation may be asymptomatic for years, with slow development of left ventricular failure with exertional dyspnea, fatigue, syncope, palpitations, and atypical chest pain.

Aortic stenosis tends to develop gradually, with ventricular hypertrophy overcoming the impedance to outflow. Eventually, hypertrophy leads to ischemia and clinical manifestations develop, including reduced systolic blood pressure and narrowed pulse pressure.

The diagnostic workup for valvular problems may include a chest x-ray that provides information about chamber size. An electrocardiogram may show hypertrophy and dysrhythmia. An echocardiogram is the recommended procedure that provides information about the severity and progression of disease, chamber responses to volume overload, determines left ventricular function, the direction of blood flow, and the size of the atria and ventricles. Color Doppler detects changes in blood flow. A transesophageal echocardiogram improves the image.

The severity of the valve dysfunction and capacity of the heart to compensate determine the degree of incapacity and the manifestations. The manifestations relate both to the compensatory mechanisms and diminished cardiac dysfunction.

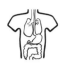

TREATMENT

Valvular dysfunction may be treated with cardiotonic medications, fluid volume control, blood pressure control, and prophylactic antibiotics before invasive procedures. Surgical repair or prosthetic valve replacement may be necessary. The valve may be replaced with a mechanical or a biological prosthesis. The mechanical prosthesis predisposes to the risk of thromboembolism and requires chronic anticoagulation. A biological prosthesis, such as porcine, bovine, or cadaver, does not require chronic anticoagulation but does require eventual replacement of the valve over time.

Table 40-1 Clinical Manifestations of Valvular Stenosis and Regurgitation

Manifestation	Aortic Stenosis	Mitral Stenosis	Aortic Regurgitation	Mitral Regurgitation	Tricuspid Regurgitation
Cardiovascular outcome*	Left ventricular failure	Right ventricular failure	Left heart failure	Left heart failure	Right heart failure
General symptoms	Fatigue	Fatigue, weakness		Fatigue, weakness	Peripheral edema (with heart failure)
Respiratory effects	Dyspnea on exertion	Dyspnea on exertion, orthopnea, paroxysmal, nocturnal dyspnea, predisposition to respiratory infections, hemoptysis, pulmonary hypertension, edema	Dyspnea with effort	Dyspnea; occasional hemoptysis	Dyspnea
Central nervous system effects	Syncope, especially on exertion	Neural deficits only associated with emboli (e.g., hepatomegaly)	Syncope	None	None
Gastrointestinal effects	None	Ascites; hepatic angina with hepatomegaly	None	None	Ascites, hepatomegaly (with heart failure)
Pain	Angina pectoris	Chest pain	Chest pain (anginal)	None	Palpitations
Heart rate, rhythm	Bradycardia, dysrhythmias (with heart failure)	Palpitations (atrial fibrillation)	Palpitations, waterhammer pulse	Palpitations	Atrial fibrillations
Heart sounds	Systolic murmur	Diastolic murmur, accentuated first heart sound, opening snap	Diastolic and systolic murmurs	Murmur throughout systole	Murmur throughout systole
Most common cause	Congenital, rheumatic fever	Rheumatic fever	Bacterial endocarditis; aortic root disease	Floppy valve; coronary artery disease	Congenital

*Untreated disease

Reprinted with permission from Huether, S., & McChance, K. (2000). Understanding pathophysiology (2nd ed.). St. Louis, MO: C. V. Mosby Co.

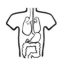

TREATMENT

Valvular dysfunction may be treated with cardiotonic medications, fluid volume control, blood pressure control, and prophylactic antibiotics before invasive procedures. Surgical repair or prosthetic valve replacement may be necessary. The valve may be replaced with a mechanical or a biological prosthesis. The mechanical prosthesis predisposes to the risk of thromboembolism and requires chronic anticoagulation. A biological prosthesis, such as porcine, bovine, or cadaver, does not require chronic anticoagulation but does require eventual replacement of the valve over time.

Table 40-1 Clinical Manifestations of Valvular Stenosis and Regurgitation

Manifestation	Aortic Stenosis	Mitral Stenosis	Aortic Regurgitation	Mitral Regurgitation	Tricuspid Regurgitation
Cardiovascular outcome*	Left ventricular failure	Right ventricular failure	Left heart failure	Left heart failure	Right heart failure
General symptoms	Fatigue	Fatigue, weakness		Fatigue, weakness	Peripheral edema (with heart failure)
Respiratory effects	Dyspnea on exertion	Dyspnea on exertion, orthopnea, paroxysmal, nocturnal dyspnea, predisposition to respiratory infections, hemoptysis, pulmonary hypertension, edema	Dyspnea with effort	Dyspnea; occasional hemoptysis	Dyspnea
Central nervous system effects	Syncope, especially on exertion	Neural deficits only associated with emboli (e.g., hepatomegaly)	Syncope	None	None
Gastrointestinal effects	None	Ascites; hepatic angina with hepatomegaly	None	None	Ascites, hepatomegaly (with heart failure)
Pain	Angina pectoris	Chest pain	Chest pain (anginal)		Palpitations
Heart rate, rhythm	Bradycardia, dysrhythmias (with heart failure)	Palpitations (atrial fibrillation)	Palpitations, waterhammer pulse	Palpitations	Atrial fibrillations
Heart sounds	Systolic murmur	Diastolic murmur, accentuated first heart sound, opening snap	Diastolic and systolic murmurs	Murmur throughout systole	Murmur throughout systole
Most common cause	Congenital, rheumatic fever	Rheumatic fever	Bacterial endocarditis; aortic root disease	Floppy valve; coronary artery disease	Congenital

*Untreated disease

Reprinted with permission from Huether, S., & McChance, K. (2000). Understanding pathophysiology (2nd ed.). St. Louis, MO: C. V. Mosby Co.

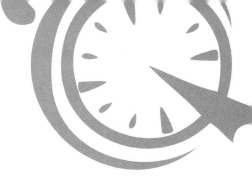

An **aneurysm** is a localized dilation of a blood vessel or cardiac chamber wall because of congenital or acquired weakness of the muscle. Because of the constant pressure it sustains, the aorta is particularly susceptible. The abdominal aorta is involved most of the time and the remaining incidence is attributable to the thoracic aorta. Peripheral arteries are less often affected. A popliteal artery aneurysm is third in order of frequency. Ventricular aneurysms may occur in the heart, and cerebral aneurysms occur in the brain. Aneurysms are potentially life threatening because rupture and hemorrhage or thromboembolism may occur.

Chronic arterial occlusive disease is a slow progressive disorder in which partial or total arterial occlusion, predominantly in the lower extremities, deprives the extremities of oxygen and nutrients. The primary cause is atherosclerosis. Varicose veins or varicosities are distended, tortuous, palpable superficial veins of the lower extremity. Veins contain valves that prevent backflow and pooling of blood. Primary varicosities originate in the superficial saphenous veins that are dilated with or without incompetent valves. Chronic venous insufficiency is inadequate venous return over time.

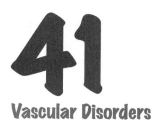

41

Vascular Disorders

TERMS
- [ ] **aneurysm**
- [ ] **dissecting aneurysm**
- [ ] **exsanguinations**
- [ ] **fusiform aneurysm**
- [ ] **saccular aneurysm**
- [ ] **true aneurysms**

Figure 41-1 Comparison of arterial and venous problems: clinical manifestations.

Chronic Arterial Insufficiency

- Intermittent claudication
- Calf pain with popliteal artery occlusion
- Hip pain with aortoiliac artery occlusion
- Chest pain in advanced cases
- Diminished, absent, or asymmetrical pulses
- Bruits
- Skin is shiny, thin, fragile, and taut
- Loss of hair
- Cool temperature
- Trophic nail changes
- Pale, blanched appearance when leg is elevated
- Dependent rubor
- Minimum edema

Acute Arterial Occlusion

- Sudden appearance of:
  Pain
  Pallor
  Pulselessness
  Paresthesia
  Poikilothermy
  Paralysis

Chronic Venous Insufficiency

- Dull discomfort worsened by standing
- Progressive edema
- Thin, shiny, atrophic skin
- Cyanotic
- Brownish pigmentation
- Eczema, weeping dermatitis
- Thick, fibrous subcutaneous tissues
- Pain with ulceration
- Varicosities
- Recurrent ulceration

Superficial Thrombophlebitis

- History of trauma or intravenous line
- Dull pain
- No significant swelling
- Induration, redness, tenderness, and warmth

Figure 41-1 *Continued.*

Deep Vein Thrombosis

- Pain in calf or thigh, though sometimes there is no pain
- History of recent surgery, inactivity, oral contraceptives, neoplasis, congestive heart failure
- Edema, tenderness, or vein
- Slight fever, tachycardia
- Local warmth, redness
- <20% have positive Homans' sign

 Aneurysms are potentially life threatening because rupture and hemorrhage or thromboembolism may occur.

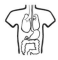

ANEURYSM

There are two major classifications of aneurysm: *true aneurysms* and *false aneurysms* or *pseudoaneurysms.* **True aneurysms** occur as a result of atrophy of the medial layer of the artery. The wall dilates but at least one wall of the artery remains intact. True aneurysms are further subdivided based on shape into a **saccular aneurysm,** a bulge with a narrow neck or spherical in shape connecting it to one side of the artery, and **a fusiform aneurysm,** circumferential and relatively uniformly shaped. Saccular aneurysms are associated with syphilis or congenital malformations. A false aneurysm involves the dissection of all the layers of the arterial wall and forms as a result of trauma, infection, or disruption of a suture line. This causes an extravascular hematoma or tamponade. Aortic dissection, sometimes referred to as **dissecting aneurysm,** occurs when a tear in the inner layer of an arterial wall allows blood to collect between layers of the wall. It is an acute, life-threatening condition requiring emergency surgery and has a high mortality rate.

Risk factors include congenital weakness of the arterial wall, atherosclerosis, hypertension, dyslipidemia, diabetes, smoking, advanced age, trauma, and infection. Syphilis, once a major cause, and other infections can also be factors. Men have a higher incidence than women, and aneurysm often occur in the seventh or eighth decade of life. There is often a genetic tendency in the development of abdominal aneurysms. Popliteal aneurysms occur almost exclusively in males. Myocardial infarction is the cause of ventricular aneurysms.

> Risk factors include congenital weakness of the arterial wall, atherosclerosis, hypertension, dyslipidemia, diabetes, smoking, advanced age, trauma, and infection.

Pathophysiology

Atherosclerosis is the cause of most degenerative arterial disease due to the deposits of plaque and the deposit of lipids, fibrin, and debris that erode the wall of the vessel. This causes degenerative changes that lead to loss of elasticity, weakness, and dilation. Smoking, hypertension, high serum lipids, and insulin resistance, all of which damage the arterial walls, can initiate plaque formation. High pressure within the vessel contributes to the weakness, dilation, and risk of rupture. With turbulent blood flow, thromboembolism may occur. The dilation of a vessel may compress surrounding structures and cause inflammation. Aneurysms can impede blood flow distally. Growth of aneurysms is unpredictable, but the larger the size, the greater the risk of rupture. An aneurysm is considered present when the diameter of the aorta is greater than 4 cm.

Rupture of an abdominal aortic aneurysm into the peritoneal cavity causes death from **exsanguination** in minutes if untreated. Retroperitoneal bleeding can produce localized tamponade, allowing more time for intervention. Cerebral aneurysms can cause focal neurological deficits due to compression of tissue or ischemia. Bleeding may occur into the subarachnoid space. Aneurysms may leak slowly rather than rupture.

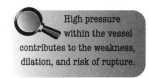

High pressure within the vessel contributes to the weakness, dilation, and risk of rupture.

Manifestations

Aneurysms are commonly asymptomatic until they rupture and cause symptoms. There may be an incidental finding during routine physical examination or x-ray, or they may also be diagnosed on computed tomography, magnetic resonance imaging, or echocardiograms.

Treatment

The goal of treatment is to prevent rupture. Surgical intervention is the only effective treatment for aneurysms and is performed any time in a

Table 41-1 Manifestations of Aneurysms

Abdominal
  May be a palpable pulsatile abdominal mass
  Vague abdominal symptoms or pain
  Pressure from enlarging aneurysm on surrounding organs
  Ileus or intestinal obstruction due to lack of blood supply to the intestines
  May be asymptomatic until they rupture
Thoracic
  Usually asymptomatic
  Generally detected on chest x-ray
  Deep back pain due to expansion of aneurysm with impending rupture
  Dyspnea or cough due to compression of respiratory structures
  Hoarseness due to recurrent laryngeal nerve compression

symptomatic individual or when the diameter is more than 5 cm in an asymptomatic individual. Blood pressure needs to be monitored and controlled. With rupture, immediate surgery is required.

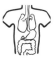

CHRONIC ARTERIAL OCCLUSIVE DISEASE

Chronic arterial occlusive disease usually occurs in the sixth through eighth decade of life but can occur at an earlier age in diabetics and is a factor in the high incidence of nontraumatic amputation in this population. It occurs more frequently in males and has a familial tendency. The most important risk factors are smoking, hypertension, diabetes, and dyslipidemia. Other risk factors include obesity and sedentary lifestyle.

Pathophysiology

Atherosclerotic plaque leads to thickening of the intima and media of arterial walls, impinging on the lumen. Primarily larger arteries and bifurcations are affected; thus, involvement is usually segmental, with normal areas between obstructed areas. The arteries most commonly affected are the aortoiliac, femoral, popliteal, tibial, and peroneal. The diminished perfusion leads to progressive oxygen deprivation or ischemia of the tissues. The byproducts of anaerobic metabolism or lactic acid stimulate pain receptors. This mostly occurs in the larger muscles such as the thighs, calves, or buttocks during exercise when an oxygen debt is incurred. With cessation of exercise and clearing of metabolic products, the pain subsides. Later, pain at rest occurs with more severe ischemia.

Ischemia leads to atrophy of tissues and poor healing capacity, infection, and tissue necrosis. Ischemic ulcers, gangrene, and amputation are the most significant complications.

Manifestations

See p. 340 for clinical manifestations.

Treatment

Treatment goals are to slow the progression of disease, improve perfusion, and prevent trauma. Reperfusion efforts may include percutaneous transluminal angioplasty, stenting, arthrectomy, arterial bypass surgery often with patch graft angioplasty, endarterectomy (rarely), and use of antiplatelet medications.

VARICOSE VEINS AND CHRONIC VENOUS INSUFFICIENCY

Varicose veins have a genetic predisposition and can also occur as a result of pregnancy, in persons who are obese, or in persons who stand for extended periods of time. Secondary varicosities are acquired or congenital and can result from any condition in which there has been a prolonged increase in venous pressure, such as a previous deep vein thrombosis or obstruction from tumors. It may also result in venous distention, pooling of blood, and valvular incompetence.

Chronic venous insufficiency generally develops secondary to deep vein thrombosis or superficial venous insufficiency. The increased venous dilation and pressure lead to changes in the skin and subcutaneous tissues.

Pathophysiology

Increased venous pressure and pooling of blood cause the veins to enlarge, stretching the valves that normally prevent the backflow of blood. The valves become incompetent, blood flow is reversed, and venous pressure and distention are further increased. There is an increase in capillary hydrostatic pressure, causing fluid and pigment to leak out with discoloration resulting in edema. Stasis pigmentation, subcutaneous induration, dermatitis, and superficial thrombophlebitis can occur. The increased tissue pressure from edema can cause circulation to become so sluggish that metabolic demands of cells for oxygen and nutrients are not met. This can lead to cell death and venous stasis ulcers.

Manifestations

The main complaint of persons with varicose veins is mainly cosmetic. Other signs and symptoms include aching in the affected extremity and/or edema, which usually resolves with elevation. See above for clinical manifestations.

Treatment

Conservative treatment of venous incompetency includes rest with affected leg elevation, compression stockings, avoidance of prolonged standing, and exercise. With inadequate response to conservative treatment or recurrent thrombophlebitis, surgical intervention to remove the vein is indicated. Unsightly superficial varicosities may be treated with sclerotherapy, which involves injection of a sclerosing agent that produces fibrosis of the lumen of the vessel.

PART VII · QUESTIONS

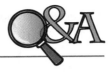

1. Which of the following heart valves is opened at the beginning of systole?
   a. The mitral valve and the aortic valve
   b. The aortic valve and the pulmonic valve
   c. The mitral valve and the tricuspid valve
   d. The aortic valve and the mitral valve

2. The community health nurse visits an elderly patient who tells her that he has been vomiting and has diarrhea. She is concerned about the possibility of his developing a decreased cardiac output and hypotension. Which of the following would be the earliest sign that his body is compensating for a diminishing cardiac output?
   a. The duration of systole is increasing.
   b. His feet are swelling.
   c. His heart rate is increasing.
   d. His urine output is decreasing.

3. In evaluating the patient's lipid profile, the nurse notes which of the following factors as *most* directly linked to atherosclerosis?
   a. High very-low-density lipoproteins (VLDL)/triglycerides (TG) and high high-density lipoproteins (HDL) cholesterol
   b. High low-density lipoprotein (LDL) cholesterol and low HDL cholesterol
   c. Low LDL cholesterol and high HDL cholesterol
   d. Low VLDL/TG and high LDL cholesterol

4. In the physical examination of an individual, which of the following factors would be evidence of atherosclerotic plaque?
   a. A bounding pulse
   b. An S_3 heart sound
   c. An arterial bruit
   d. A low blood pressure

5. Which of the following individuals is *less* likely to have classic angina pain?
    a. A young male
    b. An elderly male
    c. An alcoholic
    d. A diabetic

6. Which of the following would be indications that an individual has had a myocardial infarction?
    a. Decreased hemoglobin, elevation of white blood cells, and S-T segment elevation
    b. Decreased serum glucose, elevation of CK-MB enzymes, and S-T segment depression
    c. Elevation of serum troponin, elevation of blood sugar, and S-T segment elevation
    d. Elevation of CK-MB enzymes, decreased white blood cells, and S-T segment elevation

7. Which type of headache might be an early indication of hypertension?
    a. Progressively worsens as the day goes on
    b. Severe with visual disturbances
    c. Early morning headache that gets better as the day goes on
    d. Throbbing headache accompanied by nausea and vomiting

8. Which of the following is an indication of end-organ damage in hypertension?
    a. Positive Homans' sign
    b. Productive cough
    c. Abdominal bruits
    d. Ptosis (drooping) of the eyelid

9. Which of the following statements is *true* regarding the role of preload in congestive heart failure?
    a. Decreasing the preload is a compensatory mechanism for decreased cardiac output.
    b. Venous constriction diminishes the preload.
    c. An increase in the blood pressure causes an increase in the preload.
    d. An excessive preload can cause decompensation in heart failure.

10. Which of the following signs and symptoms indicates right-sided heart failure?
    a. Paroxysmal nocturnal dyspnea
    b. Crackles heard in the lungs
    c. Peripheral edema
    d. Frothy, blood-tinged sputum

11. What does the absolute refractory period refer to?
    a. The period in which the cardiac cells respond to the slightest stimulus
    b. The period in which the myocardial cells do not respond to any stimulus
    c. The period in which only the AV node responds to a stimulus
    d. The period when only a very strong stimulus results in depolarization

12. The patient's electrocardiogram shows a rate of 56 beats/min. What should the nurse do?
    a. Call the physician immediately.
    b. Further assess the patient.
    c. Administer oxygen via nasal prongs.
    d. Prepare atropine for administration.

13. An irregular cardiac rhythm characterized by absence of a P wave and an erratic undulating baseline is called what?
    a. Atrial fibrillation
    b. Atrial flutter
    c. Paroxysmal atrial tachycardia
    d. Premature atrial contraction

14. Which of the following is a characteristic of a second-degree atrial ventricular block type 1?
    a. No atrial impulses are conducted. The atria and ventricles contract separately.
    b. Every impulse is conducted, but conduction (P-R interval) is prolonged.
    c. Atrial impulses are dropped without antecedent prolongation of the P-R interval.
    d. AV conduction is gradually prolonged until an atrial impulse is nonconducted and a QRS complex is dropped.

15. Pericardial effusion that can occur in pericarditis has which of the following hemodynamic consequences?
   a. Decreased cardiac output and systemic venous congestion
   b. High blood pressure and pulmonary congestion
   c. Decreased cardiac output and pulmonary congestion
   d. Low blood pressure and pulmonary hypertension

16. Which type of valvular heart disease causes obstruction of the systolic ejection of blood from the left ventricle into the aorta?
   a. Mitral stenosis
   b. Mitral regurgitation
   c. Aortic stenosis
   d. Aortic regurgitation

17. A 19-year-old athlete went out for his first day of football practice. He experienced sudden cardiac death. He had no prior symptoms of cardiac disease. The cause of death was determined to be cardiomyopathy. Which form of cardiomyopathy was it most likely to be?
   a. Dilated cardiomyopathy
   b. Hypertrophic cardiomyopathy
   c. Restrictive cardiomyopathy
   d. Dystrophic cardiomyopathy

18. Which of the following is a *correct* statement regarding dilated cardiomyopathy?
   a. It is the least common form of cardiomyopathy.
   b. The ventricular myocardium is hypertrophied.
   c. The manifestations are like congestive heart failure.
   d. It is a form of diastolic dysfunction.

19. Which of the following is a manifestation of chronic venous insufficiency?
   a. Dry, necrotic ulcers in the feet
   b. Thick, deformed toenails
   c. Edema
   d. Hair loss

20. Which of the following may contribute to deep vein thrombosis?
   a. Dehydration, oral contraceptives, and high intake of calcium
   b. Immobility, diabetes, and digoxin
   c. Dehydration, immobility, and oral contraceptives
   d. Hypertension, immobility, and dehydration

21. An HDL of 35 is considered to be
   a. High
   b. Low
   c. Borderline high
   d. Borderline low

22. Coronary artery spasm is commonly known as
   a. Dressler's syndrome
   b. Frank-Starling law of the heart
   c. Prinzmetal's angina
   d. Cardiac syndrome

23. Pericarditis is often preceded by
   a. Flu-like symptoms
   b. Leukocytosis
   c. ECG changes
   d. pericardial effusion

24. Therapeutic life-style changes for hyperlipidemia include all the following *except*
   a. Dietary fat of 15%
   b. Weight loss
   c. Exercise
   d. Fiber of 10–25 g/day

25. All the following are considered risk factors for CAD *except*
   a. Premature menopause
   b. Gender
   c. High HDL
   d. Obesity

PART VII · ANSWERS

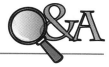

1. **The correct answer is b**. During the preceding diastolic period, the blood in the aorta and pulmonary artery has run off, so the pressure in these vessels drops. As the ventricles begin to contract at the beginning of systole, the pressure in the ventricles increases in the aorta and pulmonary artery, thus forcing the aortic and pulmonic valves open. Blood moves forward during systole into the aorta and pulmonary artery; therefore these two valves must be open.

2. **The correct answer is c**. Hypovolemia leads to a decrease in preload that then leads to a decrease in cardiac output. The falling output causes a fall in pressure that is sensed by osmoreceptors in the aortic arch and carotid bifurcation, which then causes activation of the cardioaccelerator center in the brainstem. The increased sympathetic outflow stimulates an increase in heart rate and contractility, thus increasing the cardiac output ($CO = R \times SV$). The sympathetic nervous system is the earliest compensatory mechanism to be activated.

3. **The correct answer is b**. The lipoprotein that has been identified in atherosclerotic plaque is LDL, the cholesterol-carrying lipoprotein. HDL is the lipoprotein that clears cholesterol from the blood.

4. **The correct answer is c**. The bulging of the arterial plaque into the lumen of the blood vessel creates turbulent blood flow, which results in bruits and thrills on physical examination. It may also cause a diminished pulse, and the blood pressure may rise because of the loss of distensibility of the artery.

5. **The correct answer is d**. Because of autonomic neuropathy, diabetics often have silent ischemia. Women also tend to not have classic angina symptoms but rather shoulder or abdominal discomfort rather then the typical substernal chest pain.

6. **The correct answer is c**. When infarcted myocardial cells die, they release intracellular substances into the blood that serve as a cardiac marker of MI. The stress response to an MI results in elevation of blood sugar and an elevation of the S-T segment, indicating infarction or transmural ischemia.

7. **The correct answer is c.** With hypertension, some cerebral edema develops at night when the individual is lying down. When the individual is upright during the day, venous drainage from the head decreases the edema and the headache improves. Severe headache with visual disturbances may occur with more severe levels of blood pressure.

8. **The correct answer is c.** Hypertension damages blood vessels, especially at bifurcations, thus initiating atherosclerotic plaque development. The turbulent blood flow created by the irregularity of the arterial walls causes bruits in the renal, aorta, and iliac arteries. None of the other choices indicates end-organ damage.

9. **The correct answer is d.** An increase in preload improves myocardial contractility and cardiac output to a point because an increase in venous return/blood volume in the ventricle causes increased tension in the myocardial fibers. If the preload is excessive, however, the actin and myosin if the myocardial fibers are spread too far apart and the strength of contraction is diminished.

10. **The correct answer is c.** When the right side of the heart does not adequately pump blood forward into the lungs, it backs up into the systemic venous circulation and leaks into the tissues as edema.

11. **The correct answer is b.** During depolarization and most of repolarization, the membrane potential has not been reestablished, so no stimulus causes another depolarization. During the later part of repolarization, membrane potential has been reestablished enough to enable another stimulus to cause depolarization. This is the relative refractory period.

12. **The correct answer is b.** A pulse rate of 56 constitutes bradycardia. Individuals who are sleeping or individuals who are physically fit normally have low pulse rates. With a low pulse rate the individual should be evaluated for indication of low cardiac output, such as altered mental status, poor peripheral perfusion, weakness, and low urine output.

13. **The correct answer is a.** In atrial fibrillation, totally disorganized electrical activity of the atrial myocardium results in no effective contraction, only fibrillation. The electrocardiogram reveals an erratic undulating baseline with no P wave present. Ectopic atrial foci produce between 400 and 700 impulses per minute. In atrial flutter, "saw-toothed" flutter waves are present, and in paroxysmal atrial tachycardia and premature atrial contraction P waves are present.

14. **The correct answer is d**. D describes a second-degree block type 1. Choice a refers to a third-degree block.
15. **The correct answer is a**. Pericardial effusion prevents adequate diastolic relaxation, thus impeding venous return and preventing adequate filling of the ventricles, so it diminishes cardiac output and causes systemic congestion.
16. **The correct answer is c**. The aortic valve is situated between the left ventricle and the aorta. Stenosis, which is a narrowing of the opening, impedes the flow of blood. Choice b refers to a first-degree block type 1, and choice c refers to a second-degree block type 2.
17. **The correct answer is b**. Hypertrophic cardiomyopathy often occurs in young athletic males. The first indication may be sudden death when exertion causes the hypertrophied septum to contract, blocking the aortic output.
18. **The correct answer is c**. In dilated cardiomyopathy, which is the most common form of cardiomyopathy, the thin left ventricular myocardium is unable to contract adequately during systole, resulting in the blood backing up into the lungs.
19. **The correct answer is c**. The increase in venous hydrostatic pressure, which develops when fluid accumulates in the veins, causes fluid to lead out into the tissues and causes edema. The other three choices refer to the manifestations of arterial insufficiency.
20. **The correct answer is c**. Dehydration increases the blood viscosity and immobility leads to stasis of blood. Certain oral contraceptives increase the coagulability of blood. Diabetes, hypertension, and high intake of calcium do not increase the risk of clotting.
21. **The correct answer is b**. HDL levels should be 40 or above.
22. **The correct answer is c**. Prinzmetal's angina is also referred to as variant angina due to its unpredictability.
23. **The correct answer is a**. Upper respiratory infections often serve as the primary site for pericarditis.
24. **The correct answer is a**. Saturated fat should be less than 7% of total calories per day.
25. **The correct answer is c**. High HDL is not considered to be a risk factor.

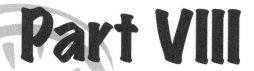

Part VIII

Gastrointestinal System

Vanessa Pomarico-Denino, MSN, APRN

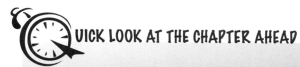

The gastrointestinal (GI) tract includes the mouth, pharynx, esophagus, stomach, and small and large intestines. These structures, together with the accessory organs of digestion—which include the salivary glands, the pancreas, and the biliary system—comprise the GI system. This system provides nutrients to the body by moving, storing, and absorbing nutrients; secreting digestive juices; and digesting food. It is also referred to as the alimentary canal.

42

Anatomy and Physiology of the Gastrointestinal System

TERMS
- ☐ chyme
- ☐ intestinal villi
- ☐ peristalsis

Figure 42-1 Diagnostic studies.

Diagnostic Studies

- Barium enema—Barium study of colon mucosa to identify structural abnormalities. It is able to show neoplasms, inflammatory bowel disease, fistulas, and diverticulitis.
- Barium swallow—Fluoroscopic examination of pharynx and esophagus, looking at filling patterns, mucosa, size, contour, and peristaltic motion.
- Brush cytology—Uses an endoscope, gastroscope, cystoscope, or bronchoscope to access the site, then a brush is used to gather cell samples for examination.
- Colonoscopy—Fiberoptic study providing visual access to the mucosa of the colon and terminal ileum to look for growths, inflammation, or bleeding and to biopsy and remove diseased areas.
- Enteroclysis—Barium study of the small bowel to determine the site of an obstruction, metastatic disease, extent of Crohn's disease, or small bowel obstruction. It is used in patients with persistent gastrointestinal (GI) bleeding but with normal upper GI and colonic studies.
- Esophageal acidity test ("Tuttle test")—A probe attached to a catheter is used to measure the pH of gastric and esophageal contents as an indicator of the integrity of the esophageal sphincter. It is often used in conjunction with esophageal manometry.
- Esophageal manometry—Uses a multilumen catheter to measure pressure along the esophagus while the patient is swallowing. It identifies abnormal peristalsis and spasms of the esophagus.
- Esophageal reflux study—A sensitive radionucleotide study to evaluate heartburn and regurgitation.
- Flat-plate x-ray—Screening film used to locate abnormalities of the GI or renal system. It can determine the size, shape, and location of vessels, structures, and gas patterns.
- GI bleeding scan—Labeled red blood cells are scanned during a period of active bleeding to find the bleeding site. Because the images are taken over a longer period of time, it is possible to locate sites that bleed either intermittently or persistently.
- Gastric acid analysis—After a substance is given to stimulate the parietal glands to secrete gastric acid, a Levin tube is inserted and specimens obtained to measure the rate and volume of gastric acid secretion. It is used to diagnose peptic ulcer disease, gastric carcinomas, gastritis, and pernicious anemia.
- Gastric emptying studies—Radionuclide study to evaluate gastric outlet obstruction due to inflammatory or neoplastic disease, dumping syndrome, or gastroparesis.
- Gastroscopy—A fiberoptic endoscope is inserted through the esophagus and the stomach up to the jejunum to visualize mucosal irregularities, varices, ulcers, perforations, or tears. It can be used to obtain brushings of gastric mucosa to identify the presence of *H. pylori*.
- Mesenteric angiography—Used with conscious sedation to localize and possibly perform therapeutic embolization of a bleeding site that does not respond to conservative therapy and cannot be visualized by endoscopy.
- Peroral pneumogram—After ingested barium has reached the cecum, air is passed into the rectum to allow for evaluation of the terminal ileum. This can be performed concurrently with an upper GI series.
- Sigmoidoscopy—A fiberoptic endoscope is inserted through the rectum to visualize the mucosa of the sigmoid colon. It can detect obstruction, carcinoma, inflammatory disease, and other irregularities.

Figure 42-1 *Continued.*

- Upper GI series—Fluoroscopic study used to evaluate the upper GI tract. Films are taken at timed intervals to observe barium as it passes through structures. Different contrast media are used depending on the diagnoses being considered. It can identify, for example, hiatal hernias, esophageal varices, carcinomas, GI perforations, and GI reflux.
- Cholescintigraphy (HIDA scan)—A radioactive dye is injected into an intravenous line to evaluate gallbladder and common bile duct function.

Laboratory Tests

- Ca 50 (carbohydrate antigen)—Tumor marker used to plot progression of many types of tumors, but it is especially useful for those of the GI tract.
- Carcinoembryonic antigen (CEA)—An antigen released during rapid proliferation of epithelial cells, particularly of the GI tract. Although not diagnostic, frequent measurement can help to guide management and evaluate success of treatment measures. Levels rise 3 months before clinical symptoms of recurrent colorectal cancer are present.
- Colorectal cancer allelotyping for chromosomes 17p and 18q—Blood and tissue samples are used to determine the presence of cellular *p53* and *DCC* genes located on chromosomes 17p and 18q, respectively. These genes are known to suppress the development of tumors in various locations. In the process of a normal cell becoming a colorectal cancer cell, predictable changes take place, including the suppression of these genes.
- Fecal fat—Stool samples are taken after ingestion of a diet with a predetermined amount of fat to measure the amount passed. It is used to diagnose conditions associated with poor fat absorption (i.e., pancreatic disorders, Crohn's disease, and hepatobiliary diseases).
- Fecal antigen assay—One test of choice to verify eradication of the *H. pylori* bacteria after treatment for the disease.
- *Helicobacter pylori*—Initially diagnosed by blood test or upper endoscopy. Breath test and stool samples obtained to determine cure.
- Ki-67 proliferation marker—Marker used to help determine prognosis and outcomes in patients with specific types of cancers, including colorectal cancer. Proliferation refers to the numbers of cells involved in a cycle and the time it takes to complete a cycle. Aggressive rapidly growing tumors have a poorer prognosis. This can also aid in managing inflammatory bowel conditions.
- Urea breath test/C-Urea—Breath samples are taken 10 to 30 minutes after ingestion of radiolabeled urea to stimulate *H. pylori* bacteria to release labeled carbon dioxide if it is present. It is noninvasive and one of the studies of choice to verify eradication of the disease after treatment.
- Vitamin B_{12} absorption test (Schilling test)—A 24-hour urine is collected after oral ingestion of Co-B_{12} and unlabeled intramuscular B_{12}; 5 days later the test is repeated with active intrinsic factor added to the oral dose. Intrinsic factor is secreted by the parietal cells in the stomach antrum, and normal ileal absorption is needed for adequate amounts of vitamin B_{12} to be absorbed into the body. Ileal disease or resection, Crohn's disease, pancreatitis, postgastrectomy, and cystic fibrosis are some conditions that affect this process.

(continued)

Figure 42-1 Continued.

Digestive Juices and Action

Source	Type	Action
Salivary glands	Bicarbonate	Moistens food
	Salivary lipase	Digests fat
Stomach	Hydrochloric acid	Digests protein
		Kills bacteria
	Pepsin	Digests protein
	Gastric lipase	Digests fat
	Intrinsic factor	Aids in absorption of vitamin B_{12} in the small intestine
	Mucus	Protects stomach lining
Liver	Bile acids	Dissolve fats
	Cholesterol	Excreted in bile
	Phospholipids	Aid in absorption of fats
	Immunoglobulins	Act as antibodies
Pancreas	Bicarbonate	Protects digestive enzymes
	Water	Neutralizes acid
	Amylase	Carries enzymes
	Lipases	Digests starch and glycogen
	Proteases	Digest fats
		Digest protein

In the mouth, food is broken down and moistened by saliva secreted from the submandibular, parotid, and sublingual salivary glands. Food then becomes a semisolid mass and is swallowed. Reflex muscular movements propel the food bolus into the pharynx, through the laryngopharynx, and into the esophagus, which is a muscular tube about 25 cm long. Strong muscular contractions and mucus secreted from epithelial cells in the lining move the bolus along. The upper esophageal sphincter prevents the food bolus from entering the trachea or posterior aspect of the pharynx. At the lower end of the esophagus near its junction with the stomach is the lower esophageal sphincter, which serves as a barrier between

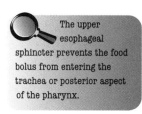

The upper esophageal sphincter prevents the food bolus from entering the trachea or posterior aspect of the pharynx.

the stomach and the esophagus. This site remains tonically constricted to prevent reflux of acidic gastric contents but relaxes during peristalsis, allowing passage of food into the stomach.

Once the bolus moves into the stomach, the reservoir that holds food, digestion continues. The stomach is divided into five anatomical areas: the cardia, which connects it to the esophagus; the fundus, the uppermost portion; the body, the largest section; the antrum, the lower section; and the pylorus, which connects the stomach to the duodenum. Here the pyloric sphincter, a muscular opening that controls gastric emptying, limits the reflux of bile from the small intestine back into the stomach. The gastric glands in the stomach contain specialized cells that act to either promote the digestive process or protect structures involved. These cells are chief cells, producing an inactivated form of the digestive enzyme pepsin, which converts proteins into proteoses and peptones; parietal cells, producing hydrochloric acid, an intrinsic factor needed for vitamin B_{12} absorption; mucous cells, producing an alkaline mucus that protects the stomach lining; and gastrin cells, which monitor pH. A 1-mm-thick layer of mucus protects the stomach lining from digestive juices.

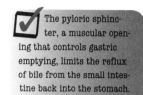

The pyloric sphincter, a muscular opening that controls gastric emptying, limits the reflux of bile from the small intestine back into the stomach.

The nutrient bolus passes from the stomach into the small intestine, which is 5 m long and divided into three sections: the duodenum, measuring 22 cm; the jejunum, measuring 2 m; and the ileum, comprising the remaining length. Circular folds line the inner walls and contain millions of finger-like projections, called **intestinal villi,** that have both digestive and absorption functions. Intestinal villi are themselves covered by their own finger-like projections called *microvilli.* The microvilli have a covering called the *brush border* containing digestive enzymes. This subdividing serves to expand the surface area of the 5 m long small intestine about 600 times. Intestinal glands found between the villi secrete fluid into the intestine for absorption by the villi. Goblet cells secrete mucus. Specialized cells found at the beginning of the duodenum secrete thicker mucus to protect that site from the gastric contents entering the small intestine. Peristaltic contractions propel the nutrient bolus through the small intestine toward the large intestine. The sphincter separating the two structures, referred to as the ileocecal valve, prevents contents in the large intestine from moving back into the small intestine.

The large intestine, which is about 1.5 m long, contains no villi. It is composed of five main sections: the cecum, to which the appendix is attached; the colon, which is subdivided into the ascending, transverse, and descending, which together form a frame around the small intestine; the sigmoid colon; the rectum; and the anus. The large intestine absorbs water and electrolytes and contains goblet cells, which produce mucus and endocrine cells.

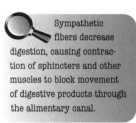

Gastrin is the major stimulus in gastric acid production and protects esophageal mucosa when acid levels are high. Cholecystokinin stimulates the gallbladder to secrete bile and the pancreas to secrete alkaline fluid, thereby decreasing gastric motility.

The GI tract's wall consists of four layers: mucosa, which is involved in absorption and secretion; submucosa, which contains loose connective tissue, blood vessels, nerves, and lymphatic tissue; muscular layer, which consists of circular and longitudinal fibers responsible for peristaltic movements; and serosa. The outer covering, called the *visceral peritoneum*, secretes a fluid that keeps the outer surface of the alimentary tube moist.

Sympathetic and parasympathetic fibers innervate the GI tract. Parasympathetic fibers increase digestive actions. Branches of the vagus nerve innervate the esophagus, stomach, pancreas, gallbladder, small intestine, and proximal large intestine. Nerves arising in the sacral region of the spinal cord innervate the distal large intestine. Sympathetic fibers decrease digestion, causing contraction of sphincters and other muscles to block movement of digestive products through the alimentary canal.

Sympathetic fibers decrease digestion, causing contraction of sphincters and other muscles to block movement of digestive products through the alimentary canal.

Gastrin and cholecystokinin are polypeptide hormones that are released in response to a food bolus action. Gastrin is the major stimulus in gastric acid production and protects esophageal mucosa when acid levels are high. It increases motility and constriction of the lower esophageal sphincter. Cholecystokinin stimulates the gallbladder to secrete bile and the pancreas to secrete alkaline fluid, thereby decreasing gastric motility and aiding in the absorption of fatty foods. Secretin, which is secreted by the mucosa of the duodenum in response to the entrance of gastric juices from the stomach, inhibits the GI tract. Gastric inhibitory peptide, secreted by the mucosa of the small intestine in response to the presence of fats and carbohydrates, slows stomach motility and emptying.

Peristalsis is the process of mixing food with digestive juices and moving it toward the anus. Peristalsis, or propulsion, is initiated by distension of the intestinal wall. New food arriving in the stomach stays close to the esophagus in the fundus. Older food moves to the walls of the stomach body, where constant pressure is placed on it. Moving next into the antrum, strong contractions mix the food, gastric secretions, and fluids into a thick, white substance called **chyme.** The liquefied and partially digested mixture moves into the small intestine, where the major part of absorption and digestion occur. Peristaltic waves, involving regular and irregularly spaced segments of contracting intestine, are intensified by the ingestion of food. They move chyme through the intestine and spread out the mucosa, facilitating the absorption of nutrients. Chyme passes through the ileocecal valve into the colon, where water and electrolytes are absorbed, and the fecal mass is stored, awaiting defecation. It takes about 3 to 5 hours for the chyme to pass from the pyloric sphincter to the ileocecal valve.

Segmental mixing movements in the out-pouchings of the colon wall expose the contents of the large intestine to mucosa for the absorption of water. About 500 mL of chyme enters the colon each day—400 mL of water

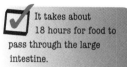
It takes about 18 hours for food to pass through the large intestine.

are absorbed and 100 mL of feces are left for elimination. It takes about 18 hours for food to pass through the large intestine.

Carbohydrate digestion begins in the mouth by action of salivary amylase and continues in the stomach and small intestine under the action of pancreatic amylase. The brush borders of the intestine secrete maltase, sucrase, and lactase to aid in the process. Digested carbohydrates are absorbed as glucose and galactose across the intestinal epithelium, as fructose absorbed by facilitated diffusion, and as monosaccharides via the bloodstream to the liver.

Lipids are acted on in the small intestine by the action of enzymes from the liver and pancreas. Without enzymes to emulsify lipids into a form that can be acted on by pancreatic lipase, fat absorption is decreased by about 25%. This seriously affects the absorption of fat-soluble vitamins A, D, E, and K.

Without enzymes to emulsify lipids into a form that can be acted on by pancreatic lipase, fat absorption is decreased by about 25%. This seriously affects the absorption of fat-soluble vitamins A, D, E, and K.

Protein digestion begins in the stomach by the action of pepsin and continues in the small intestine by the action of the pancreatic juices and the brush border–secreting peptidases. Digestion breaks protein down into different types of amino acids that are transported via different carrier systems into the bloodstream and to the liver.

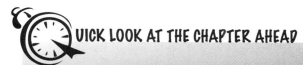
Gastritis is a documented inflammation of the gastric mucosa. It has many causes, can occur as either an acute or chronic problem, or can be related to a specific condition of which it is a symptom.

43

Gastritis

TERMS
☐ intrinsic factor
☐ metaplasia
☐ pernicious anemia
☐ petechiae
☐ urease

Figure 43-1 A hypothesis of how *H. pylori* produces chronic gastritis and peptic ulcer disease (PUD).

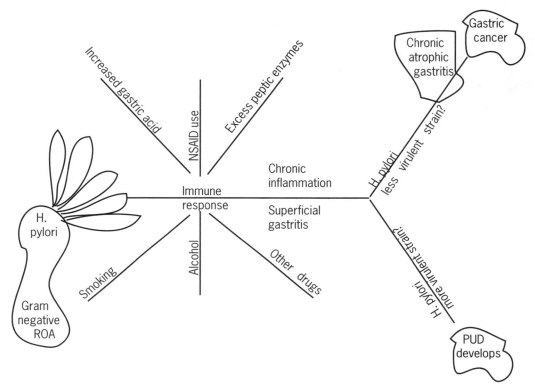

Schematic drawing that hypothesizes how *H. pylori* produce chronic gastritis and peptic ulcer disease (PUD). The organism invades the mucous layer of the gastric mucosa, causing an antiinflammatory response. Other factors can also cause an inflammatory response. Any one of these factors can enhance or maintain another, producing a chronic superficial gastritis. A more virulent strain of *H. pylori* goes on to cause PUD. A less virulent strain maintains the gastritis, which eventually causes mucosal atrophy and epithelial metaplasia—the precursor to gastric cancer.

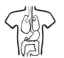

CHRONIC GASTRITIS

Pathophysiology

Chronic gastritis is defined as the presence of chronic mucosal inflammatory changes of the superficial and glandular portions of the gastric mucosa that, if left untreated, lead to the development of mucosal atrophy and epithelial **metaplasia.** Typical inflammatory changes include lymphocytic and plasma cell infiltrate in the lamina propria and inflammation of mucosal pits. There are also loss of glands and mucosal atrophy.

The two types of chronic gastritis are type A (fundal), which is autoimmune and associated with pernicious anemia, and type B (antral), which is more common and caused by *Helicobacter pylori.* Chronic gastritis can also be a combination of both types A and B with persistent presence of lymphocytes and plasma cell involvement. Type A has positive antibodies to parietal cells, and approximately 20% of those afflicted are 60 years of age or older. Other populations affected by type A are those with Addison's disease or vitiligo. Approximately half of those with type A test positive for thyroid antibodies.

Type B is more common. The increased inflammation is directly correlated with the level of causative organisms found. Pan-gastritis develops over a period of 15–20 years and increases with age. Most patients improve with treatment. Only about 15% of those infected with the organism actually develop gastritis. In some areas of the world it is almost endemic. For example, it has been found in almost 80% of Puerto Ricans; however, most remain asymptomatic all their lives.

The early phase of chronic gastritis is a superficial gastritis that is limited to the lamina propria. Atrophic gastritis is an inflammation that extends deeper into the mucosal layer with progressive destruction of cells. Gastric atrophy occurs as a result of the loss of glandular structures when the mucosa is thinned, as seen by endoscopy with visualization of the blood vessels.

The most common pathogen responsible for gastritis in Western countries is the gram-negative rod *H. pylori.* This organism can be transmitted by a number of routes. As it has been identified in dental plaque, an oral route is one mode thought to occur by kissing or sharing utensils, food, or drink. The gastric–oral route occurs via vomitus and the fecal–oral route via poor hand-washing techniques. It is believed to be transmitted in childhood and remains dormant until later in life when an unknown factor causes it to become active.

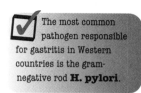

The most common pathogen responsible for gastritis in Western countries is the gram-negative rod **H. pylori.**

When activated, *H. pylori* begins as an acute infection, with nausea and/or vomiting and abdominal pain that appears to resolve in a few days. The organism does not disappear, however, but rather remains and produces an enzyme called **urease** that decomposes the byproduct of protein metabolism, urea, to produce ammonia. Ammonia neutralizes gastric acid, allowing the organism to thrive. It colonizes areas safely tucked beneath the gastric mucosa adjacent to the gastric epithelial cells, producing an inflammatory response. Some organisms burrow deeper into the gastric glands, causing the glands to atrophy. It is thought that chronic gastritis is a result of the ammonia and other byproducts of the organism damaging the mucosal surface. Most people infected with *H. pylori* are asymptomatic, but the infection is strongly associated with the development of peptic ulcer disease. Those infected are at risk for adenocarcinoma and low-grade B-cell gastric lymphoma due to the chronic T-cell stimulation caused by the organism that increases cytokinin production. Increased cytokinin promotes B-cell tumor formation, leading to lymphoma. With treatment of *H. pylori,* there is noted tumor regression.

> ✓ Most people infected with **H. pylori** are asymptomatic, but the infection is strongly associated with the development of peptic ulcer disease.

Pernicious anemia gastritis, also a form of type A chronic gastritis, is an autoimmune disorder of the stomach's fundic glands that results in an absence of free hydrochloric acid in the stomach and malabsorption of vitamin B_{12}. It is caused by an autoantibody response to gastric gland parietal cells, leading to destruction of the glands, mucosal atrophy, and loss of the acid and **intrinsic factor** they produce. Inflammation destroys the acid-secreting parietal cells and the zymogenic cells that produce intrinsic factor. The loss of intrinsic factor leads to the development of pernicious anemia. Without the acid-inhibiting gastric G cells, a severe hypergastrinemia develops, producing an intestinal metaplasia in which gastric epithelium is replaced by columnar and goblet cells of the intestinal variety. Metaplasia of this type of cell is known to give rise to the development of gastric carcinoma. Patients with pernicious anemia have a threefold increase in the incidence of adenocarcinoma and should have regular endoscopies.

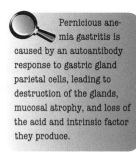

> 🔍 Pernicious anemia gastritis is caused by an autoantibody response to gastric gland parietal cells, leading to destruction of the glands, mucosal atrophy, and loss of the acid and intrinsic factor they produce.

Patients with pernicious anemia have a threefold increase in the incidence of adenocarcinoma and should have regular endoscopies.

Treatment is aimed at sequelae and not at level of inflammation. Antibiotics are used to treat *H. pylori* and are 85% effective. After treatment, antibody levels remain high for another 6 to 12 months despite eradication of the organism. Relapse is associated with reinfection with the organism. Those with pernicious anemia require B_{12} supplementation long term. (Treatment for pernicious anemia is discussed in Chapter 12.)

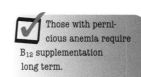
Those with pernicious anemia require B_{12} supplementation long term.

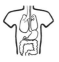

ACUTE GASTRITIS

Pathophysiology

Acute erosive gastritis is a transient secondary inflammation of the gastric mucosa that, although short-lived, can result in either a mild or severe bleeding state. It is most commonly caused by nonsteroidal anti-inflammatory drugs (NSAIDs) or aspirin or excessive ingestion of alcohol, but it is also seen in critically ill patients as part of a stress response to a bacterial infection. If left untreated, it can lead to chronic gastritis.

NSAIDs such as aspirin, ibuprofen, and naproxen are widely used to treat musculoskeletal and other chronic pain disorders. They act by suppressing the synthesis of prostaglandins. One source of prostaglandin production is from the gastric epithelial cells, which produce prostaglandins to protect the stomach mucosa from gastric acid. Without prostaglandins, the mucosa is susceptible to the effect of the gastric acid. The condition is often asymptomatic, with complaints, if any, being anorexia, nausea, vomiting, and epigastric pain. Vomiting of material resembling coffee grounds or the discovery of blood in a nasogastric tube aspirate is the most common initial manifestation of a problem. On endoscopy, superficial injury to the mucosa is found, including small hemorrhages, **petechiae,** and erosion. These lesions can vary in size and number and may be located at a single site or scattered throughout the stomach. The extent of the injury is not related to the amount of bleeding. Only the mucosa is affected; the submucosa and muscularis mucosae are not penetrated, as is the case with peptic ulcer disease. Endoscopy hemostasis techniques are not effective in treating the gastritis because the bleeding is usually diffuse.

NSAID-induced gastritis can be reduced by discontinuing the medication, reducing the dosing amount, and/or scheduling the lowest effective dose. Taking the medication with meals is helpful to some patients. Symptoms can be further controlled by using sucralfate or an H_2 receptor antagonist. Endoscopy should be performed if symptoms persist.

 Vomiting of material resembling coffee grounds or the discovery of blood in a nasogastric tube aspirate is the most common initial manifestation of a problem.

A stress-induced gastritis usually occurs within the first 18 hours of the onset of the illness episode. Critically ill patients who experience respiratory failure are put on mechanical ventilation; those who develop a coagulopathy are at high risk. Although not causing death, the development of gastritis is associated with a high mortality rate.

For stress-induced gastritis, treatment is aimed at prevention by administering sucralfate or H_2 receptor antagonist prophylaxis routinely to those patients who fall in the categories of those likely to suffer from stress-induced gastritis.

A stress-induced gastritis usually occurs within the first 18 hours of the onset of the illness episode.

Alcoholic gastritis accounts for 20% of all upper gastrointestinal bleeding in that population. Because alcohol is a gastric irritant that stimulates gastric acid secretion, the individual must completely stop drinking alcohol for any kind of recovery to be possible.

Other causes of gastritis are acute bacterial infections, viral infections with cytomegalovirus commonly seen in those with human immunodeficiency virus or after organ transplant, fungal infections with *Candida* seen in immunocompromised patients, and granulomatous gastritis caused by a variety of systemic diseases such as Crohn's disease, tuberculosis, and sarcoidosis. Acute bacterial infections that cause gastritis can be life threatening, especially in the elderly or immunocompromised. The causative organisms include streptococci, staphylococci, *Escherichia coli, Proteus,* and *Haemophilus,* and may lead to a gastrectomy.

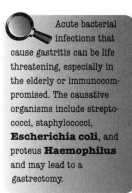
Acute bacterial infections that cause gastritis can be life threatening, especially in the elderly or immunocompromised. The causative organisms include streptococci, staphylococci, **Escherichia coli**, and proteus **Haemophilus** and may lead to a gastrectomy.

Figure 43-2 (a) Multiple, small (<1 cm), superficial erosions occur, which may be transient and asymptomatic or cause mild symptoms and superficial bleeding. (b) Mucosa atrophies and parietal and chief cells are lost. They are replaced by intestinal epithelium (intestinal metaplasia), a precursor to gastric cancers. (c) *H. pylori* bacteria located on the superficial layer of the gastric mucosa. If left untreated, this will progress to an acute and then chronic gastritis.

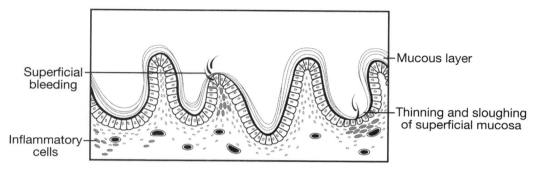

(a)

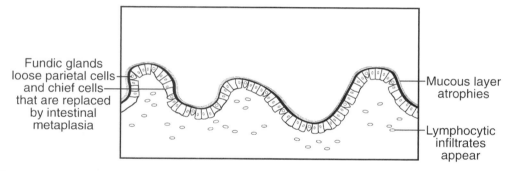

(b)

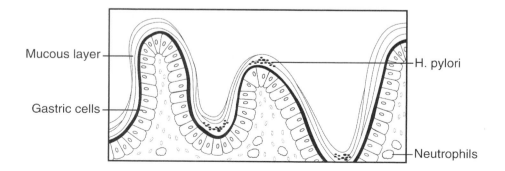

(c)

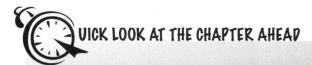

Despite a decreasing incidence since the 1950s, peptic ulcer disease (PUD) remains a serious health concern. In developing countries it is common among children, but in the United States it is rarely seen until after age 15. About 500,000 new cases are diagnosed each year in the United States; another 4 million individuals experience recurrence of the disease. Fifteen percent of the United States population is thought to be diagnosed with it at some point in their lives. PUD has a slightly higher frequency in males and peaks at age 50 and then again at about age 75.

Peptic Ulcer Disease

TERMS
- [ ] flagella
- [ ] hematemesis
- [ ] hematochezia

Figure 44-1 Factors affecting the mucosa.

Factors Affecting the Mucosa

Aggressive Factors

- Pepsin—Causes proteolytic and mucosal damage
- Bile—Mucosal damage with motility or abnormal gastric anatomy disorders
- Alcohol—Increases production of gastric acid
- Tobacco—Decreases production of bicarbonate, a protective factor
- Caffeine—Acts with histamine to stimulate the production of gastric acid
- *H. pylori*—Invades gastric mucosa, producing an inflammatory response and allowing erosion and ulceration to develop
- Nonsteroidal antiinflammatory drugs (NSAIDs)—Cause topical irritation and inhibit the production of prostaglandins

Protective Factors

- Mucus—Forms protective barrier over the epithelial lining
- Bicarbonate—Helps neutralize stomach acid
- Mucosal blood flow—Provides well-oxygenated environment for the gastric and duodenal mucosa
- Prostaglandins—Enhance mucosal blood flow, inhibit gastric acid secretion, inhibit histamine release, inhibit parietal cells from producing H^+, and are active in daily repair of gastric epithelium
- Genetics—Enhance or retard development of peptic ulcer disease (PUD); threefold increase in those with a first-degree relative with the disease

Medications Used in Treatment of PUD

Antacids

- Decrease symptoms, promote healing, reduce recurrences
- Capacity to neutralize stomach acid varies with product, amount taken, and individual response
- Available over the counter
- Liquids more effective than tablets

Types

Absorbable

- Rapidly and completely neutralize gastric acid
- Sodium and calcium bicarbonate strongest
- Are absorbed into blood and can upset acid–alkaline balance, producing alkalosis

Nonabsorbable

- Fewer side effects
- Combine with stomach acid and stay in stomach, relieving symptoms
- Can interfere with absorption of other drugs (i.e., digitoxin, iron)

(continued)

Figure 44-1 *Continued.*

Aluminum hydroxide

- Commonly used
- Can decrease blood phosphate levels
- Should not be taken by those on dialysis, those with kidney disease, or alcoholics

Magnesium hydroxide

- More effective than aluminum hydroxide
- Can cause diarrhea in large doses

Other Ulcer Drugs

Sucralfate

- Forms protective coat in base of ulcer
- Alternative to antacids
- Few side effects

H$_2$ antagonists

- Reduce acid and digestive enzymes in the stomach
- Once or twice daily dosing
- Available over the counter

Proton pump inhibitors

- Inhibit acid secretion
- Long lasting
- Promote greater healing in less time than H$_2$ antagonists

Antibiotics

- To treat *H. pylori*
- Combination therapy with bismuth subsalicylate, tetracycline, and metronidazole or amoxicillin
- Proton pump inhibitors (omeprazole) and an antibiotic also used

Misoprostol

- Used in prevention of gastric ulcers when NSAIDs must be used

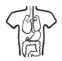

PATHOPHYSIOLOGY

Ulcers are a disruption in the gastric mucosa (stomach and/or duodenum) greater than 5 mm, causing chronic inflammation. Chronic ulcers can be found anywhere in the gastrointestinal tract and are named according to their location or etiology (gastric or stress ulcers). Peptic ulcer disease, however, refers to those occurring in the stomach or duodenum. An ulcer begins as a superficial erosion of the mucosa that is then subjected to the presence of pepsin and hydrochloric acid. The acid erodes the tissue as it attempts to heal itself and forms scar tissue at the base of what is now a developing ulcer. There is a decreased incidence of duodenal ulcers due to the eradication of *Helicobacter pylori.*

There are aggressive and defensive factors within the stomach and duodenum that balance each other to maintain a state of homeostasis. Aggressive forces are acid producers, whereas defensive forces are mucosal protectors. All people produce acid that is needed for digestion, but they can be separated into high, medium, or low acid producers. However, people who are high acid producers do not develop PUD at any greater rate than low acid producers. An imbalance between the aggressive and protective factors causes formation of an ulcer. Once considered a chronic disease, PUD is now thought to be caused by three major factors: *H. pylori,* nonsteroidal antiinflammatory drugs (NSAIDs), and Zollinger-Ellison syndrome. Other contributory risk factors include corticosteroid use, anticoagulants, cigarette smoking and alcohol abuse.

H. pylori

This microorganism is a small, curved, gram-negative rod with **flagella** found in 95% of patients with duodenal ulcers and in 75% with gastric ulcers. It is transmitted by an oral–oral or fecal–oral route. There are various strains of the organism, with some more virulent than others. Those acquiring a less virulent strain tend to develop gastritis rather than actual PUD. Infection with *H. pylori* does not always cause PUD to develop.

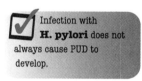

Infection with **H. pylori** does not always cause PUD to develop.

 H. pylori is transmitted by an oral–oral or fecal–oral route.

What triggers the organism's attack on the mucosal lining is not known. It gains access to the gastric mucosa through the epithelial cells protecting it. In the mucosa the bacteria release toxins, stimulating an inflammatory response that causes tissue injury and the release of antibodies that can be detected in the blood or stool. The organism mainly invades the gastric mucosa, but it is unclear how it causes duodenal ulcers to form. It is presumed that the duodenum has patches of gastric cells, which allows bacteria to colonize, or that excessive production of gastric acid in the stomach causes erosions, allowing the organism to take hold. Most people infected with *H. pylori* are asymptomatic, but their risk of developing gastric cancer is three to six times higher than noninfected people.

> In the mucosa the bacteria release toxins, stimulating an inflammatory response that causes tissue injury and the release of antibodies that can be detected in the blood or stool.

NSAIDs

This class of medications act by inhibiting the enzyme cyclooxygenase (COX), preventing the production of prostaglandins. COX has two forms, each with a different function. COX-1 helps maintain homeostasis of the gastric mucosa, whereas COX-2 is responsible for the inflammatory response from an injury stimulus. Both NSAIDs and aspirin inhibit the effects of COX-2. If COX-1 is inhibited, ulcers form because the protective mechanism cannot work. Individuals who routinely take NSAIDs produce less mucus and bicarbonate and have a 20% prevalence of gastric ulcers and a 5% prevalence of duodenal ulcers. They have three times the rate of serious complications of non-NSAID users. Risk is greatest during the first 3 months of use and in those who also smoke, drink alcohol, or take steroids. Newer COX-2 inhibitor NSAIDs, such as Celebrex or Bextra (Pharmacia, Peapack, NJ), are less likely to cause ulcers because they spare the gastric mucosa while still affecting prostaglandin synthesis. However, the U.S. Food and Drug Administration called for a mandatory revised labeling to include the increased risk of cardiovascular events and serious gastrointestinal bleeding with the use of COX-2 inhibitors.

Because most NSAIDs can be purchased over the counter, it is important to always inquire about their use when taking a health or medication history. The elderly are especially at risk, because with arthritic and other musculoskeletal conditions they tend to be NSAID users.

Zollinger-Ellison Syndrome (Gastrinomas)

This syndrome consists of hypersecretion of gastric acid, PUD, and non–beta-islet cell tumors of the pancreas. The gastrinomas, 50% to 75% of which are malignant with a 40% rate of metastasis, produce the hypersecretion. This syndrome accounts for about 1% of PUD, has a genetic predisposition, and is seen in 40- to 75-year-olds.

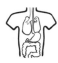

DUODENAL ULCERS

Most PUD occurs in the duodenum, with 95% located in the first portion of the duodenum and 90% located within 3 cm of the junction of the pyloric and duodenal mucosa. Lesions are usually 1–6 cm with sharp margins and rarely become cancerous. The mechanisms for development are most likely high gastric acid production and *H. pylori* infection. Risk factors include smoking, alcoholic cirrhosis, and chronic renal disease. There is also a familial tendency to develop them and no evidence that psychological factors play a role. Patients with duodenal ulcers experience sharp, burning, or gnawing epigastric pain in a fasting state that can awaken them from sleep. Eating or using antacids neutralizes the acid and relieves the pain.

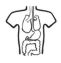

GASTRIC ULCERS

Although less common than duodenal ulcers, gastric ulcers have a higher mortality rate because of their increased association with a malignancy, unless they are NSAID-related or due to abuse of aspirin. They generally occur between the ages of 55 and 65. The ulcer is deep, penetrates beyond the mucosal layer, and tends to involve surrounding tissue. They are thought to be caused by a breakdown of mechanisms that normally protect the gastric mucosa coupled with changes in the output of gastric acid that increases exposure to bile salt. Bile salt decreases cell membrane potential, potentiating cell membrane disruption. Although acid production remains at normal or slightly below normal levels, gastric emptying is sluggish, allowing acid to bathe the area for a prolonged period of time, predisposing to ulcer development. Direct injury contributes to gastric ulcers as with the regurgitation of bile secondary to delayed gastric emptying or NSAID use.

Although *H. pylori* does attack the gastric mucosa, it is less likely to be involved here than in the duodenum. Smoking and steroid use also predispose to gastric ulcers. Pain from gastric ulcers is less severe than with duodenal ulcers and is relieved by food or antacids. Pain is increased when the stomach is empty due to gastric acid secretion. Gastric acid secretion after eating may produce increased pain in people with severe ulcers.

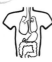

CLINICAL MANIFESTATIONS

Patients with PUD typically present with abdominal pain, most specifically epigastric pain, described as burning or aching, approximately 90 minutes after eating. It is relieved with over-the-counter antacids or H_2 antagonists. Pain associated with gastric ulcers is generally relieved with eating and causes more nausea and weight loss than with duodenal ulcers. The pain may awaken patients from sleep when gastric acid secretions are at their peak. Anemia, blood in stools, and **hematochezia** are not uncommon.

> Patients with PUD typically present with abdominal pain, most specifically epigastric pain, described as burning or aching, approximately 90 minutes after eating.

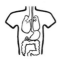

DIAGNOSIS

Hemoccult testing confirms the presence of occult blood in stool. Barium studies, although still used, may reveal anatomical deformities or associated conditions. Flexible endoscopy, an invasive test that requires mild anesthesia, allows visualization of the gastric mucosa and evaluation of dysplastic changes. It also allows biopsy of questionable tissue. Testing for *H. pylori* is routinely performed.

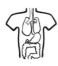

COMPLICATIONS

About 25% of those with PUD experience one of the following complications:

1. Hemorrhage—Most commonly found in those with *H. pylori* who are taking NSAIDs. The ulcer erodes through a blood vessel with the amount of bleeding dependent on the size of the involved vessel. Small vessels present with chronic slow bleeding as evidenced by dark tarry stools positive for occult blood, **hematemesis,** and anemia. Sudden onset of major bleeding, hypotension, and tachycardia occurs and carries a high mortality rate. Treating *H. pylori* significantly decreases a recurrence of hemorrhage.

2. Perforation—An ulcer can erode through the wall of the stomach or duodenum, allowing its contents to leak into the peritoneal cavity and causing peritonitis. This presents with acute onset of severe abdominal pain, rebound tenderness, fever, and hypotension.

3. Obstruction—As gastric ulcers heal, they produce scars that can be large enough to obstruct the gastric outlet, preventing food from passing through into the duodenum. This presents with a feeling of being bloated or full, weight loss, a palpable abdominal mass, and vomiting after eating.

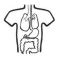

MANAGEMENT

Nonpharmacological management consists of stopping or at least reducing the use of aspirin and NSAIDs as well as smoking cessation. Pharmacotherapy consists of H_2 receptor antagonists to decrease acid production by up to 90% and cytoprotective agents such as sucralfate or alginic acid. Proton pump inhibitors, which are the most powerful inhibitors of acid secretion, are considered the agent of choice for control of symptoms and healing of inflammation. Antacids neutralize acid and should be a combination of aluminum and magnesium hydroxide to avoid side effects of constipation or diarrhea. Sodium bicarbonate antacids should be avoided in patients with hypertension or congestive heart failure. Magnesium-based antacids should not be used in those with chronic renal failure. Antibiotics treat *H. pylori* and consist of "triple therapy": bismuth, metronidazole, and amoxicillin or tetracycline. Other new combination therapy includes ranitidine and bismuth citrate. There is no evidence to support using milk or not eating spicy foods in the treatment of PUD.

Sodium bicarbonate antacids should be avoided in patients with hypertension or congestive heart failure. Magnesium-based antacids should not be used in those with chronic renal failure.

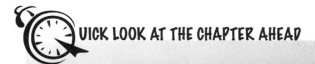

Irritable bowel syndrome (IBS) is a chronic functional gastrointestinal (GI) disorder characterized by periods of exacerbation often associated with stress. It is an alteration in bowel habits and abdominal pain without any structural abnormalities. In the United States it is more common in women, usually beginning in late adolescence or early adulthood. It is the most common GI disorder found in the primary care setting, accounting for 50% of all visits to gastroenterologists. Most patients are able to function with little or moderate difficulty, whereas only 5% are seriously debilitated by the disorder.

45

Irritable Bowel Syndrome

TERMS
- [ ] **constipation**
- [ ] **defecation**
- [ ] **diarrhea**
- [ ] **flatus**

Figure 45-1 Manning criteria.

Manning Criteria

A least 6 months of recurrent symptoms of the following:
- Abdominal pain or discomfort that is (at least one of the following):
    Relieved by defecation
    Associated with a change in stool frequency
    Associated with a change in stool consistency
                            and
- Two or more of the following, at least 2 days per week:
    Altered stool frequency (greater than three bowel movements a day or less than three movements
        a week
    Altered stool form (lumpy/hard or loose/watery)
    Altered stool passage (straining, urgency, or feeling of incomplete passage)
    Passage of mucus
    Bloating or feeling of abdominal distension

Differences Between Inflammatory Bowel Disease and Irritable Bowel Syndrome

	Inflammatory Bowel Disease		Irritable Bowel Syndrome
	Ulcerative colitis	Crohn's disease	
Epidemiology	Abrupt onset	Insidious onset	Late teens/early
	Peak ages 15 to 30/60	15 to 40	adulthood
	Caucasian>African	Female>Male	Female>Male
	American		
	Female>Male		
Pathology	Possible autoimmune	Possible autoimmune	Cause unknown
	infection may	infection may precipitate	Bowel has increased
	precipitate familial	genetic predisposition	response to stimuli
	tendency	Skipping ulcerations	and visceral
	Continuous, irregular	involving mucosal	hypersensitivity
	superficial	and submucosal	Altered perception
	inflammation of	layers along the	of CNS
	mucosal layer	entire GI tract;	
	of colon	50% involve small	
	and rectum	intestine/colon	
		Strictures/fistulas	
		common	

(continued)

Figure 45-1 *Continued.*

Signs and Symptoms

Abdominal pain	Intermittent, mild crampy tenderness	Crampy or steady Periumbilical or right lower quadrant	Sharp, burning; may be diffuse or left lower quadrant (LLQ)
Mass present	No	Common	No
Bleeding	Common	Occasionally	No
Diarrhea	Frequent watery stools with blood and mucous	Chronic, reccurent, may have some blood	Intermittent, predominant Symptom varies with individual
Perianal lesions	No	One third develop perianal abscesses or fistulas	No
Weight loss	With severe diarrhea	Common	No
Fever/malaise	During severe exacerbation	With exacerbation and abscess formation	No
Psychological	As result of longstanding disease	As result of longstanding disease	Exacerbation with stressful situations
Course/ prognosis	75% to 80% relapse after first attack; most have mild to moderate disease Routine colonoscopy with biopsy after having the disease for 7 to 8 years because of increase colon cancer risk	Recurrent, progressive Typically need surgery after 7 years to treat/repair fistulas or abscesses; shortened life span	Chronic, intermittent Rare functional limitations

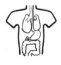

PATHOPHYSIOLOGY

IBS is a poorly understood chronic condition that causes abdominal pain relieved by **defecation.** It is associated with changes in bowel habits (either **constipation** or **diarrhea** predominate) and abdominal distension. The etiology of IBS is unknown and it cannot be diagnosed with laboratory, endoscopic, or radiological studies. The condition is diag-

Table 45-1 Rome III Criteria

Twelve weeks within 12 months (need not be consecutive) of abdominal pain or discomfort that has two of three features: 1. Relieved by defecation 2. Onset associated with changes in stool frequency 3. Onset associated with changes in stool form or appearance Symptoms that support diagnosis of IBS: • Abnormal stool frequency (>3/day or <3/week) • Abnormal stool form (lumpy and hard or watery and loose) • Abnormal stool passage (straining, urgency, feeling of incomplete evacuation) • Passage of mucus • Bloating or feeling of abdominal distention

nosed by excluding other conditions, most notably the inflammatory bowel disorders, and by the Rome III criteria (Table 45-1), a pattern of symptoms that must be present for 12 weeks within 12 months, but does not need to be consecutive.

Although there are no findings on examination, it is postulated that patients with IBS experience a heightened response to stimuli such as meals or stress with increased intestinal motility and prolonged contractions in discrete areas of the intestine. Patients also have low sensation and pain thresholds in the smooth muscle of the ileum and colorectum, causing them to respond to stimuli to which people without IBS do not respond.

 In the United States IBS is more common in women, usually beginning in late adolescence or early adulthood.

 It is postulated that patients with IBS experience a heightened response to stimuli such as meals or stress with increased intestinal motility and prolonged contractions in discrete areas of the intestine.

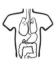

CLINICAL MANIFESTATIONS

Bowel movements are characterized by recurrent or persistent symptoms that include abdominal pain, urgency, **flatus,** and a feeling of incomplete evacuation. Abdominal pain varies in intensity and location and may be episodic, crampy, or a dull ache, all of which may interfere with a persons' day to day activities. Symptoms of IBS do not awaken them from sleep (a pertinent negative classically associated with functional bowel disorder) and may be exacerbated by eating or emotional stress. Symptoms are relieved with flatus or passage of stool. Pencil-thin hard stool may be present if spasms are occurring in the rectosigmoid region. No blood is found in the stool, but it may contain mucus. Diarrhea-predominant IBS consists of small volumes of loose stools, whereas constipation-predominant IBS has episodes of constipation interrupted by episodes of diarrhea. Pain may be in any quadrant of the abdomen, but its location is fairly consistent for an individual. The pain is sharp or burning and does not radiate. Weight loss does not occur.

Patients generally complain of much discomfort, but the severity of the symptoms experienced is not proportionate to the degree of motility and contraction actually occurring in the intestines. More recently, it was found that the syndrome has constipation variant and diarrhea variant subsets. Those with constipation variant IBS appear to have an abnormality in vagal (cholinergic) function. Those with diarrhea variant IBS may have a sympathetic adrenergic dysfunction.

Intolerance of selected foods is common, particularly gas-forming foods and those containing sorbitol, lactose, or gluten. Those with diarrhea variant IBS have difficulty with fatty foods and are generally intolerant of fast food. Women, on entering menopause, report that symptoms were first noted in relation to their menstrual cycle but had thought them to be a normal component and did not recognize them as a separate entity.

Although no direct effect of psychological stress has been documented, the correlation of symptoms with the occurrence of stressors has been noted. Because of the close connection of the central nervous system and the GI tract, it can be expected that those with significant psychological distress have some GI complaints. This, however, does not support a causal relationship between the two events.

Stressful life events—whether they are related to family, work, economic, or environmental factors—frequently precede an exacerbation of the disorder because stress alters normal sensory thresholds. Those with mild symptoms generally manage these events without outside help but report symptoms of IBS when questioned. Those with moderate symptoms have a higher incidence of anxiety and somatization disorders and often present with recurrent GI complaints that cannot be satisfactorily managed without attending to the associated emotional problems as well. The small percent severely impaired by IBS have a much higher incidence of major depression and panic attacks and are usually being treated for these disorders. The IBS symptoms may be thought to be a part of the emotional disorder but cannot be managed by treating the emotional disorder only. It has also been found that women with a history of physical or sexual abuse, when questioned, report a greater incidence of IBS than do women who have no such history.

Stressful life events—whether they are related to family, work, economic, or environmental factors—frequently precede an exacerbation of the disorder because stress alters normal sensory thresholds.

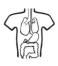

DIAGNOSIS AND MANAGEMENT

Diagnosis is based on clinical symptoms and exclusion of other bowel and psychogenic disorders. Treatment is aimed at management of symptoms using antidiarrheals, laxatives, and antispasmodics depending on the dominance of symptoms. Diet should provide adequate fluids and fiber while eliminating foods that cause symptoms. Antispasmodics are used to decrease intestinal spasm. Opiate-derived antidiarrheals are used for diarrhea-predominant IBS to decrease fecal transit. Antidepressants, selective serotonin reuptake inhibitors, and tricyclics are also used. Cognitive-behavioral therapy to identify triggers and stress reduction techniques also help. Relaxation training such as yoga or meditation can help individuals decrease smooth muscle tension and autonomic arousal. Some may benefit from short-term psychotherapy. Those more severely stressed may need long-term psychotherapy and medication.

Figure 45-2 Effect of stress on development of IBS.

Effect of Stress on Development of IBS

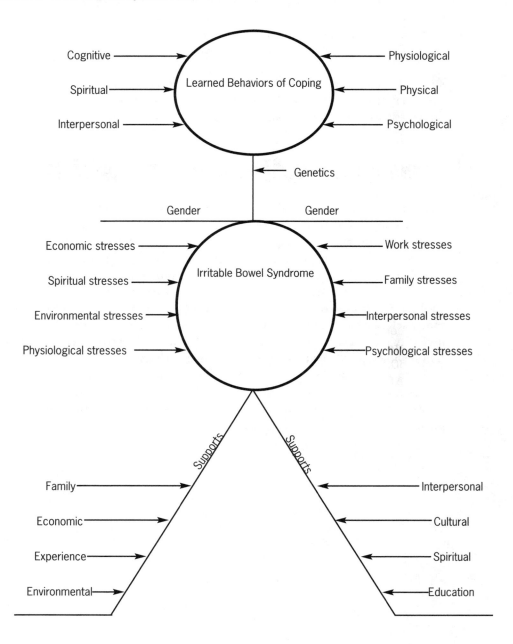

Inflammatory bowel disease (IBD) includes two disorders: ulcerative colitis (idiopathic proctocolitis) and Crohn's disease (regional enteritis). Both conditions are chronic and characterized by periods of exacerbation and remission. Although both diseases share many commonalities, each is distinctive in terms of its level, extent, and area of involvement. Exact etiology and pathogenesis are unknown, but a genetically associated autoimmune disorder activated by an infectious process is suspected. The changes produced by IBD result when immunocyte cells located in the mucosal layer are stimulated to release inflammatory mediators such as histamine, prostaglandins, leukotrienes, and cytokines. These act on the secretory and smooth muscle cells of the gastrointestinal tract, altering its functions and neuronal activity. Gastrointestinal salt and water transportation and the absorption and excretion of nutrients, salt, water, and electrolytes are affected. Onset of IBD occurs in late adolescence/young adulthood or around age 60. It occurs more commonly in whites than in African Americans or Asians, more commonly in Jewish than in non-Jewish persons, and more commonly in women than men. The incidence of ulcerative colitis is increased 40% among smokers. There is a familial component affecting approximately 10% of those with a first-degree relative who has IBD.

Ulcerative colitis is discussed here, and Crohn's disease is discussed in Chapter 47.

46

Inflammatory Bowel Disease: Part I

TERMS
- ☐ **crypt abscesses**
- ☐ **proctitis**
- ☐ **tenesmus**

Figure 46-1 Ulcerative colitis.

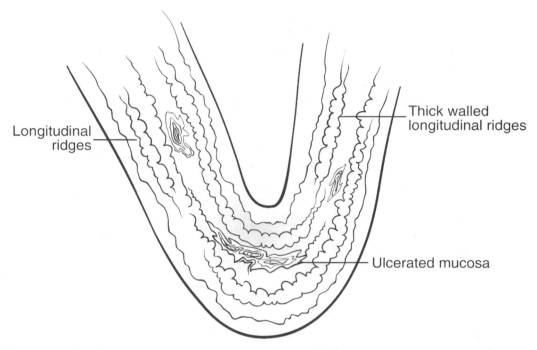

Longitudinal ridges

Thick walled longitudinal ridges

Ulcerated mucosa

Ulcerative colitis. This segment of colon shows long ridges of thickened wall separated by depressions of ulcerated mucosa.

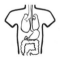

PATHOPHYSIOLOGY

Ulcerative colitis, the more common of the two inflammatory disorders, is a chronic, recurrent disease confined to the rectum and colon. The inflammatory action is confined to the mucosal layer of the gut and produces a progressive loss of epithelium with resulting surface erosion and ulceration. The characteristic pattern of ulceration

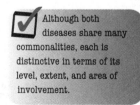

Although both diseases share many commonalities, each is distinctive in terms of its level, extent, and area of involvement.

lesions begins in the mucosal layer of the rectum and then extends proximally in a continuous fashion and can involve the entire colon. The disease is confined to the rectosigmoid region in most patients.

Less than 20% have involvement of the entire colon. Necrosis of epithelial tissue can result in abscess formation, known as **crypt abscesses,** with adjacent abscesses joining to form large areas of ulceration. Seventy-five percent of people have repeat attacks after an initial episode.

There is a familial component affecting approximately 10% of those with a first-degree relative who has IBD.

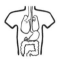

CLINICAL MANIFESTATIONS AND DIAGNOSIS

Onset may be acute with episodes of nocturnal or postprandial diarrhea and abdominal pain that generally increase in frequency and severity. Bloody diarrhea is the hallmark of the disease, with the amount varying according to the location and extent of the disease. Patients experience rectal discomfort, **tenesmus,** and urgency with active disease. Stool may be mucous- or blood-tinged and accompanied by **proctitis.** There may be spasm and stasis of stool, resulting in constipation with distal colon inflammation or fecal incontinence.

Bloody diarrhea is the hallmark of the disease, with the amount varying according to the location and extent of the disease.

Ulcerative colitis is characterized by remissions and exacerbations. Most patients have mild disease with few, if any, physical findings. Endoscopic findings are subtle, showing only mucosal edema, loss of normal vascular patterns, and erythema. Moderately ill people present with symptoms that may include slight weight loss, abdominal tenderness, and low grade fever. Severely ill patients experience weakness, dehydration, tachycardia, and significant abdominal tenderness. Endoscopic findings demonstrate mucosal granularity, friability, ulceration, bleeding, pseudopolyps, and mucopurulent exudate. Absent bowel sounds and abdominal distension suggest a perforation or megacolon.

Ulcerative colitis is characterized by remissions and exacerbations.

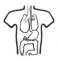

TREATMENT

Treatment depends on the extent of disease and symptoms. Medications include 5-acetylsalicylic acid compounds (mesalamine, olsalazine) or cyclosporine. Topical administration of 5-acetylsalicylic acid is available in suppository or enema form. Steroid therapy is sometimes used to decrease symptoms of severe disease. Surgical intervention with ileostomy is required in those who do not respond to conservative management. Mild or moderate symptoms may be controlled with avoidance of triggers such as caffeine, lactose products, or gas-producing foods. Fiber supplementation is used to provide bulk and form to stool.

Figure 46-2 Ulcerative colitis. Microscopic view of a pseudopolyp found with ulcerative colitis.

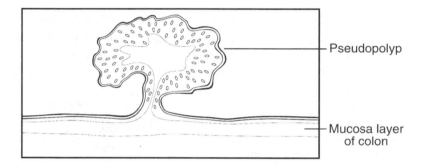

Figure 46-3 Ulcerative colitis. Pseudopolyps of the sigmoid colon.

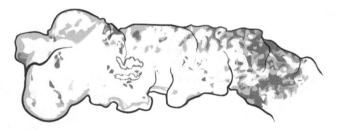

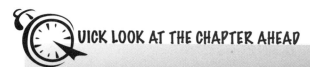
Crohn's disease, a disease that is characterized by periods of exacerbations and remissions, can involve any segment of the bowel. The etiology of this disease is largely unknown. Exacerbations are painful and sometimes require surgery or hospitalization. Management is aimed at providing symptomatic relief.

47

Inflammatory Bowel Disease: Part II

TERM
☐ **Crohn's disease**

Figure 47-1 Areas (shaded) frequently affected by Crohn's disease.

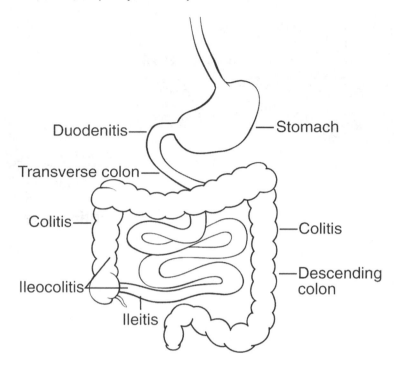

Duodenitis— ——Stomach

Transverse colon—

Colitis— —Colitis

—Descending colon

Ileocolitis—

Ileitis

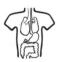

PATHOPHYSIOLOGY

Crohn's disease is an insidious, slow-developing, chronic, progressive disorder that involves the full thickness of the bowel wall. The pattern of ulceration is linear and penetrating, skipping over regions of normal tissue. Typically occurring in the distal colon, 30% of cases involve the small intestine alone and 40% the proximal ascending colon alone. Ulceration and inflammation can, however, involve any segment of the

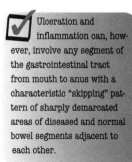

Ulceration and inflammation can, however, involve any segment of the gastrointestinal tract from mouth to anus with a characteristic "skipping" pattern of sharply demarcated areas of diseased and normal bowel segments adjacent to each other.

gastrointestinal tract from mouth to anus with a characteristic "skip-ping" pattern of sharply demarcated areas of diseased and normal bowel segments adjacent to each other.

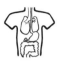

CLINICAL MANIFESTATIONS

Crohn's disease is a recurrent disease of the intestines that causes right lower quadrant or periumbilical pain, especially after eating. It is characterized by a colicky pain relieved with defecation. Patients present complaining of low-grade fever, abdominal pain, a number of liquid bowel movements per day, abdominal tenderness, malaise, weight loss, and fatigue. The diarrhea is nonbloody and intermittent. A palpable mass may be present in the lower abdomen because of inflamed and thickened loops of intestine. Recurrent bouts of diarrhea and progressive disease produce weight loss and malabsorption syndromes that include anemia from inadequate absorption of iron, folate, vitamin B_{12}, and other vitamin deficiencies.

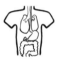

DIAGNOSIS

Stool cultures are obtained to rule out any bacterial or viral infection that may cause diarrhea. Barium studies determine the extent of disease or presence of fistulas. Sigmoidoscopy and colonoscopy provide direct visualization of affected tissues with the ability to biopsy questionable tissue. Computed tomography detects masses or abscesses. A plain frontal supine radiograph of the abdomen shows thickening and dilatation of the colon.

Endoscopy shows focal mucosal ulcers resembling canker sores, edema, and loss of normal mucosal texture. As the disease progresses, ulcers coalesce in a linear manner along the long axis of the bowel with relatively disease-free areas between the ulcerative streaks. Noncaseating granulomas and fissures, which develop into fistulas, are common. Transmural ulceration and inflammation can result in submucosal thickening and may involve the adjacent mesentery and lymph nodes. Fissure formation and submucosal thickening produce a characteristic "cobblestone" appearance. Strictures, abscess or fistula formation, perforation, adhesions, track formation, and small intestine obstruction are frequent complications. Bleeding from deep ulcerations may occur and can be insidious or massive.

Narrowing of the small bowel may occur as a result of inflammation and spasm, producing intestinal obstruction. Fistula formation can result in abscess formation with fever, chills, leukocytosis, and a tender abdominal mass. Fistulas can occur between the colon and small intestine or bladder or vagina with invasion of these structures by colonic bacteria. One-third of patients develop anal and/or perianal fistulas, whereas one-third develop systemic manifestations, including inflammatory disorders of the eye, skin, and mucous membranes of the mouth or renal disorders, especially nephrolithiasis from increased oxalate absorption associated with steatorrhea.

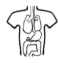

MANAGEMENT

When the cause of a disorder is unknown, management must be aimed at providing symptomatic relief. The goals of all management techniques are to control symptoms and to bring about a remission, which then is carefully protected. It is far easier to maintain remission than to achieve one.

Pharmacological therapy seeks to control diarrhea and discomfort with antidiarrheals and antispasmodics. The underlying problem of inflammation is treated with aminosalicylates, sulfasalazine, and mesalamine. 6-Mercaptopurine, cyclosporine, anti–tumor necrosis factor antibodies, and infliximab are also used in the treatment of moderate to severe Crohn's disease that is unresponsive to first-line therapies. Antibiotic therapy (metronidazole) is used for abscess formation and bacterial contamination of the gut. It takes a combination of therapeutics to achieve remission, and patients must be strongly cautioned to continue with therapy to prevent repeat flare-ups.

> It takes a combination of therapeutics to achieve remission, and patients must be strongly cautioned to continue with therapy to prevent repeat flare-ups.

Adequate nutritional status is critical for patients with inflammatory bowel disease. Because it is absorbed by the jejunum, an elemental diet may also effect remission in up to 90% of patients with colon or distal small bowel involvement. Once remission is achieved, a low residue diet with any possible trigger foods eliminated works best. Nutritional supplements like Ensure (Abbott Laboratories, Columbia, OH) or Sustacal (Bristol Myers, Evansville, IN) may be needed for healing and repair. Nutritional therapy for ulcerative colitis is less effective, with a low residue diet and multivitamin supplemental therapy working best.

Surgery is used for about 30% of patients with ulcerative colitis because of dysplasia, hemorrhage, strictures, perforation, or cancer. Surgical intervention is related to the site of involvement and duration of disease. The only procedures that cure ulcerative colitis are ileostomy and total proctocolectomy, which is generally unacceptable to most patients.

Lifestyle changes needed include education about and commitment to a therapeutic regimen that supports remission. Although there is no psychological basis for inflammatory bowel disease, the problems that chronicity brings may be helped with psychotherapy and/or support group involvement.

Figure 47-2 Mucosal and transmural lesions of Crohn's disease.

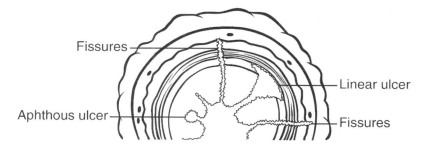

Figure 47-3 Crohn's disease of the ileum showing narrowing of the lumen, bowel wall thickening, serosal extension of mesenteric fat ("creeping fat"), and linear ulceration of the mucosal surface.

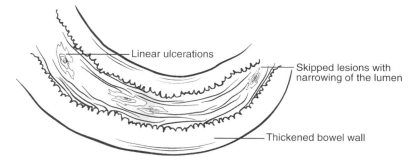

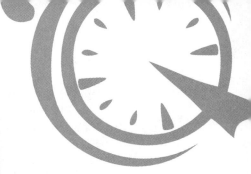

By age 80, more than 50% of the U.S. population has acquired the condition called **diverticulosis** in which individual outpouchings, or diverticula, present in the mucosa and submucosa of the muscular wall of the large intestine herniate through weak sites. Most cases are asymptomatic and are discovered incidental to colonoscopy or barium enema. It is believed to be caused by a diet low in fiber, resulting in chronic constipation. Because of dietary factors, it is a condition seldom found in developing countries, where a more fibrous diet is the norm. Poor bowel habits, such as ignoring the urge to defecate, contribute to the development of diverticular disease. Approximately 20% of all people with diverticulosis develop symptomatic disease.

48

Diverticulitis

TERMS
- [ ] **anastomosis**
- [ ] **diverticulitis**
- [ ] **diverticulosis**
- [ ] **obstipation**

Figure 48-1 Diverticula are small pouches of mucosa that bulge outward into the mesentery through weak spots in the muscle wall of the sigmoid colon. A cross-section of the colon and multiple diverticula are shown.

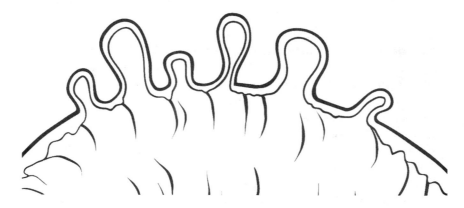

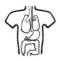

PATHOPHYSIOLOGY

The three types of diverticular disease are true, false, and pseudodiverticula. Most diverticula occur in the distal sigmoid colon in the presence of long-standing constipation. From the prolonged effort of moving small, hard stools along, the muscular layer becomes hypertrophied, rigid, thick, and fibrous. High intraluminal pressure is needed to propel stool through the colon, but this same pressure can force the mucosa through a preexisting area of weakness in the wall, producing a diverticula. Most individuals are asymptomatic and require no treatment except for a high fiber diet or fiber supplements such as bran. Some may complain of abdominal pain lasting hours to days and relieved by passing flatus or feces. Because these events are often accompanied by either diarrhea or constipation, a constellation of symptoms also found with the condition of irritable bowel, it is speculated that there may be a relationship between the two diseases.

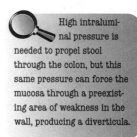

High intraluminal pressure is needed to propel stool through the colon, but this same pressure can force the mucosa through a preexisting area of weakness in the wall, producing a diverticula.

There are two common complications of diverticulosis: bleeding and diverticulitis. **Diverticulitis** is caused by retention of fecal matter within the diverticular sac. Blood vessels may be compromised or erode, causing perforation or bleeding. Bleeding of a diverticular sac occurs because of the proximity to branches of the colonic intramural arteries. Typically, it occurs in an older individual taking nonsteroidal antiinflammatory drugs. The person is asymptomatic and experiences an episode of acute bleeding with no warning. The individual complains of abdominal cramping followed by the passage of a large quantity of bright red or maroon blood mixed with clots. Depending on how much blood is passed, there may be symptoms of shock. Bleeding can persist for hours or days before a spontaneous remission occurs. Eighty percent of persons with diverticular bleeding have a single episode and require no further treatment. Persistent or recurrent bleeding requires colonoscopy, computed tomography, or magnetic resonance imaging studies to identify the site, followed by surgery to repair it.

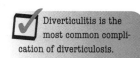

Diverticulitis is caused by retention of fecal matter within the diverticular sac. Blood vessels may be compromised or erode, causing perforation or bleeding.

Diverticulitis is the most common complication of diverticulosis. It develops when either an obstruction, usually fecal matter, or a perforation leads to inflammation. Intraabdominal infection can range from mild to severe, complete with abscess formation, development of sinus tracks, and/or peritonitis. More commonly, a microperforation occurs, resulting in a localized inflammation and infection with complaints of mild to moderate aching and abdominal pain, usually in the left lower quadrant.

Diverticulitis is the most common complication of diverticulosis.

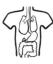

CLINICAL MANIFESTATIONS

Patients present with a low grade fever, left lower quadrant tenderness, constipation, nausea, vomiting, a palpable mass, and leukocytosis. **Obstipation,** abdominal distention, and peritonitis may also occur. Depending on the size of the perforation or the severity of inflammation, symptoms vary accordingly.

Patients present with a low grade fever, left lower quadrant tenderness, constipation, nausea, vomiting, a palpable mass, and leukocytosis.

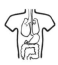

DIAGNOSIS AND MANAGEMENT

Computed tomography of the abdomen reveals a thickened sigmoid colon and presence of abscesses. A colonoscopy is not indicated in acute disease secondary to risk of perforation.

Treatment depends on the severity according to Hinchey staging (Table 48-1). Mild disease is treated conservatively with antibiotics and a low residue diet, which includes 15–30 g of fiber daily and avoidance of nuts, seeds, and popcorn. Antibiotic therapy includes quinolones and metronidazole for gram-negative coverage for 7–10 days. Ampicillin may be added if the patient is not responding. Severe cases require hospitalization, a nasogastric tube, intravenous IV fluids, and intravenous antibiotics.

If there is no rapid improvement on oral medications or for those with complicated disease, anastomosis or a temporary colostomy is performed until the infection and inflammation have cleared, at which time the colostomy is reversed and the colon reconnected. Local abdominal abscesses are treated with a percutaneous catheter for drainage and antibiotic therapy. Recurrent attacks occur in about one-third of patients and require elective surgery for removal of the affected site and anastomosis of the colon.

Table 48-1 Hinchey Staging

Stage I: nonoperative management of isolated or perforated diverticulitis with confined abscess
Stage II: perforated diverticulitis that has closed over abcess. Surgical resection for recurrent symptoms on distant abscesses
Stage III: perforated diverticulum with fecal peritonitis. Surgery with Hartman's procedure (primary anastomosis and proximal diversion)
Stage IV: perforation and communication with peritoneum causing fecal peritonitis

Figure 48-2 The protrusion of the mucosa and submucosa through the muscle wall.

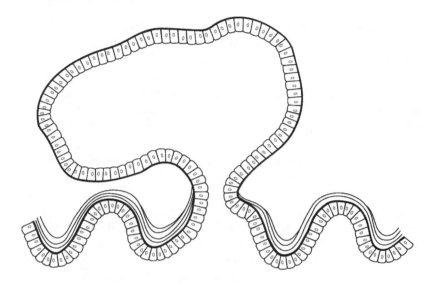

Figure 48-3 A view of the diverticulum from inside the colon itself.

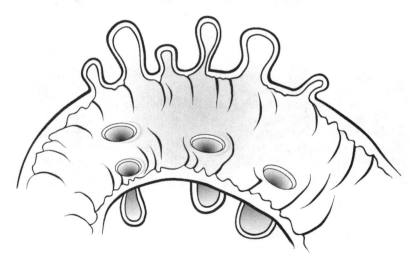

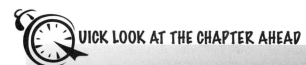

Paralytic ileus and intestinal obstruction are caused by tumors, adhesions, or can occur due to effects of certain drugs or anesthesia on the bowel. Onset of symptoms may be insidious.

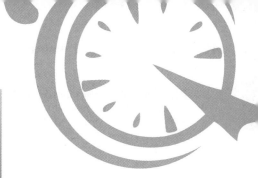

49

Intestinal Obstruction and Paralytic Ileus

TERMS
- [ ] **borborygmi**
- [ ] **intussusception**
- [ ] **volvulus**

401

Figure 49-1 Adhesions, or bands of connective tissue, sometimes form after abdominal surgery. Structures that have not yet twisted or looped are still under tension from pulling.

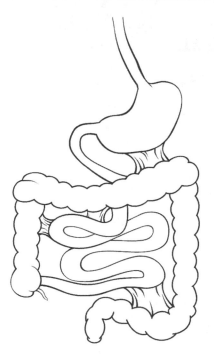

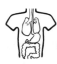

INTESTINAL OBSTRUCTION

A blockage in either the small or large intestine stops the movement of abdominal contents through the intestine. It is caused by a mechanical obstruction due to hernias (75%), **volvulus, intussusception,** tumors, or adhesions that impede bowel motility. The severity of symptoms is related to the site and degree of obstruction. Most obstructions block the intestinal lumen, resulting in distention and dehydration, which is the loss of large amounts of fluids.

Most obstructions block the intestinal lumen, resulting in distention and dehydration, which is the loss of large amounts of fluids.

Pathophysiology

Distention of the abdomen is caused by a buildup of gas and intestinal contents proximal to the area of blockage. When the patency of the lumen is compromised, buildup of saliva, gastric juices, and biliary and pancreatic secretions occur along with electrolytes and serum proteins. As the bowel attempts to accommodate increasing pressure from the excess of fluid, abdominal distention and pain occur. Necrosis then begins as blood flow to the intestine is impaired. Peritonitis develops when intestinal contents are released into the abdomen as a result of increased pressure on the lumen.

 As the bowel attempts to accommodate increasing pressure from the excess of fluid, abdominal distention and pain occur.

Adhesions, which are bands of connective tissue that form after abdominal surgery, are the most common cause of intestinal obstruction. They can pull, twist, loop, or compress a section of bowel, causing an obstruction. Hernias develop when a loop of bowel protrudes through a weak abdominal wall. Inguinal hernias are common in men; femoral and umbilical hernias occur in both sexes. The peritoneum along with a loop of bowel is pushed through the opening, preventing the passage of abdominal contents. Stasis and edema increase the size of the loop, leaving it trapped or incarcerated and the blood supply threatened or compromised. When drainage leads to infarction of the bowel loop, it is said to be strangulated.

A volvulus usually occurs in the sigmoid colon. The degree of twist determines how much, if any, abdominal content can pass along. Intussusception is the telescoping of one section of bowel into another segment, producing an obstruction. It may result from a tumor that is pulling the bowel wall it is attached to into the segment with it or because vigorous peristalsis drags it through. The latter is more common in children. Neoplasms of the colon are a rare cause of intestinal obstruction, but if left undetected they can grow to a size that partially or completely occludes the lumen, causing an obstruction.

Clinical Manifestations

Symptoms include acute onset of crampy, periumbilical pain as peristaltic waves try to force abdominal contents through the obstructed site. The pain is initially colicky in nature, lasting seconds to minutes, but eventually

Figure 49-2 Intussusception: the telescoping of one section of intestine into another structure, producing an obstruction.

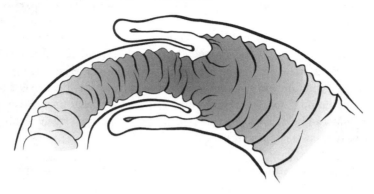

becomes constant and severe. **Borborygmi** are present early on but are absent as the condition progresses. Severe vomiting occurs within minutes of the onset of pain, causing dehydration and electrolyte imbalance.

Similar but less severe symptoms occur when the obstruction site is in the distal colon. Vomiting does not occur for several hours after the onset of pain and may be bilious or feculent. Abdominal distension is more pronounced. Patients may also have diarrhea if there is a partial obstruction. Hypovolemia occurs due to the shift in fluid from the intestines and vomiting. If rupture occurs, peritonitis may lead to sepsis.

 Vomiting does not occur for several hours after the onset of pain and may be bilious or feculent.

Diagnosis and Treatment

Diagnosis is based on clinical history and physical examination. A plain frontal supine radiograph of the abdomen detects presence of air. Computed tomography of the abdomen or abdominal ultrasound may confirm obstruction. Treatment depends on the cause of obstruction. Initial treatment in all cases is aimed at restoring fluid and electrolyte balance. Decompression of the bowel through the use of a nasogastric tube along with nasogastric suctioning relieves vomiting and abdominal distension. Encouragement of ambulation is particularly helpful in promoting return of peristalsis. Surgery is needed to relieve the obstruction.

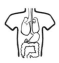

PARALYTIC ILEUS

This disorder is a neurogenic and peristaltic failure of the intestine. It is seen most commonly in patients hospitalized with acute pancreatitis, appendicitis, or gastroenteritis. It is also more likely to be seen in those patients with any of the following: abdominal surgery (due to anesthesia effects), peritoneal irritation, hemorrhage, intestinal ischemia, or severe medical illness. It is also likely to be seen in those taking medications that can affect intestinal activity, such as anticholinergics or opioids.

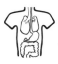

It is also more likely to be seen in those patients with any of the following: abdominal surgery (due to anesthesia effects), peritoneal irritation, hemorrhage, intestinal ischemia, or severe medical illness. It is also likely to be seen in those taking medications that can affect intestinal activity, such as anticholinergics or opioids.

PATHOPHYSIOLOGY

During the first 24 hours of a functional obstruction of the bowel, decreased blood flow from the lumen is followed by sodium and water passage into the lumen, causing distention and fluid loss. Intracellular pressure increases, causing decreased blood supply and occlusion. Impaired blood supply leads to bacterial infection, peritonitis, and necrosis. It can occur in either the small or large intestine.

Clinical Manifestations

Characteristic symptoms include intermittent, crampy, midabdominal pain that is moderate to severe progressing to abdominal distension and continuous abdominal pain accompanied by nausea and vomiting. High-pitched bowel sounds initially are absent as ileus progresses and are signs of peritoneal irritation. Pain becomes more localized, and failure to pass flatus occurs as the ileus worsens. Late signs include shock, tenderness, abdominal rigidity, and fever.

High-pitched bowel sounds initially are absent as ileus progresses.

Diagnosis and Treatment

Diagnosis includes white blood cells that reveal a left shift and increased serum amylase. A plain frontal supine radiograph of the abdomen and barium enema confirm ileus. Sigmoidoscopy or colonoscopy determine the site of obstruction but is contraindicated if perforation is suspected. Treatment focuses on the underlying problem. Patients are maintained on intravenous fluids, on a nothing-by-mouth diet, and have a nasogastric tube until bowel sounds return and resolution of symptoms has occurred as well as absence of gas on x-ray, at which time oral fluids can be resumed.

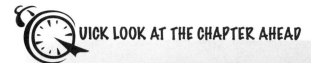

Gastroenteritis is an inflammation of the gastrointestinal system. It is a sudden onset on symptoms and can be caused by viral, bacterial or parasitic infections. Acute gastroenteritis is one of the most common illnesses afflicting people, second only to the common cold. It is the most common gastrointestinal disorder worldwide. An infectious illness common during childhood, it spreads rapidly through sites where people gather, such as day care centers, schools, nursing homes, and prisons. Diarrhea, which is often accompanied by vomiting, is the leading cause of death in young children in developing countries.

Diarrhea is defined as a change from normal bowel habits evidenced by increased frequency, amount, and water content of stools. It can be classified as acute or chronic and is attributable to a multitude of causes. Acute diarrhea is self-limiting to its cause, but chronic diarrhea is considered when symptoms last longer than 3–4 weeks.

50

Gastroenteritis: Part I

TERMS
- [ ] **endotoxins**
- [ ] **large-volume diarrhea**
- [ ] **motility diarrhea**
- [ ] **norwalk virus**
- [ ] **osmotic diarrhea**
- [ ] **rotaviruses**
- [ ] **secretory diarrhea**
- [ ] **small-volume diarrhea**

Table 50-1 Differentiating Types of Diarrhea

Type of	Characteristics	Incidence	Duration
Acute Gastroenteritis			
Viral			
Norwalk virus (most common in adults)	Most common type; small bowel secretory form; seen in family/school outbreaks especially during winter and summer; water-borne, person-to-person, and food-borne; prodrome of malaise then abrupt onset of diarrhea, nausea/vomiting, abdominal cramps, headache, low grade fever; resolves spontaneously; in adults is mild illness with diarrhea predominating; can be serious in children with vomiting predominant	Norwalk 12–60 hrs	Norwalk 12–72 hrs
Rotavirus (most common in children)		Rotavirus 1–3 days	Rotavirus 4–8 days
Bacterial			
Salmonella	From contaminated food or water; can passed by asymptomatic carrier	3–10 days	3–6 weeks
Shigella	Contaminated food and water	1–2 days	3–7 days
Camplyobacter jejuni	Most common of bacterial causes	1–3 days	1 week
Staphylococcus	No prodrome; no fever; severe N/V; severe diarrhea, abdominal cramps; moderately common	1–6 hours after ingesting contaminated foods, especially meats	12–36 hours
	All bacterial causes produce watery stools containing mucus, pus, and leukocytes; all occur after eating foods, especially meats, that also made others sick; and there is a high relapse rate		
Traveler's Diarrhea	Small bowel, secretory diarrhea caused by action of a toxin contaminating food or water; watery diarrhea with with stools; contains blood, pus and leukocytes	Found in persons who are in or have returned from a tropical environment	1–2 days

Table 50-1 *Continued.*

Type	Characteristics	Incidence	Duration
Chronic			
Inflammatory bowel	Bloody stools, abdominal pain, weight loss, fever, arthralgias. Extraintestinal symptoms involving skin, joints, liver and/or heart		
Irritable bowel	Motility disorder; alternating bouts of constipation and diarrhea. Loose stools after bout of abdominal pain which defecation relieves; early morning evacuation; tenesmus; rectal urgency; mucus on stool surface		
Giardiasis lamblia	Can have an acute or gradual onset with explosive diarrhea; abdominal discomfort; distention; watery, foul smelling stools; flatulence; anorexia, nausea; weight loss	Most common parasitic diarrheal infection in United States and overseas; endemic to Rocky Mountains; history of drinking water contaminated by human waste; hikers and campers are at high risk	Days–months
Chronic pseudo-membranous enterocolitis	Osmotic diarrhea caused by taking antibiotics, especially clindamycin or ampicillin, that kill normal bacteria present in the colon that metabolize carbohydrates that have not been absorbed; when not metabolized this material draws water to itself, producing a profuse, watery diarrhea and abdominal pain; allows a clostridium difficile superinfection to occur	3 days–6 weeks	3–10 days
Lactase deficiency	Onset is usually adulthood with bloating, abdominal cramps, and diarrhea after ingesting more than customary intake of milk or milk products, which raises the lactose load; can cause failure to thrive in in children	Seen in Asians, Africans, and Jews and can occur in infants	

> Acute diarrhea is self-limiting to its cause, but chronic diarrhea is considered when symptoms last longer than 3–4 weeks.

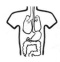

ACUTE GASTROENTERITIS

Pathophysiology

Gastroenteritis is an inflammation of the lining of the stomach and intestine accompanied by fever, nausea, vomiting, watery diarrhea, and abdominal cramping. It is usually caused by viruses or bacteria. Incubation is 12 to 72 hours, with a duration of 12 to 60 hours. Associated viruses are generally transmitted by the fecal–oral route in crowded areas with poor hygiene. The diarrhea and vomiting that accompany it are discussed in Chapter 51 also.

Rotaviruses are the most common cause of infectious diarrhea in children under age 3 years in whom it can be a serious, even life-threatening, illness. In adults it produces only mild symptoms or is completely asymptomatic. It has an incubation period of 1 to 3 days and a duration of 4 to 8 days. The tetravalent vaccine was introduced in 1998, but the Centers for Disease Control and Prevention advised against its use because of the increased incidence of intussusception. The vaccine was then removed from the market.

Enteric adenovirus, also transmitted by a fecal–oral route, is the second leading cause of diarrhea in children under age 3. **Norwalk virus,** which is highly infectious, is responsible for one-third of all viral gastroenteritis cases and affects all age groups. It is passed by a fecal–oral route via either contaminated water or food through infected food handlers or from shellfish, and it is the chief cause of outbreaks in adult communities, such as nursing homes and prisons, but it can also affect children, especially those attending camp. Norwalk virus can be transmitted by contact with infected vomitus or through aerosolization. It is the most common form of gastroenteritis found on cruise ships today.

> ✓ Norwalk virus can be transmitted by contact with infected vomitus or through aerosolization. It is the most common form of gastroenteritis found on cruise ships today.

Viruses act by invading and killing cells of the intestinal villi, disturbing the structural integrity of the region so that foods cannot be completely digested. Instead, food molecules act as osmotic agents, pulling large amounts of water, electrolytes, and intestinal fluids to themselves, which are passed along as watery diarrhea. Normally, the host's immune system quickly responds, and because the lifetime of mature intestinal cells is only about 3 to 5 days, the illness is usually self-limiting. Infected cells slough away and are replaced by new cells with anti-bodies to the invaders. If the individual, especially the young child, can be supported through the illness episode, he or she can emerge with a defense against the organism should it invade again with future exposure.

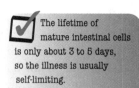

The lifetime of mature intestinal cells is only about 3 to 5 days, so the illness is usually self-limiting.

Bacterial causing acute gastroenteritis includes *Campylobacter jejuni*, which is found in unpasteurized milk, infected animals, contaminated meat, or humans infected with the bacteria. It can also be transmitted from cutting boards and countertops that have been contaminated by these products. A bacterial source is usually suspected when other individuals who have shared the same food or water source as the patient become ill at the same time with similar symptoms. Illness within 12 hours up to 5 days of ingestion is likely due to a bacterial source. The host's response depends on prior exposure to the organism, age, and nutritional and immune status.

> A bacterial source is usually suspected when other individuals who have shared the same food or water source as the patient become ill at the same time with similar symptoms.

Bacteria entering the body must overcome its normal defensive mechanisms. They must survive stomach acidity and normal bacteria in the gut; however, most do not. Some bacteria secrete **endotoxins** into food so that even if the organism dies its toxin is left behind to cause illness. An example of this is *Staphylococcus aureus* growing in unrefrigerated foods containing mayonnaise that are typically found at picnics. Surviving bacteria find their way into the gut by either attaching themselves to intestinal epithelium where they secrete their endotoxin or by invading intestinal mucosa, producing cellular inflammation and death. Endotoxins act on cells, enhancing fluid secretion and retarding fluid and electrolyte absorption from the gut.

Clinical Manifestations

Acute onset of fever, abdominal cramps, anorexia, watery diarrhea, and malaise occur in the early hours of infection. Symptoms peak after 12 to 60 hours, and the patient's symptoms progressively improve.

Diagnosis and Management

Diagnosis is based on clinical history and presentation. Stool cultures are obtained for white blood cells, ova, and parasite culture for specific bacteria. Treatment is aimed at prevention through careful hygiene and replacing fluids lost during the acute phase and immediately thereafter. Sips of clear liquids and avoidance of dairy products is recommended. Diet may be advanced as tolerated. In severe cases in very young or old patients, oral rehydration therapy with specially formulated fluids or intravenous therapy may be needed to reestablish fluid and electrolyte balance.

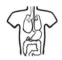

DIARRHEA

Diarrhea is defined as a change from normal bowel habits evidenced by increased frequency, amount, and water content of stools. It can be classified as acute or chronic and is attributable to a multitude of causes. Acute diarrhea is self-limiting to its cause, but diarrhea is considered chronic when symptoms last longer than 3–4 weeks.

Pathophysiology

Diarrhea has many causes, some inconvenient and some serious, but all are associated with an increase in the water content of the stools. This increase is caused by an increase in the amount of fluid secreted, a decrease in the amount of fluid absorbed, or an alteration in the motility of the bowel. Acute diarrhea is generally caused by viral or bacterial infections, medications, or food intolerance. Chronic diarrhea is attributable to inflammatory bowel diseases, malabsorption syndromes, thyroid or endocrine disorders, or from chemotherapy and radiation. The three types of diarrhea are osmotic, secretory, and motility.

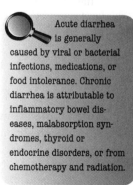

Acute diarrhea is generally caused by viral or bacterial infections, medications, or food intolerance. Chronic diarrhea is attributable to inflammatory bowel diseases, malabsorption syndromes, thyroid or endocrine disorders, or from chemotherapy and radiation.

An increase in the amount of fluid secreted (**secretory diarrhea**) occurs when increased amounts of fluids are transported out of epithelial cells. Caused by inflammation, an enterotoxin, or hormonal changes, secretory diarrhea continues even if the individual fasts. The amount of fluids absorbed is decreased when there is either an abnormality in the absorptive surface of the intestinal mucosa or when some unabsorbed material in the intestinal lumen acts as an osmotic force, drawing water to itself. Fasting improves this condition. When the motility of the bowel increases, intestinal contents have less contact time with the mucosal surface so that adequate fluids cannot be absorbed. This can occur as a result of a vagotomy or with hypergastrinemia.

Osmotic diarrhea is a result of increased stool weight and volume due to the osmotic effect of the intestine drawing excess water into itself. This produces **large-volume diarrhea**. **Motility diarrhea** occurs when the intestines have been surgically repaired or compromised or because of formation of fistulas. Gallbladder disease, biliary dyskinesia, and diabetes can also affect motility.

When the diarrhea originates in the small bowel, stools are large, loose, and provoked by eating either a meal or a specific food. It is often accompanied by pain in the right lower quadrant or periumbilical region. When it originates in the large bowel, usually the left or rectosigmoid colon, small volume diarrhea is passed frequently accompanied by crampy left lower quadrant pain and tenesmus.

Acute diarrhea is usually infectious in origin and accompanied by abdominal cramps, fever, chills, nausea, and vomiting. Chronic diarrhea is defined as the passage of more than 200 g of loose stool per day for more than 3 weeks. This is associated with some type of chronic condition with the diarrhea being symptomatic.

Diagnosis and Management

Diagnosis is based on clinical symptoms, physical examination, and history. Stool cultures to rule out infectious pathogens are recommended. Workup for inflammatory bowel diseases should be considered if symptoms are chronic and should include endoscopy and colonoscopy. Opium-based drugs such as diphenoxylate and loperamide decrease intestinal motility and stimulate absorption of fluid and electrolytes. Over-the-counter medications containing kaolin and pectin should be reserved for short-term treatment. Patients should be advised that products containing bismuth will turn stools a dark black color. Low fiber diets and increased fluids contribute to adding bulk to stool and help to decrease any risk of dehydration from diarrhea. The patient should be advised to seek medical therapy if symptoms do not resolve in 3–4 weeks. Chronic diarrhea requires diagnosis of the cause followed by corrective and supportive therapy.

 Patients should be advised that products containing bismuth will turn stools a dark black color.

 The patient should be advised to seek medical therapy if symptoms do not resolve in 3–4 weeks.

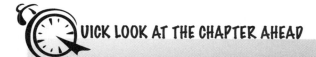

Nausea and vomiting are common problems with a variety of causes. Nausea is defined as an unpleasant sensation described as "feeling sick" or "queasy." It is frequently followed by **vomiting**, or emesis.

51

Gastroenteritis: Part II

TERMS
- ☐ **projectile vomiting**
- ☐ **vomiting**

Table 51-1 Differentiating Types of Vomiting

Type	Characteristics	Other Findings/Diagnostics
Gastroenteritis (vital or bacterial)	Most common cause in all age groups; acute onset; may be accompanied by diarrhea, mild fever, crampy abdominal pain, and muscle aches; may be associated with indigestion of contaminated food	Hyperactive bowel sounds; minimal abdominal tenderness on palpation
Gastritis	Acute or chronic nausea/vomiting (N/V) occurs after eating; can be induced by alcohol ingestion or drugs or be associated with ulcers that result from irritation, spasm, and edema of the pyloric muscle	
Pancreatitis	Repeated episodes of N/V, abdominal pain that radiates to the back; associated with excessive alcohol intake	Elevated serum amylase
Appendicitis	Anorexia, N/V early symptoms in most patients; pain precedes vomiting	Elevated leukocytes
Binge drinking	Excessive alcohol consumption; early morning N/V and dry heaves	
Esophogeal obstruction	Vomiting of undigested food, odorless, early AM or after meals	Endoscopy
Pyloric obstruction	In children: persistent projectile vomiting of large amounts of food, especially in infants <3 months; in adults: associated with tumor or scar formation from an ulcer	Palpable mass; weight loss
Lower bowel	Abdominal distension with no or very small amount of stool; green bile in vomitus; breath may have fecal odor	Decreased/absent bowel sounds
Labyrinthine disorders	N/V accompanied by vertigo, tinnitus, and motion sickness	Nystagmus
ICP	Sudden, forceful vomiting not accompanied by nausea; headache; symptoms get progressively worse over hours or days	Positive neurological findings; changes in mentation; motor function
Morning sickness	N/V occurring in early morning during first trimester of pregnancy that usually ends by the fourth month	Last menstrual period > 6 weeks ago Elevated human chorionic gonadotropin (HCG) level

Table 51-1 *Continued.*

Type	Characteristics	Other Findings/Diagnostics
Bulimia	Self-induced vomiting after binge eating; usually in young women with poor self-image and preoccupation with being thin; may be accompanied by laxative abuse	
Metabolic etiologies	Seventy-five percent of those with diabetic ketoacidosis Ninety percent of those with Addison's crisis	Check blood sugar levels
Drug induced	Associated with cancer treatment either drug (especially cisplatin) or radiation therapy, producing pever N/V caused by serotonin released from cells activating receptors an stimulating the vomiting center and chemoreceptor trigger zone; with opiate drug withdrawal, vomiting begins 36 hours after last dose, accompanied by sweats, chills, and restlessness; peaks at 72 hours	

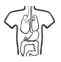

PATHOPHYSIOLOGY

Nausea precedes vomiting with hypersalivation and tachycardia. Abdominal muscles contract, creating intraabdominal pressure and allowing the lower esophageal sphincter to relax. Simultaneously, spasms occur in the stomach and duodenum, leading to retching.

Vomiting may be induced by stimulation of any of the following: afferent vagal or splanchnic fibers stimulated by biliary or gastrointestinal distension, peritoneal or mucosal irritation, or infection; the vestibular system affected by motion or infection; the higher central nervous system affected by sights, smells, or emotions; or the chemoreceptor trigger zone in the area of the medulla, which is affected by drugs, chemotherapeutic agents, uremia, toxins, acidosis, hypoxia, or radiation therapy.

Vomiting is a symptom. The cause of vomiting may be indicated by the type and pattern of vomiting (Table 51-1). Acute vomiting without significant abdominal pain is likely due to drugs, infectious gastroenteritis, or food poisoning. **Projectile vomiting** is not preceded by any symptoms and can be caused by metabolic or pathological disturbances.

Acute vomiting with abdominal pain is indicative of peritoneal irritation, intestinal obstruction, or pancreatic and/or biliary disease. Persistent vomiting may be due to pregnancy, gastric outlet syndrome, psychogenic causes, or systemic disorders. Vomiting immediately after eating is associated with bulimia. Vomiting undigested food within a few hours of eating may be caused by gastric outlet syndrome or gastroparesis. Consequences of vomiting include dehydration, electrolyte imbalance, metabolic acidosis, and aspiration.

 Projectile vomiting is not preceded by any symptoms and can be caused by metabolic or pathological disturbances.

 Consequences of vomiting include dehydration, electrolyte imbalance, metabolic acidosis, and aspiration.

MANAGEMENT

Acute vomiting is treated with rest and rehydration. Dehydration and electrolyte imbalances are treated accordingly. Persistent and psychogenic vomiting is managed by treating the underlying cause.

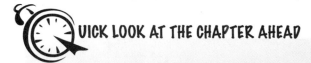

Esophageal tumors are almost always malignant, accounting for 6% of all gastrointestinal cancers and 1% of all new cancers, and their incidence is rising at an alarming rate. It is more common in persons over 60 years of age, and it is the seventh leading cause of death among men.

Gastric cancer, one of the most common cancers worldwide, is more prevalent in developing countries among lower socioeconomic groups in urban settings. Japan, China, South America, and Eastern Europe have a high incidence, whereas the United States and Canada have a low incidence, approximately 1–2% of all new cancer cases annually. Immigrants acquire the same risk as natives, pointing to environmental factors in its development. Cancers in the antrum and body have been declining, whereas those of the cardia and gastroesophageal junction are increasing at an alarming rate. Causes are thought to be chronic **Helicobacter pylori** infection, genetic predisposition, and diet, especially diets with foods high in nitrates (bacon or hot dogs) and smoked, salted, or pickled foods. Other considered causes for gastric cancer include smoking and alcohol abuse.

Adenocarcinoma, also called colorectal cancer, is the second leading cause of cancer death in the United States and the most common type of cancer of the large bowel. Since the promotion of early detection, 5-year survival rates have risen to 60% but are much lower for low income groups, especially African-American males.

52

Cancers of the Gastrointestinal Tract

TERMS
- [ ] atypia
- [ ] Barrett's esophagus
- [ ] dysphagia
- [ ] dysplasia

Figure 52-1 Carcinoma of the stomach.

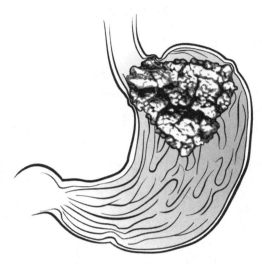

Carcinoma of the stomach arising from the gastric mucosa (see arrow) and extending into the esophagus. Risk factors include the following:

Dietary

- Smoked foods
- Pickled foods
- Nitrates (contained in preservatives of prepared meats and in some drinking water supplies)
- High salt intake

Nondietary

- Chronic gastritis with intestinal metaplasia due to either *H. pylori* or pernicious anemia
- Altered anatomy after subtotal gastrectomy

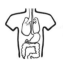

ESOPHAGEAL CANCER

Pathophysiology

Two types of cancer predominate. Squamous cell carcinoma, associated with the use of tobacco and alcohol, is more common in African-American males. Patients usually seek help because of progressive **dysphagia** for solids and then liquids, by which time the tumor is already inoperable.

Adenocarcinoma arises from columnar epithelium tissue and is associated with **Barrett's esophagus,** which is a complication of chronic gastric esophagitis. This is found more commonly in whites in the distal one-third of the esophagus. Patients seek help for persistent gastroesophageal reflux that progresses to dysphagia. The tumor gradually narrows the

> Adenocarcinoma arises from columnar epithelium tissue and is associated with Barrett's esophagus, which is a complication of chronic gastric esophagitis.

lumen of the esophagus, infiltrates the surrounding tissues, and can invade the trachea, causing a tracheoesophageal fistula (Figure 52-1). Risk factors for esophageal cancer include cigarette smoking, alcohol abuse, gastroesophageal reflux, and poor diet.

Diagnosis and Management

Endoscopy and biopsy are the most reliable methods for diagnosing. Barium studies may be performed to determine extent of tumor growth.

Surgery is the treatment of choice for tumors of the lower one-third of the esophagus, whereas radiation is the treatment for the upper two-thirds. Surveillance of known or suspected cases of Barrett's esophagus is paramount. It is suggested that those with Barrett's esophagus undergo annual endoscopy surveillance.

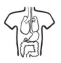

STOMACH CANCER

Pathophysiology

Gastric cancers have several morphological types, including polypoid intraluminal masses, ulcerating masses, diffuse and spreading through the submucosa, and superficial confined to the mucosa or submucosa with or without lymphatic involvement—the only type with a good prognosis. Most individuals, up to 90%, do not seek help until the disease is very advanced, having relied on over-the-counter medications for what had been mild but persistent abdominal complaints they mistook for indigestion.

Clinical Manifestations

Vague symptoms include loss of appetite, indigestion unrelieved by medications, unexplainable weight loss, and change in bowel habits.

Anemia may present because of occult blood loss. Advanced cases also complain of persistent abdominal pain. Half of those with advanced disease have a palpable mass. Tumors of the cardia and gastrointestinal junction present with dysphagia and weight loss caused by anorexia and early satiety.

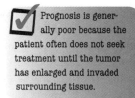
Prognosis is generally poor because the patient often does not seek treatment until the tumor has enlarged and invaded surrounding tissue.

Prognosis is generally poor because the patient often does not seek treatment until the tumor has enlarged and invaded surrounding tissue.

 Vague symptoms include loss of appetite, indigestion unrelieved by medications, unexplainable weight loss, and change in bowel habits.

Diagnosis and Management

Diagnosis is made by endoscopic cytology brushings and biopsy of suspected lesions. All patients are surgical candidates unless there is clear evidence of metastasis or the individual is considered a poor surgical risk. Chemotherapy is used for nonsurgical candidates, radiation therapy to treat complications such as obstruction, and stent placement and nutritional support provide some palliative care. Eighty-five percent of patients experience recurrence within 2 years of surgery. Preventing the disease points to dietary changes, the need to monitor and eradicate *H. pylori,* and carefully monitoring those with a strong family history. Early intervention is critical.

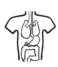

COLORECTAL CANCER

Adenomas are precursors of most colorectal cancers (Figure 52-2). Although the reason for this is unknown, strong environmental and genetic links are recognized. Dietary factors include high calorie, high fat, and high red meat content and alcohol consumption. Other lifestyle factors include obesity, lack of exercise, and long-term exposure to cigarette smoke. It is estimated that one-half of colorectal cancers could be prevented by lifestyle modifications alone. There are clearly established links between the development of this cancer and familial adeno-

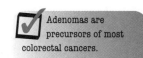
Adenomas are precursors of most colorectal cancers.

Figure 52-2 Colon.

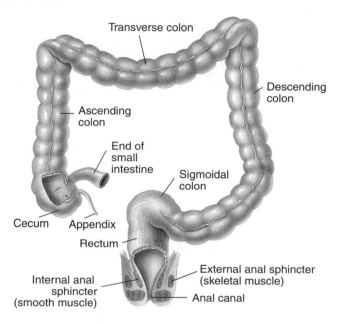

Transverse colon

Descending colon

Ascending colon

End of small intestine

Sigmoidal colon

Cecum   Appendix

Rectum

Internal anal sphincter (smooth muscle)

External anal sphincter (skeletal muscle)

Anal canal

matous polyposis (most common), nonpolyposis colorectal cancer, and nonadenomatous polyposis. A history of inflammatory bowel disease also increases risk, with a duration of 10 to 15 years of active disease and extensive involvement of the disease being the important factors. Colorectal cancers associated with inflammatory bowel diseases arise from the ulcer craters and are difficult to detect (Figure 52-3).

Pathophysiology

Benign adenomatous polyps, which are precursors of colorectal cancer, are generally detected and excised on screening examinations (Figure 52-4). All have some degree of **dysplasia** as determined by cytology **atypia** and architectural abnormality. Those classified as mild dysplasia have few characteristics of cancer; those classified as severe dysplasia have many cancer characteristics but remain noninvasive. A malignant polyp contains cancer cells and is invasive. It appears to take about 10 to 15 years for a benign polyp to become malignant with genetic mutations occurring in a predictable order. *Ras* oncogene mutations are seen in 50% of adenocarcinomas, and 75% have alterations in the tumor suppression genes, especially

Figure 52-3 Adenocarcinoma of the colon. Risk factors include adenomatous polyps and inflammatory bowel disease.

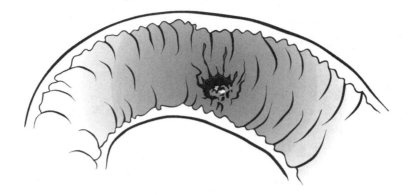

Figure 52-4 Adenomatous polyp of the colon.

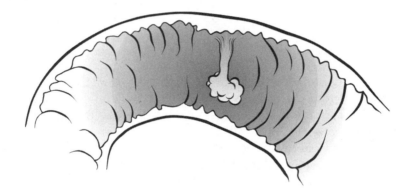

those involving chromosomes 17 and 18. Several other types of benign polyps can be found, but these do not become malignant.

Most colorectal cancers present as ulcerative, infiltrating, or nodular lesions in either the rectum, sigmoid, or descending colon. Metastasis occurs via either lymphatic invasion to the mesentery lymph nodes or through the portal system to the liver, and eventually through systemic circulation to the lung and other body sites. Tumor staging is based on the depth of invasion and extent of lymphatic involvement. Stage I tumors have a 97% 5-year survival rate; stage IV tumors a 4% survival rate. The loss of DCC or *p53* tumor suppressor genes indicate poor prognosis, as do findings of differentiated histology, abnormal DNA content, and invasion into adjacent structures or elevation of carcinoembryonic antigen. Tumor size does not predict prognosis.

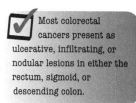

Most colorectal cancers present as ulcerative, infiltrating, or nodular lesions in either the rectum, sigmoid, or descending colon.

Adenomatous polyps are generally asymptomatic. Symptoms of cancerous tumors are dependent on their size and location.

Clinical Manifestations

Cancer of the right (ascending) colon presents with occult bleeding, iron deficiency anemia, and some complaints of pain. A mass may be palpable in the right lower quadrant. Tumors here and in the cecum do not generally cause obstruction because the lumen is large and stools are soft in this area of the bowel. Cancers of the transverse colon usually present as an obstruction. Those of the left (descending) and sigmoid colon present with rectal bleeding and symptoms of bowel obstruction (such as crampy abdominal pain, change in bowel habits, and changes in stool size and consistency). Cancers of the rectum rarely produce symptoms until they have been present for a long time. Small amount of bright red bleeding is an early symptom and is the reason people seek medical care. It may be followed or accompanied by urgency, change in bowel habits, or incomplete evacuation. Advanced cancers produce perianal pain, hematuria, urinary frequency, and vaginal fistulas. They can perforate into the peritoneum, producing a local abscess or peritonitis. Metastasis to liver and surrounding lymph nodes is common.

 Small amount of bright red bleeding is an early symptom and is the reason people seek medical care.

Diagnosis and Management

Screening examinations and lifestyle changes have a major impact on the development and cure rates of colorectal cancer. Diagnosis is made by computed tomography or magnetic resonance imaging of the abdomen followed by colonoscopy and biopsy. Surgical resection is the only potentially curative treatment for those diagnosed with the disease. Chemotherapy and radiation improve prognosis. Chemotherapy is the treatment of choice for those with metastasis. Individuals with diagnosed adenomas require surveillance colonoscopy every 3 years. Prevention includes consuming a low-fat diet rich in fruits, vegetables, and whole grains along with a regular program of exercise.

 Prevention includes consuming a low-fat diet rich in fruits, vegetables, and whole grains along with a regular program of exercise.

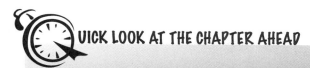

The liver is an organ that receives blood flow from gallbladder, pancreas, intestines and spleen and is responsible for carbohydrate and fat metabolism as well as filtration of toxic substances in the body. Along with the many functions of the liver, it is able to regenerate itself.

53

Liver and Biliary Anatomy and Physiology

TERM
☐ jaundice

Figure 53-1 Diagnostic studies and laboratory tests.

Diagnostic Studies

- Endoscopic retrograde cholangiopancreatography (ERCP)—Using a flexible fiberoptic endoscope, a contrast medium is instilled into the duodenal papilla or ampulla of Vater to view the hepatic tree and pancreatic ducts. After viewing, the endoscope can be used to drain cysts, remove stones from the common bile duct, or place stents across biliary or pancreatic structures.
- Hepatic angiography—Assessment of hepatic vasculature commonly used before transplantation, to place a transjugular intrahepatic portosystemic shunt, or after trauma.
- Hepatobiliary scan (HIDA)—A radionuclide study that shows hepatic parenchyma; extrahepatic bile ducts; gallbladder; normal passage into the intestine; and the size, shape, and position of the liver. A series of images permits visualization of the gallbladder and determines the patency of the biliary system. It is used to evaluate biliary leaks, cholecystitis, and biliary atresia; to differentiate obstructive from nonobstructive jaundice; and to evaluate upper abdominal pain.
- Liver biopsy (percutaneous liver biopsy)—A needle is inserted through the abdominal wall into the liver to obtain tissue samples to diagnose or confirm liver disease and responses to therapy and to evaluate transplant allografts.

Laboratory Tests

- Hepatitis screen—Five major types of hepatitis have thus far been identified, with two new viruses, hepatitis F and G, which are non-ABCDE viruses. These two new types are currently undergoing genetic testing. Because they present with common symptoms, a hepatitis screen can be used to determine the presence, type, stage, and progress of the disease. Each type of hepatitis has specific markers that rise and fall in a predictable pattern. Markers specify the type of hepatitis (i.e., HAV for hepatitis A; HBcAb or HBsAg for hepatitis B; anti-HCV for hepatitis C; HDAg for hepatitis D; and IgM anti-HVE for hepatitis E). The form of immunoglobulin found indicates that an infection is in the early stages (i.e., IgM or later stages IgG). Use of the prefix "anti" explains that the body has produced an antigen to the virus. Finally, because some types of the hepatitis virus have various layers or components, different names are used to represent the identified component (i.e., HBcAg means the hepatitis B core antigen, anti-HBs means the antibody to the hepatitis B surface antigen). Once the particular type of hepatitis is known, the specific kind and pattern of hepatitis markers for that virus can be consulted.

Hepatitis A markers:

- HAV-Ab (hepatitis A antibody)
- IgM—Acute infection
- IgG—Postinfection, previous exposure, immunity

Hepatitis B markers

- Anti-HB (hepatitis B core antibody)—Rises within 2 weeks of contracting virus, rises again during chronic phase, and remains present for life.
- Anti-HBc, HBeAb (hepatitis B antibody)—Indicates resolution of infection; if found in the presence of chronic hepatitis B surface antigen, it indicates an asymptomatic healthy carrier.

Figure 53-1 *Continued.*

- HBs-AB (hepatitis B surface antibody)—Represents clinical recovery and immunity to virus; if present with hepatitis B surface antigen, indicates a poor prognosis.
- HBsAg: HAA (hepatitis B surface antigen)—Indicates active hepatitis B either acute or chronic; is early indicator and can be present before clinical symptoms; if present with hepatitis B surface antigen, it indicates a poor prognosis.

Hepatitis C markers

- Anti-HCV (hepatitis C antibody)—Identifies total antibodies of the IgG close to the hepatitis C virus.

Hepatitis D markers

- HDAg (hepatitis delta antibody)—Identifies total antibodies of the IgG close to the hepatitis D virus; this virus requires the presence of HBsAg to express itself.

Hepatitis E markers

- IgM anti-HVE—Antibodies to hepatitis E virus.
- Liver enzymes/liver function panel (LFTs)—Panel usually consists of aspartate aminotransferase, alanine aminotransferase, alkaline phosphatase, bilirubin, and albumin; other tests are also included here.
- Alanine aminotransferase (ALT)—Intracellular enzyme involved in amino acid metabolism; found in large concentrations in the liver and smaller concentrations in heart muscle and kidney; released with tissue damage; used to diagnose liver disease and to monitor course of hepatitis, cirrhosis, and drug therapy; helps differentiate between hemolytic jaundice and jaundice due to liver disease.
- Aspartate aminotransferase (AST)—Intracellular enzyme involved in amino acid metabolism; found in large concentrations in the liver, skeletal muscle, heart, brain, and red blood cells; released into blood when tissue, especially liver, is damaged.
- Lactate dehydrogenase (LDH)—Intracellular enzyme found in almost all body tissues; is released after tissue damage but is not specific as to site.
- Alkaline phosphatase (ALP)—Enzyme found in bone, liver, intestine, and placenta; rises during periods of bone growth, liver disease, or bile duct obstruction.
- γ-Glutamyltransferase/transpeptidase (GGT/GTTP)—A biliary excretory enzyme that assists in transferring amino acids and peptides across cellular membranes; used to evaluate liver disease and hepatic metastasis and screen for alcoholism.
- Albumin—Major component of plasma proteins; influenced by nutritional state and hepatic functioning; gives indication of severity in chronic liver disease; low levels occur because of decreased hepatic synthesis.
- Bilirubin is produced in the liver, spleen, and bone marrow; is a byproduct of hemoglobin metabolism; total bilirubin is broken down into direct (conjugated) normally excreted from the gastrointestinal tract; and indirect (free) bilirubin circulating in the blood; total bilirubin rises with any kind of jaundice; direct rises with obstructive or hepatic jaundice and is excreted by the kidneys; indirect bilirubin rises in hemolytic jaundice with increased amount of present in the blood.
- 5'-Nucleotide—A plasma membrane enzyme found in hepatic parenchyma and bile duct cells; is elevated in liver cancer; when occurs with accompanying elevation in alkaline phosphatase indicates liver metastasis.

(continued)

Figure 53-1 *Continued.*

- Ornithine carbamoyltransferase (OCT)—A liver enzyme involved in urea metabolism, elevations are specific and sensitive to liver cell disease.
- Leucine aminopeptidase (LAP)—Enzyme found in liver, bile, and urine; helps with differential diagnosis when client presents with elevated alkaline phosphatase because it is normal in bone disease.
- Amylase—Enzyme produced in pancreas and salivary glands that aids in digestion of complex carbohydrates; elevated in blood 2–3 days after acute pancreatitis attack; stays elevated in urine for 7–10 days.
- Lipase—Pancreatic enzyme that digests fats and triglycerides; elevated in association with amylase but is more specific than amylase.

The liver, which is the largest organ in the body, is located below the diaphragm in the upper right quadrant of the abdomen. It has a dual blood supply, in which one-third of the total is oxygenated blood under high pressure arriving from the hepatic artery. The remaining two-thirds of the total comes via the portal vein and brings blood rich in nutrients under low pressure from the stomach, intestines, spleen, and pancreas. These two sources mix as they begin to flow through the liver and collect in the left and right hepatic veins, which then drain into the inferior vena cava.

The functional unit of the liver is the lobule, in which hepatocyte cells are organized around a central vein in a spoke-like fashion to form a hexagon. At the corners of the hexagon are the portal tracts where branches of the hepatic artery, portal vein, and lymphatic vessels converge. Blood flows from these tracts through vascular spaces called *sinusoids* toward the central vein. Lining the walls of the sinusoids are various one-layer-thick cells: hepatocytes, which are responsible for carbohydrate and fat metabolism, blood detoxification, and initial bile formation; bile duct cells, which add to the composition of bile and propel it; endothelial cells, which help filter blood; perisinusoidal cells, which aid in lipid and vitamin A metabolism, production of proteins, and liver regeneration; and Kupffer cells, which are phagocytes. Because the outer portion of the hexagon has initial contact with well-oxygenated nutrient-rich blood, it is less vulnerable to injury and circulatory disturbances than cells located near the central vein.

Via these structures and processes, the liver converts fructose and galactose to glucose; removes excess glucose from the blood in response to insulin; makes and stores glycogen, which reconverts into glucose when circulating glucose levels fall; builds and breaks down phospholipids, triglycerides, and cholesterol as needed; manufactures bile to send to the gallbladder for use as needed; makes ketone bodies as needed; removes excess amino acids from the blood and deaminates them or converts them to other amino acids; stores iron, copper, and vitamins, including B_{12}; synthesizes plasma proteins needed for blood clotting such as albumin, which holds water in the blood vessels, fibrinogen, and prothrombin; digests bacteria and toxic substances to cleanse the blood; detoxifies substances such as urea from amino acid metabolism; converts ammonia to urea for excretion by the kidneys; produces the bases for nitrogen containing compounds needed to make DNA and RNA; and forms lymph.

The liver is capable of renewing itself. Hepatocytes generally live up to 120 days but can survive for months or years. They can proliferate rapidly in response to injury and cell loss.

Bile duct epithelial cells can also do this. Hyperplasia of hepatocytes occurs in response to significant metabolic alterations in carbohydrate or lipid metabolism. Hypertrophy can occur when there is a need for increased chemical transformation, as with drug detoxification. Cell death is characterized by shrinkage, cytoplasmic condensation, nuclear loss, and disappearance of individual hepatocytes as they slide down the sinusoids and are carried away via blood into the central vein. The liver loses cells and mass with age, so that by age 90, about two-thirds of the hepatic mass is lost. Fat accumulates, cells shrink, and functions are compromised.

Liver cells may be injured by drugs, alcohol, chemicals, or viruses. The result is cellular death, accumulation of fat within liver cells, or a combination of the two. With mild injury, liver cells can regenerate, but repeated episodes of even mild disease are cumulative and can lead to scarring and permanent damage. Chronic, progressive diseases have the same effect. With severe disease and the death of large numbers of liver cells, it may be impossible for regeneration to occur. Postnecrotic scarring can change liver architecture to such a degree that normal functioning is impossible. Some substances (especially alcohol), obesity, diabetes, and malnutrition can produce excessive accumulations of fats in the liver. This probably results from an imbalance between the amount of fats arriving and the ability of the liver to mobilize very-low-density lipoproteins as triglycerides. With abstinence and good nutrition this condition can be reversed.

Bile is formed when blood passes through the liver. There bilirubin, the yellow-orange colored iron-free heme present from red blood cell breakdown, is removed from it. Bilirubin is combined with water and other substances excreted by the liver (i.e., bile salts, lecithin, cholesterol, and minerals) to form bile. Bile travels in the opposite direction as blood and collects in bile canaliculi located at the periphery of the hexagon. These collecting ducts gradually increase in size and eventually end in the left and right hepatic ducts that join to form the common hepatic duct. This duct and the cystic duct of the gallbladder together form the common bile duct. Bile is constantly secreted, concentrated, and stored in the gallbladder. Bile contains no enzymes but acts as a digestive detergent, emulsifying fat into small globules so that more surface area can be acted upon by pancreatic enzymes.

The pancreas is located across the abdomen behind the stomach with its head fitting into the curve of the duodenum, where the pancreatic duct empties. It operates as a dual gland. As an exocrine gland, the pancreas releases the following digestive enzymes: amylase, which breaks down carbohydrates; trypsin and chymotrypsin, which break down protein; and lipase, which breaks down fat. As an endocrine gland, small clusters of cells, called *Langerhans' cells*, discharge secretions into the blood. Langerhans' cells are composed of different types of cells: alpha cells, which secrete glucagon; beta cells, which secrete insulin when blood glucose levels rise after eating; and delta cells, which secrete somatostatin, which inhibits the secretion of both glucagon and insulin.

Jaundice is a condition in which the skin, tissues, and conjunctiva become yellow because of the excess bilirubin in the blood. This may be caused by an obstruction such as a tumor, a gallstone in the duct, or a congenital defect. It may also be present in liver diseases like hepatitis or cirrhosis. Because bile does not reach the duodenum, stools are light colored, and because the bilirubin-loaded blood is filtered by the kidneys, the urine becomes very dark. Without bile aiding digestion, digestion of fats is compromised and fat-soluble vitamins are not absorbed.

Hemolytic jaundice is very different and develops in the presence of hemolytic anemias in which red blood cells are hemolyzed with excessive amounts of bilirubin released. Physiological jaundice in newborns may develop shortly after birth because the liver is too immature to manage the bilirubin already in the blood. Normally, this condition only lasts a few days and is not usually serious.

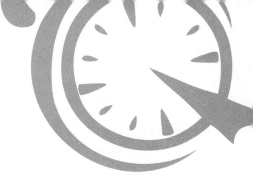

Hepatitis may be caused by a viral infection, or it may result from sensitivity to a hepatotoxic drug or chemical, from chronic excessive alcohol consumption, or from autoimmune factors. It can be acute, chronic, or fulminant. People with viral hepatitis can be carriers in that they transmit the virus but have no evidence of infection themselves. Hepatitis may also be in an active or dormant state. There are currently five types of viral hepatitis known, and two types are currently undergoing further research. Hepatitis and its sequelae affect more than 500 million people worldwide. Both sexes and all age groups are equally affected. Hepatitis can cause cirrhosis or liver cancer, and it is the underlying basis for most liver transplants.

54

Hepatitis

TERMS
- [ ] **icteric phase**
- [ ] **preicteric period**
- [ ] **pruritus**
- [ ] **superinfection**

Table 54-1 Viral Hepatitis: Important Characteristics

Characteristic	Type A	Type B	Type C	Type D	Type E
Mode of transmission	Waterborne Fecal-oral Venereal	Perinatal Blood/skin Venereal	Venereal Blood/skin	Venereal Blood	Waterborne Fecal-oral
Incubation period (range in days)	15 to 42	42 to 160	14 to 160	28 to 49	14 to 56
average	30	90	50	35	40
Onset	Abrupt	Insidious	Insidious	Insidious	Abrupt
Symptoms					
Fever	Common	Uncommon	Uncommon	Common	Common
Nausea/ vomiting	Common	Common	Common	Common	Common
Jaundice	More common in adults than children	Occasionally	Uncommon	Common	Common
Outcome					
Severity	Mild	Moderate	Mild	Moderate to Severe	Severe
Fulminating hepatitis	>.5%	<1%	Rare	3% to 4% with coinfection with hepatitis B	.3% to 3% 20% in pregnant women
Mortality rate	Low (<1%)	Low (1% to 3%)	Low (2%)	High (5%)	Moderate; high with pregnancy
Chronic hepatitis	No	Yes (5% to 10%)	Yes (80%)	<5% with coinfection 80% with superinfection	No
Carrier state	No	Yes (1 million in United States)	Yes	Yes	No
Relapse	Yes	Yes	Persistent	Unknown	Unknown
Carcinoma	No	Yes (25% to 40%)	Yes (25% to 30%)	No increase above that for hepatitis B	Unknown but not likely
Develop cirrhosis	No	40%	30%	Yes, with superinfection	No

Table 54-2 Clinical Manifestations of Hepatitis

Prodromal phase: viral symptoms such as nausea, vomiting, malaise, anorexia, low-grade fever, headache; 2 weeks after exposure to virus, which ends with the onset of jaundice

Icteric phase: jaundice, dark tea-colored urine or clay-colored stools, hepatomegaly and right upper quadrant pain; begins 1–2 weeks after prodromal phase and lasts up to 6 weeks

Recovery phase: resolution of jaundice approximately 6–8 weeks after exposure; liver may remain enlarged for up to 3 months

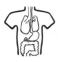

PATHOPHYSIOLOGY

Acute hepatitis is usually caused by one of the hepatotropic viruses (see Table 54-1). These viruses specifically affect hepatocyte cells, causing the cell membrane to rupture and contents to leak out. Each virus type differs in its mode of transmission and incubation, ability to become asymptomatic, and the degree to which it causes liver damage. Macrophages consume the destroyed cells. Cell necrosis can occur in isolated clusters with large regions developing as clusters enlarge and connect with each other, disrupting the normal architecture of the area. Cell damage can extend into the parenchyma, causing inflammation, disrupting the bile channel structure, and resulting in pooling of bile and engorgement of the liver.

Acute hepatitis has four distinct periods: period of incubation, symptomatic preicteric period, symptomatic period with jaundice and sclera icterus referred to as the **icteric phase,** and period of convalescence. The individual is most infectious during the last days of incubation and early days of acute symptoms. The symptomatic **preicteric period** is marked by nonspecific constitutional changes common to most viral syndromes, such as malaise, fatigue, anorexia, low-grade fever, and muscle aches. There is no evidence of jaundice.

The symptomatic preicteric period is marked by nonspecific constitutional changes common to most viral syndromes, such as malaise, fatigue, anorexia, low-grade fever, and muscle aches. There is no evidence of jaundice.

Some patients with hepatitis B also experience rash, fever, and arthralgias. Jaundice does not occur with every type of hepatitis but is common in adults with hepatitis A and about half of those with hepatitis B. Jaundice generally does not develop with hepatitis C. When jaundice develops, it is caused by conjugated hyperbilirubinemia and results in dark-colored urine, light-colored stools, and **pruritus** as bile salts are retained. It can take weeks to months for jaundice and other symptoms to resolve.

Chronic hepatitis is diagnosed by symptomatic, serological, or histological evidence of continuing or relapsing hepatic disease lasting more than 6 months. It may be caused by hepatitis virus (usually B or C), alcoholism, or drugs. Outcome is determined by the histological pattern that develops rather than the etiology of the disease. An individual may have only elevated enzyme; a single complaint, usually fatigue; or severe systemic symptoms associated with cirrhosis or hepatic failure. With mild or slowly progressing disease, the liver architecture is usually well preserved and function remains essentially intact. More severe or rapidly progressing disease results in more serious changes. Coalescing areas of necrosis extending into the parenchyma cause disruption of hepatic structures and functioning. Irreversible liver damage is characterized by deposits of fibrous tissue first in the portal tracts, later in the adjacent tissues, and finally enveloping whole lobules. Cirrhosis develops with large, irregularly shaped nodules and broad bands of scarring. The individual can live for years with chronic hepatitis; however, when architectural changes, fibrous scars, and cellular death make even minimal liver functioning impossible, transplantation is the only option.

Fulminant hepatitis is a rapidly progressive form of the disease that causes rapid liver failure and can end with hepatic encephalopathy or death within 2 to 3 weeks. Uncommon but extremely serious, it is usually caused by superinfection of hepatitis D in a person with existing chronic hepatitis B or as a complication of hepatitis E in pregnant women. It may also result from drugs or chemicals, such as acetaminophen, isoniazid, halothane, or toxic mushrooms. Rapid and massive loss of liver tissue occurs after initial symptoms of viral hepatitis are recognized. Progressive destruction of liver function, jaundice, and abdominal pain from hepatomegaly are followed by ascites and

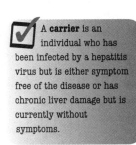
A **carrier** is an individual who has been infected by a hepatitis virus but is either symptom free of the disease or has chronic liver damage but is currently without symptoms.

gastrointestinal bleeding. Initial serologies may be negative for hepatitis viruses, making diagnosis and treatment extremely difficult.

A *carrier* is an individual who has been infected by a hepatitis virus but is either symptom-free of the disease or has chronic liver damage but is currently without symptoms. In both states the individual harbors the hepatitis virus and is able to transmit it to others. Up to 95% of those affected with hepatitis B at birth become carriers. Most persons with hepatitis C are carriers.

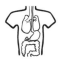

HEPATITIS VIRUSES

Hepatitis A is typically acquired as part of a local epidemic associated with shellfish harvested from contaminated water. It can be transmitted by the fecal–oral route, with an increased incidence among people in large institutions, poor hygiene, or among day care attendees. Individuals are usually asymptomatic or only mildly ill; the incubation period is as little as 2 weeks to 30 days. It may go unrecognized in children. About 50% of adults in the United States are seropositive for hepatitis A, many never realizing they have ever had it. Peak titers of IgM anti-HAV occur during the first week of clinical disease and usually disappear within 3 to 6 months. Titers of IgG anti-HAV peak 1 month and may persist for years. Recovery without complications is common; lifelong immunity to hepatitis A is conferred by one episode. Management is symptom supportive. Vaccination for hepatitis A is recommended to anyone traveling to certain parts of the world where sanitation is poor or for those who have high-risk exposure.

> Vaccination for hepatitis A is recommended to anyone traveling to certain parts of the world where sanitation is poor or for those who have high-risk exposure.

Hepatitis B virus (HBV), one of most serious hepatitis viruses, is present in all body fluids except stool. Most individuals are infected during passage through the birth canal of an infected mother. More than 90% of those infected as children become hepatitis B carriers, with many going on to develop cirrhosis or hepatocellular carcinoma. More than one million people in the United States have chronic HBV infection.

Infected hepatocytes synthesize and secrete massive quantities of a noninfective surface protein that appears in cells and serum as HBeAg. This indicates the disease is present. HBeAg appears shortly thereafter, indicating that active viral replication is taking place, infectivity is high, and progression to a chronic hepatitis state is likely. HBV has a longer incubation period (60–80 days) than other hepatitis viruses and is transmitted through blood or serum and oral or sexual contact, with a significant incidence among intravenous drug abusers, men having sex with men, or those with multiple sexual partners.

> HBV has a longer incubation period (60–80 days) than other hepatitis viruses and is transmitted through blood or serum and oral or sexual contact, with a significant incidence among intravenous drug abusers, men having sex with men, or those with multiple sexual partners.

Management is aimed chiefly at prevention by vaccination against the disease. Hepatitis B immunoglobulin may be protective if given in large doses within 7 days of exposure and if followed by initiation of the hepatitis B vaccine series, which provides long-term protection against acquisition of the virus. The vaccine is recommended for all health care workers, staff members of large institutions for the mentally disabled or incarcerated, all contacts (household and sexual) of HBV carriers, intravenous drug abusers, and those with multiple sexual partners. Viral replication can be diminished in about 30% of cases by interferon therapy continued for at least 4 months. Other treatment is aimed at symptom management.

> The vaccine is recommended for all health care workers, staff members of large institutions for the mentally disabled or incarcerated, all contacts (household and sexual) of HBV carriers, intravenous drug abusers, and those with multiple sexual partners.

Hepatitis C, the most common cause of chronic hepatitis, often goes unnoticed and is discovered by following up on routine blood tests that initially show elevated alanine aminotransferase and/or aspartate aminotransferase. Originally part of a viral group known as non-A, non-B hepatitis, hepatitis C is now thought to be responsible for 80% to 90% of these viruses. The mode of transmission often cannot be identified, but it is believed that about 50% of cases have a past history of intravenous drug use. Recent data suggest that as many as one in three people with tattoos or body piercing have been infected with the virus by that process.

 Recent data suggest that as many as one in three people with tattoos or body piercing have been infected with the virus by that process.

Persistent infection and chronic hepatitis are common. Cirrhosis can be present at the time of diagnosis or develop within 5 to 10 years. Because hepatitis C mutates at a rapid rate, it is expected that a vaccine against it will not be found. Interferon and interferon derivatives, which boost the body's immune response, have had great success in decreasing viral load. Other treatment is supportive.

Hepatitis D is able to persist only in the presence of hepatitis B. It can occur either as a coinfection or as a **superinfection** and is managed by managing the hepatitis B.

Hepatitis E is thought to be transmitted via contaminated drinking water and is found in almost half of adults in Third World countries. It is usually a self-limiting illness, causing symptoms similar to hepatitis A, resulting in neither chronicity nor carrier state. In pregnant women, however, it can result in fulminating hepatitis, with a 20% mortality rate. It is endemic to parts of Africa, Mexico, and Southeast Asia.

Cases of non-A, non-B hepatitis have resulted in the identification of other hepatitis viruses, most notably C and D, but also others about which little is known. A single case of hepatitis F suggests that the virus may not even exist. Hepatitis G has been seen with blood transfusions and causes cirrhosis as documented by liver biopsy.

Cirrhosis is a condition of chronic, progressive, irreversible damage to the liver resulting in compromised hepatic functioning due to a variety of causes. The seventh leading cause of death in the United States, it affects about 11 million Americans. Although caused by many different conditions, in the United States cirrhosis is most often caused by chronic alcohol consumption. In Third World and developing countries, it usually results from chronic hepatitis, either B, C, or D. Biliary cirrhosis is due to inflammation and scarring of the bile ducts and liver. There is a genetic component to this type of cirrhosis. Other types of cirrhosis include postnecrotic cirrhosis from hepatitis infection and metabolic cirrhosis from diseases such as Wilson's disease, glycogen storage disease, or α_1-antitrypsin deficiencies. Symptoms are similar regardless of the cause. Fifty percent with an established diagnosis of cirrhosis survive for 2 years; 35% survive 5 years. About 40% of cases are discovered on autopsy.

55

Cirrhosis

TERMS
- [ ] ascites
- [ ] cirrhosis

Figure 55-1 Cross-section of a liver lobule.

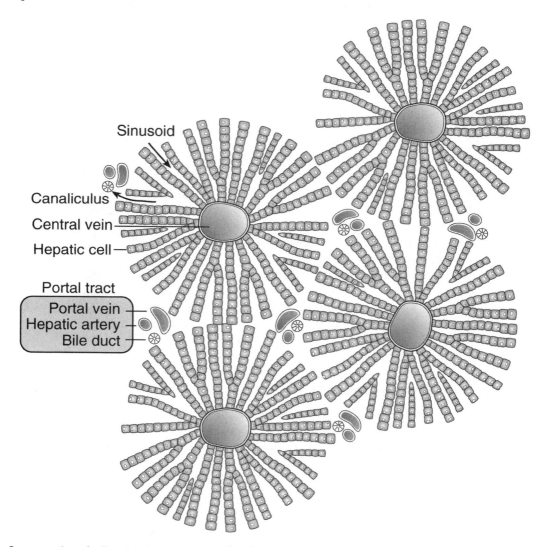

Cross-section of a liver lobule showing the direction of blood flow in sinusoids toward the central vein and of bile toward the bile duct.

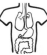
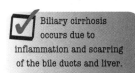

PATHOPHYSIOLOGY

The architecture of the liver is precisely arranged, with each cell and structure having a specific function to perform. If only small areas are affected, the liver can maintain vital functions, but as larger sections are destroyed, its abilities are taxed beyond repair. Damaged liver cells are replaced by tissue that is thick, rigid, inflexible, and incapable of performing any of the functions of healthy hepatocytes. This formation of scar tissue contracts, shrinking the organ and producing nodules in the hepatic parenchyma that is surrounded by fibrotic tissue with an irregular surface appearance that interferes with the normal vascular and bile pathways. Pressure gradients are affected, compromising blood flow in and out of the organ and backing up the bile. Bile stasis irritates and inflames hepatocytes, causing additional damage. Symptoms develop as the liver is first compromised and then fails.

> Biliary cirrhosis occurs due to inflammation and scarring of the bile ducts and liver.

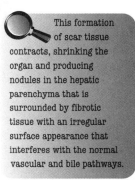

> This formation of scar tissue contracts, shrinking the organ and producing nodules in the hepatic parenchyma that is surrounded by fibrotic tissue with an irregular surface appearance that interferes with the normal vascular and bile pathways.

Portal Hypertension

When the intrahepatic branches of the hepatic artery and portal vein are constricted by scar tissue, high pressure develops in the blood vessels leading to the liver. Veins swell, producing varices, especially in the abdomen and esophagus. Organs connected to the liver via circulation, such as the spleen, pancreas, and stomach, enlarge as pressure rises. Collateral circulatory pathways develop to shunt as much blood as possible around the obstruction and back into the systemic circulation. Anastomosis develops to shunt blood from high-pressure portal veins to lower-pressure systemic vessels. However, veins of the systemic system are not structurally equipped to deal with the volume of blood that is diverted or blood arriving under such high pressure. They dilate and form varicosities.

Hemorrhage, or a slow, persistent bleed, is possible anywhere along the circulatory pathway. The vessels in the esophagus are particularly vulnerable because of the fragility of their walls and are prone to rupturing. There is a 70% risk of death from a single esophageal bleed. Recurrence is common within 2 weeks of the first episode. Anastomosing varicosities in the abdominal cavity produce a temporary reduction of pressure in the portal system but cause changes that are not always obvious until it is too late to rectify them. Superficial abdominal varicosities are common.

 Hemorrhage, or a slow persistent bleed, is possible anywhere along the circulatory pathway.

Ascites

Ascites is the accumulation of fluid in the peritoneal cavity. First, it occurs because high pressure within the obstructed portal system forces fluids to back up into the abdominal cavity. Second, the damaged liver is unable to produce a sufficient supply of albumin, a protein responsible for maintaining normal osmotic pressure and holding fluid in the capillaries. Without albumin, fluid leaks out of the capillaries, collecting in the abdomen. A similar process results in edema, particularly of the lower extremities.

Without albumin, fluid leaks out of the capillaries, collecting in the abdomen. A similar process results in edema, particularly of the lower extremities.

Jaundice

Changes in liver structure impair its ability to manufacture and move bile. Surviving cells continue to produce bile but cannot move it through the collecting system. Bile accumulates in the liver, causing inflammation and necrosis, whereas some enters into the bloodstream, causing jaundice. Without bile, fats cannot be digested and fat-soluble vitamins cannot be absorbed. Stools become clay colored. Excess bile in the blood is excreted by the kidneys, producing dark urine. Bile salts accumulate, causing intense pruritus.

Estrogen Build-up

Small amounts of estrogen are normally secreted by the adrenal gland in both sexes. A normal liver inactivates it, but a cirrhotic liver cannot. The hormone builds up, producing feminine characteristics in the male (gynecomastia, feminine distribution of body hair, testicular atrophy, and impotence). Females experience irregular menses.

Hepatic Encephalopathy

Severely damaged hepatic cells cannot detoxify blood; numerous poisons accumulate. One of them, ammonia, produces neurological manifestations, including confusion, disorientation, and a characteristic hand tremor called liver flap. A gastrointestinal tract bleed can significantly increase protein levels, causing the rapid onset of encephalopathy. Excessive protein ingestion, infection, or renal failure can also increase protein levels. Death is common.

 Ammonia produces neurological manifestations, including confusion, disorientation, and a characteristic hand tremor called liver flap.

Metabolic Dysfunction

Hepatocyte destruction produces metabolic dysfunction. Changes in protein metabolism result in decreased production of protein clotting factors, muscle wasting, hyperlipidemia, and hypoalbuminemia. Impaired metabolism of glucose results in either hyperglycemia or hypoglycemia. Reduced bile salts make absorption of fat-soluble vitamins from the gastrointestinal tract difficult. Osteomalacia develops from lack of vitamin D, and bleeding tendencies from lack of vitamin K. Without hepatocytes, the liver cannot metabolize and/or clear substances like drugs and toxins.

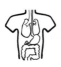

DIAGNOSIS AND MANAGEMENT

Liver damage is irreversible, but its progression can be delayed or halted. Diagnosis is based on clinical history and manifestations. Liver function tests, including amylase and lipase, and liver biopsy confirm diagnosis of cirrhosis. Management depends on the cause and is aimed at preventing further dysfunction and treating complications. Hepatitis-related disease may involve the use of interferon for viral hepatitis and corticosteroids for autoimmune hepatitis. Bile acid–binding drugs are used for pruritus. Alcohol- or drug-induced cirrhosis requires complete

Figure 55-2 Normal liver tissue.

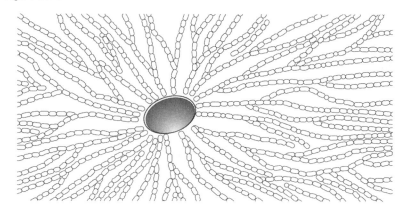

Figure 55-3 Cirrhotic liver. Note the bands of fibrous tissue and regenerating parenchyma.

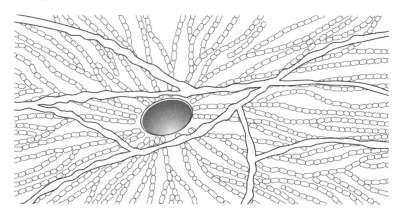

abstinence. Nutritional management is essential to correct imbalances, manage complications, and promote health. Portal hypertension is treated with surgical intervention to position shunts where commonly needed: hepatorenal, transjugular, or peritovenous. Ascites/edema is treated with fluid restriction, low-sodium diet, diuretics, and paracentesis, if needed. Esophageal varices are treated with endoscopy to band, shunt, or sclerose and are then used in combination with octreotide, a somatostatin.

Encephalopathy treatment seeks to find and eliminate the underlying cause. Dietary proteins are eliminated, and the colon is evacuated to

Figure 55-4 Effects of hepatic failure and portal hypertension.

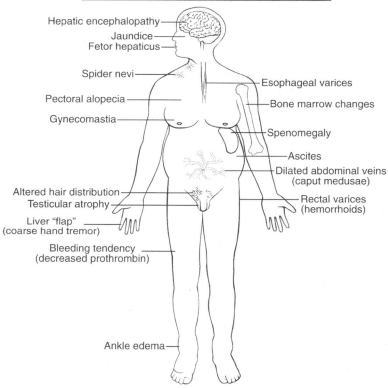

Effects of Hepatic Failure and Portal Hypertension

eliminate sources of protein breakdown. Antibiotics are given to suppress intestinal flora and decrease endogenous sources of ammonia production. Lactulose promotes the excretion of ammonia in the stool.

Transplantation is an option for some patients with severe cirrhosis, but wait time is long and not all patients are candidates. Alcoholics, who are not considered good candidates, must refrain from any drinking for at least 6 months to be eligible. Patients with hepatitis often have a return of their infectious disease after transplant. Individuals with any evidence of malignancy are not considered candidates for transplantation.

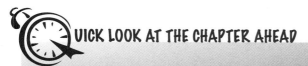
The functions of the pancreas and gallbladder are closely related. The gallbladder secretes bile; the pancreas secretes enzymes that aid in digestion. When one organ is not functioning optimally, it is not uncommon for it to affect the other organ.

56

Pancreas and Gallbladder Diseases

TERMS
☐ **cholecystitis**
☐ **pancreatitis**

Figure 56-1 Carcinoma of the tail of the pancreas.

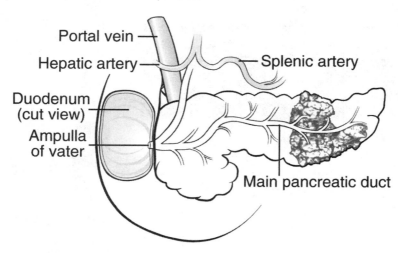

Carcinoma of the tail of the pancreas. Most pancreatic tumors arise in the pancreatic ducts. Small carcinomas of the head of the pancreas usually obstruct the internal pancreatic ducts so that the parenchyma of the exocrine pancreas then undergoes atrophy distal to the obstruction. Carcinomas of the body and/or tail are larger lesions that quickly invade adjacent organs (i.e., the spleen, colon, and adrenals) and metastasize to regional lymph nodes. Hepatic metastasis follows once the spleen is invaded.

Major Etiologies of Acute Pancreatitis

- Metabolic
- Alcohol consumption
- Hyperlipoproteinemia
- Hypercalcemia
- Mechanical
- Gallstones
- Trauma
- Vascular
- Shock
- Atheroembolism

Table 56-1 Causes of Pancreatitis

Gallstones: leading cause, usually ≥ 6.5 mm
Alcohol abuse
Biliary dyskinesia: functional motility disorder involving sphincter of Oddi
Hepatotoxic drugs
Increased triglycerides (≥1,000)
Post-endoscopic retrograde cholangiopancreatography and manometry
Trauma

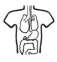

PANCREATITIS

Pancreatitis is a self-limiting inflammation of the pancreas with spontaneous regression in 3–7 days. It is more common in men than in women and usually occurs after age 40. It may be acute or chronic and has a high correlation with alcoholism and biliary tract abnormalities.

Pathophysiology

Specific enzymes are needed for digestion and help provide optimal gastric pH. Gastric acid stimulates secretion of secretin, an enzyme necessary for stimulation of pancreatic juice. Cholecystokinin is secreted from the duodenum and jejunum and is triggered by long-chain fatty acids. It is controlled by the parasympathetic nervous system.

The leading cause of acute pancreatitis is a gallstone (>6.5 mm diameter) causing an obstruction of the pancreatic duct at its entrance to the duodenum. As the common bile duct and the common pancreatic duct enter into the duodenum through a common channel (the ampulla of Vater), a stone lodged in the ampulla causes pancreatic juices to back up. Eventually, the pressure in the pancreatic ducts results in their rupture, and pancreatic enzymes leak into the surrounding pancreatic tissues. The enzymes cause autodigestion, inflammation, edema, and necrosis of pancreatic cells.

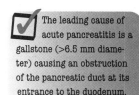
The leading cause of acute pancreatitis is a gallstone (>6.5 mm diameter) causing an obstruction of the pancreatic duct at its entrance to the duodenum.

A second cause is excessive alcohol consumption. Alcohol forms plugs in the pancreatic ducts, causing edema and spasm of the pancreatic sphincter in the ampulla of Vater. It also activates the release of proteolytic enzymes. The obstruction of the duct and the excessive production of enzymes have the same result as above. Together, gallstones and alcohol account for about 80% of acute pancreatic attacks. Other causes include infection, hyperlipidemia, trauma, an idiosyncratic reaction to drugs, and heredity.

> ✔ Eighty percent of patients with chronic pancreatitis are alcoholics, but only 5% to 10% of alcoholics develop chronic pancreatitis.

Eighty percent of patients with chronic pancreatitis are alcoholics, but only 5% to 10% of alcoholics develop chronic pancreatitis. Alcohol causes insoluble pancreatic proteins to be released, which calcify and occlude the large pancreatic duct.

Clinical Manifestations

There are three acute phases: edematous, which is mild and self-limiting; necrotizing, which depends on the degree and severity of attack; and hemorrhagic, which is usually due to trauma, neoplasm, or congestive heart failure. The chronic phase is associated with diabetes, B_{12} deficiencies, and malabsorption syndromes.

Acute states produce symptoms that include severe, colicky abdominal pain progressing to constant pain located in the epigastric area with radiation to the right upper quadrant. Pain is relieved with sitting up and forward in a "tripod position." Pain increases with supine positioning. Other symptoms include low-grade fever, tachycardia, and hypotension. Jaundice is rare and usually secondary to pancreatic head edema

> ✔ Pain increases with supine positioning.

with compression of the common bile duct. Bowel sounds are diminished or absent. With chronic pancreatitis, patients may present with steatorrhea.

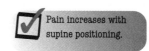

Acute states produce symptoms that include severe, colicky abdominal pain progressing to constant pain located in the epigastric area with radiation to the right upper quadrant.

Recurrent episodes of acute pancreatitis produce inflammation and scarring, damage to the ductal system, and high blood pressure. It becomes a self-perpetuating disease, with repeated episodes of acute pancreatitis eventually leading to endocrine and exocrine insufficiency.

Without lipid enzymes, fats cannot be digested. Foul-smelling, greasy stools and vitamin B$_{12}$ malabsorption develop because undigested fats and fat-soluble vitamins cannot be absorbed. Patients may present with weight loss due to maldigestion. The persistent, severe pain not uncommonly leads to an addiction to narcotics.

Diagnosis and Management

Elevated liver function tests with an increase in serum amylase and lipase occur within 48–72 hours of onset of symptoms. Abnormalities in alkaline phosphate, aspartate aminotransferase, and alanine aminotransferase also occur. Leukocytosis (15–20K) is common, along with increased blood sugar secondary to decreased insulin release. A plain frontal supine radiograph of the abdomen is taken to rule out other underlying disease. Computed tomography with contrast determines presence of neoplasm. Hydroxy iminodiacetic acid (HIDA) scans evaluate common bile duct function. An endoscopic retrograde cholangiopancreatography (ERCP) is the diagnostic tool of choice with manometry that measures pressures within the common bile duct and pancreatic duct.

Treatment

Patients are placed on nothing-by-mouth status and intravenous fluids, or a nasogastric tube is inserted if severe. Analgesics and pain management are extremely important. Antibiotics are used for necrotizing pancreatitis. A low-fat diet is prescribed. Pancreatic enzymes may be used for those with malabsorption syndrome. Abstinence from alcohol is imperative. Surgery is indicated for those with obstruction due to fibrosis or formation of cysts with the potential for rupture.

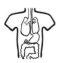

PANCREATIC CANCER

Adenocarcinoma of the pancreas is found more often in males, is relatively common, and has a high mortality rate. About 75% of cases involve the head of the pancreas, which is defined as the ampulla of Vater; the distal common bile duct; and the duodenum. This gives rise to symptoms that occur earlier than cancer of the body or tail of the pancreas, which can be well advanced before being detected.

The onset of symptoms is usually insidious. Cancer of the head of the pancreas causes obstructive jaundice and impairs digestion due to the inability of the bile and digestive enzymes to enter into the duodenum. Patients are unable to digest fats, leading to malabsorption of nutrients and weight loss. Increased blood sugar is an early sign of altered pancreatic function. Lack of

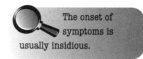

The onset of symptoms is usually insidious.

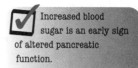

Increased blood sugar is an early sign of altered pancreatic function.

bile produces clay-colored stools. Cancer of the body or tail generally presents as diffuse, vague, epigastric pain radiating to the back and diarrhea due to the malabsorption of nutrients.

Pancreatic cancer is diagnosed based on spiral computed tomography or abdominal ultrasound and liver function tests. ERCP may be performed if all tests are negative but a high index of suspicion is present. Treatment is surgical resection of tumor if possible, chemotherapy, and pain management. It has a poor prognosis.

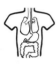

CHOLELITHIASIS

Biliary calculi, also known as *gallstones,* are very common in both sexes and all races, with their incidence increasing with age. They occur in about 20% of the population and are found in about one-third of those with sickle-cell anemia because of the repeated episodes of hemolysis. Women and the obese both have a greater incidence, because each excretes more cholesterol in the bile than do males and people of normal weight. Women with a history of multiple pregnancies are more likely to have stones because of the excessive amounts of estrogen produced by the placenta. Those on oral contraceptives are also prone because the synthetic estrogen saturates the gallbladder, increasing cholesterol production in the bile.

Gallstones are classified according to their chemical composition: cholesterol or pigmented. In the United States and Europe, most are cholesterol stones. Eighty percent to 90% of the solids in bile consist of conjugated bile salts, lecithin, and cholesterol. Both cholesterol and lecithin are insoluble in water, but the presence of bile salts with lecithin enables the cholesterol to become soluble. When this process fails, cholesterol microcrystals form and eventually become gallstones.

Figure 56-2 Types of gallstones.

Cholesterol

- Can be small or large, single or multiple, with small ones likely to enter the biliary tree, causing obstruction, pain (biliary colic), and jaundice
- More common in women >20 and men <60
- Strong association with female hormones (i.e., increased incidence with female gender, pregnancy, use of oral contraceptives)
- Increased incidence with obesity, those on crash diets, and those with hyperlipidemia syndromes

Bilirubin (Pigmented)

- Usually multiple, small, black stones that pass through the cystic duct into the common bile duct
- More common in Asians and those with chronic illnesses such as hemolytic syndromes, cystic fibrosis, and Crohn's disease

Mixed

- The most common type; usually found in large numbers
- Layers of stones form with a bilirubin nucleus surrounded by cholesterol and calcium deposits, which add on one at a time so that the size of the stone reveals something about its age

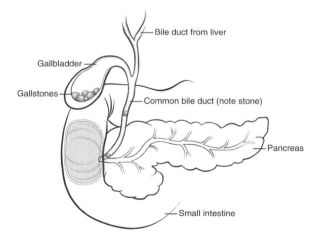

Gallstones. Note those in the gallbladder itself, the common bile duct, and at the ampule of Vater.

The stones do not in and of themselves cause symptoms, and the condition can be entirely asymptomatic and detected only on radiograph or incidental to surgery or autopsy. It is when they move into the cystic duct or common bile duct and become impacted that they cause symptoms. They cause the smooth muscle of the duct to contract in an attempt to forcefully dislodge the stone. This produces a characteristic severe right upper quadrant abdominal pain called *biliary colic.*

The gallbladder can contain one or many stones, with each being large or small. If a stone blocks the common bile duct, bile can no longer be excreted into the duodenum and accumulates in the blood, causing obstructive jaundice.

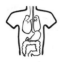

CHOLECYSTITIS

Cholecystitis is an inflammation of the gallbladder and is usually caused by an obstruction, either gallstone or tumor, that makes it impossible for bile to leave the gallbladder. The bile becomes increasingly concentrated, irritating the lining and causing inflammation. The gallbladder becomes edematous, and pain is felt in the right upper quadrant radiating to the shoulder and/or through to the back. The client develops symptoms of infection with fever, chills, nausea, and vomiting.

Treatment includes having the patient take nothing by mouth to stop the release of bile and using intravenous fluids to maintain hydration, analgesics for pain, and antibiotics for the infection. Treatment is surgical intervention to remove the obstruction. Although this can be accomplished during the acute attack, it is generally preferable to wait until the inflammation subsides before intervening surgically.

Complications of acute cholecystitis occur depending on where the obstruction occurs. Tissues die and gangrene develops without blood flow. An inflamed gallbladder can rupture, causing peritonitis. Bile can accumulate in the liver ducts, damaging liver cells and producing biliary cirrhosis.

Individuals with chronic cholecystitis have nausea and indigestion after eating fatty foods. Fat in the duodenum stimulates the gallbladder to contract and release the bile, which produces the pain described previously. Treatment is dietary to control symptoms, but surgical intervention is needed for permanent relief. Once the gallbladder is removed, bile flows directly from the liver into the duodenum, with the flow increasing when fatty foods are digested.

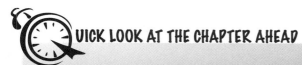
Celiac disease (also known as celiac sprue) is a malabsorption of nutrients found predominantly in whites. The etiology is unknown, but it is thought to have immunological and genetic components (10% in first-degree relatives). The incidence is approximately 1:13, and onset of symptoms varies from the first year of life to the eighth decade.

57

Celiac Disease

TERM
☐ **celiac disease**

PATHOPHYSIOLOGY

Gluten is composed of gliadin, a substance found in wheat, barley, and rye products. Celiac disease is an immune-mediated disorder that develops as a result of ingestion of those products. Those with the disease have increased levels of antibodies that have an inflammatory response manifested by loss of intestinal villi. (It is unknown whether antibodies are produced primarily or secondarily to tissue damage.) This causes malabsorption and can lead to severe malnutrition in infants and elderly. People with eating disorders who have celiac disease are especially at risk.

> This causes malabsorption and can lead to severe malnutrition in infants and elderly. People with eating disorders who have celiac disease are especially at risk.

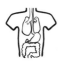

CLINICAL MANIFESTATIONS

The degree of symptoms directly corresponds to the amount of dietary gluten and intestinal changes. Diarrhea, steatorrhea, weight loss, metabolic bone disease, and decreased levels of iron and folate are common.

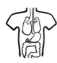

DIAGNOSIS AND TREATMENT

The hallmark of this disease is found on duodenal biopsy, which reveals abnormalities. Celiac sprue serologies and correlation of clinical presentation help in accurately diagnosing this disease. Spontaneous remission occurs in approximately 20% of the population. Most people (90%) are well controlled by eliminating gluten products from their diet. The use of rice products and rice flour and label reading are of critical importance in control of celiac disease. Glucocorticoids are used in severe refractory disease. There is an increased incidence of intestinal lymphoma and nongastrointestinal neoplasm among those who do not respond to treatment for celiac disease.

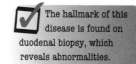

The hallmark of this disease is found on duodenal biopsy, which reveals abnormalities.

PART VIII • QUESTIONS

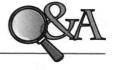

1. Where are nutrients primarily absorbed?
   a. Stomach
   b. Small intestine
   c. Large intestine
   d. They are absorbed in each of these sites.

2. Gastric secretions include all the following *except*
   a. Bicarbonate
   b. Pepsin
   c. Hydrochloric acid
   d. Mucus

3. What is the most common cause of chronic gastritis?
   a. Excessive alcohol intake
   b. Stress response
   c. *Helicobacter pylori*
   d. Pernicious anemia

4. Treatment for acute gastritis associated with stress response includes which of the following?
   a. Antacids
   b. Sucralfate
   c. Beta-blockers
   d. Foods containing lactose

5. What is the most significant factor in the development of gastric ulcers?
   a. NSAIDs
   b. *H. pylori*
   c. Excess gastric acid
   d. Spicy foods

6. Factors that protect the gastric mucosa include all the following *except*
   a. Mucus
   b. Prostaglandins
   c. Pepsin
   d. Bicarbonate

7. How does *H. pylori*, a bacterium, cause ulcers?
a. It increases production of gastric acid.
b. It causes an inflammatory response that destroys tissue.
c. It directly erodes sites in the mucosal wall.
d. All of the above.

8. What is the underlying pathology experienced by people with irritable bowel syndrome?
a. Changes in mucous cell structure
b. Excessive gastric secretions
c. Hypersensitive responses to ordinary stimuli
d. Impaired colonic reflexes

9. Which of the following statements about the relationship of IBS and psychiatric disorders is correct?
a. People with IBS have poor coping skills.
b. Women who have been sexually or physically abused may also have IBS.
c. Anxiety and depression cause IBS.
d. People with IBS often have psychiatric histories.

10. Jane S., 24, comes to the emergency room complaining of abdominal pain and bloody stools since yesterday afternoon. This has never happened to her before, and she is very alarmed. While talking with her, she remembers that her aunt and grandmother both had similar complaints at times. She says neither of them ever ate fresh fruit for that reason. She has no fever but complains that she constantly feels as if she is going to have a bowel movement regardless of how often she goes. What do you suspect she has?
a. Ulcerative colitis
b. Irritable bowel disease
c. Crohn's disease
d. Infectious diarrhea

11. Pharmacological management of Crohn's disease may include the use of which of the following?
a. Steroids
b. Antibiotics
c. Antidiarrheals
d. All of the above

12. What is thought to cause diverticulitis?
 a. Genetics
 b. Infection
 c. Environmental factors
 d. Diet

13. Which of the following is a complication of diverticulitis?
 a. Abscess formation
 b. Peritonitis
 c. Local inflammation
 d. All of the above

14. An intestinal obstruction usually results in which of the following?
 a. Massive fluid and electrolyte imbalances
 b. Life-threatening peritonitis
 c. Bowel infarction
 d. All of the above

15. Which of the following is *not* associated with a bacterial gastroenteritis?
 a. Others who have shared the same food and water source are ill with similar symptoms.
 b. The source of contamination is unwashed surfaces or undercooked food.
 c. Individuals become ill within 12 hours of ingesting the contaminated product.
 d. It is highly contagious and spreads rapidly among children and the elderly.

16. Diarrhea is always accompanied by an increase in the water content of the stools. All of the following are responsible for this *except*
 a. Increased fluid ingestion
 b. Increased fluid secretion
 c. Decreased fluid absorption
 d. Alteration in bowel motility

17. Adenocarcinoma of the esophagus is associated with which of the following?
 a. Gastritis
 b. Iron excess
 c. Alcoholism
 d. Barrett's esophagus

18. From what do colorectal cancers most often arise?
a. Ulcerated tissue
b. Adenomas
c. Lipomas
d. Diverticula

19. The liver receives blood from two sources, each with a different pressure gradient. This becomes important when the liver is not functioning properly. Which of the following is correct?
a. Hepatic artery under high pressure; portal vein under low pressure
b. Hepatic artery under moderately high pressure; portal vein under low pressure
c. Mesenteric artery under high pressure; mesenteric vein under low pressure
d. Mesenteric artery under moderately high pressure; mesenteric vein under low pressure

20. What do alanine aminotransferase and aspartate aminotransferase measure?
a. Pancreatic damage
b. Hepatic damage
c. Hepatitis antibodies
d. Gallstones

21. Jeanette tells you that several friends with whom she shared a beach house for 2 weeks a month ago have recently been diagnosed with hepatitis. She says she has been vaccinated against hepatitis and was not sexually active with anyone in this group. She asks if she is likely to get hepatitis too. How do you respond?
a. No, the vaccination will protect you.
b. No, not if you did not have unprotected sex.
c. Possibly, the source may be from shellfish or poor hand washing.
d. Possibly, but it has been a month and if you have not contracted it already, it's unlikely that you will.

22. Anitha and Vivic are a married couple. Both have hepatitis B and are now carriers of the disease. Which of the following statements about hepatitis B is *true?*
    a. Carriers cannot infect others if they are not having symptoms themselves.
    b. They probably infected each other.
    c. Their children will not be affected by their illness.
    d. They are both at risk for developing cirrhosis and carcinoma of the liver.

23. Cirrhosis may be caused by which of the following?
    a. Alcohol
    b. Hepatitis
    c. Obstruction
    d. All of the above

24. Esophageal varicosities are a result of which of the following?
    a. Ascites
    b. Portal hypertension
    c. Hepatic encephalopathy
    d. Metabolic dysfunction

25. Elevated levels of which substance produce hepatic encephalopathy?
    a. Nitrates
    b. Glucose
    c. Ammonia
    d. Albumin

26. Pancreatitis is commonly associated with which chronic disease?
    a. Multiple sclerosis
    b. Alcoholism
    c. Rheumatoid arthritis
    d. Diabetes

27. How are fatty foods digested after surgical resection for cholecystitis?
    a. By bile flowing directly from the liver into the duodenum
    b. By bile stored in the pancreatic ducts into the duodenum
    c. Fatty foods must be avoided to remain comfortable
    d. By dietary supplements or bile enzymes taken by mouth to digest fatty foods

28. A patient with a nasogastric tube is at increased risk for
   a. Chronic gastritis
   b. *H. pylori*
   c. B_{12} deficiency
   d. Stress-induced gastric ulcer

29. Altered bowel habits, bloating, and abdominal pain that occur when a person's stress level is increased are characteristic of
   a. Crohn's' disease
   b. IBS
   c. Ulcerative colitis
   d. Diverticulosis

30. *H. pylori* produce release of urease. This enzyme is necessary for
   a. Inhibition of ammonia production that decreases gastric acid
   b. Prevention of formation of adenocarcinomas
   c. Inhibition of cytokinin production
   d. Formation of B_{12}

31. Clinical manifestations of diverticulitis include
   a. Left lower quadrant pain
   b. Constipation
   c. Leukocytosis
   d. All of the above

32. Signs and symptoms of ulcerative colitis include all of the following *except*
   a. Periumbilical pain
   b. Relief with defecation
   c. Bloody diarrhea
   d. Weight loss

33. Your patient was recently diagnosed with celiac sprue. Which of the following foods would you tell her to avoid?
   a. Rice
   b. Wheat flour
   c. Nuts
   d. Fiber

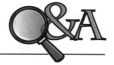

PART VIII • ANSWERS

1. **The correct answer is b.** Most nutrients are absorbed in the small intestine. The stomach helps prepare food for digestion by the action of its enzymes. The food then passes into the small intestine, where it undergoes further digestion and is absorbed by the microvilli. Water and electrolytes are absorbed by the large intestine.

2. **The correct answer is a.** The stomach is very acidic as it works to initiate digestion of proteins, fats, and carbohydrates. Bicarbonate neutralizes acid and would work against this process if it was in the stomach.

3. **The correct answer is c.** This pathogen is responsible for most chronic gastritis, peptic ulcer disease, and ultimately stomach cancers. It infects almost half of the population but is asymptomatic in most individuals and does not manifest itself until about age 60 in those who do develop symptoms.

4. **The correct answer is b.** This is a complex salt of sucrose sulfate and aluminum hydroxide. In the acid environment of the stomach, it becomes a gel-like substance that binds to both defective and normal mucosa and acts as a physical barrier to acid, pepsin, and bile acids. It also increases prostaglandin and mucus production. It has few side effects and is well tolerated.

5. **The correct answer is a.** Gastric ulcers are more common in people older than age 55 and most common in people older than age 75; these individuals frequently take large amounts of NSAIDs to control arthritis pain, making it the primary cause of ulcers. *H. pylori* are associated with peptic ulcer disease and in 90% of cases affect the duodenum. An imbalance of protective and aggressive factors, not excess stomach acid, is associated with the development of gastric ulcers. Spicy foods do not cause ulcers.

6. **The correct answer is c.** Pepsin is an enzyme that causes mucosal injury in the intestine; all of the other choices protect the mucosa.

7. **The correct answer is b.** The exact mechanism is not known, but it is thought that *H. pylori* releases toxins that produce an inflammatory response. This in turn damages tissues, allowing ulcer formation to occur.

8. **The correct answer is c.** The etiology of IBS is not known, but studies have consistently shown that those with the syndrome respond to low levels of stimuli. The response produces increased motility, spasms, bloating, and discomfort.

9. **The correct answer is b.** There is no causal relationship between psychiatric disorders and IBS. However, the central nervous system when stimulated by fear, sadness, anger, and so on produces a variety of gastrointestinal symptoms such as nausea, vomiting, diarrhea, and pain. People who experience panic attacks, have high anxiety, or are sad or fearful have their central nervous systems overstimulated for long periods of time and, as a result, are likely to have such symptoms. If they have a hypersensitive gut, they can have a recurrent and prolonged response and IBS symptoms. Women who have been assaulted have been found to have a higher incidence of IBS than the general population. This is probably due to the long-term psychological trauma caused by such assaults. This places continued stress on the central nervous system and all other body systems.

10. **The correct answer is a.** Ulcerative colitis is characterized by abrupt onset and bloody diarrhea plus abdominal pain. There is a familial tendency to develop the disease. *Tenesmus* is the term for discomfort caused by inflammation of the rectum, producing a feeling of incomplete emptying of the bowel. Some people with ulcerative colitis find that eating fresh fruits and vegetables exacerbates the symptoms.

11. **The correct answer is d.** Management of Crohn's disease includes all of those listed plus antispasmodics, immunosuppressive, and bulk agents, depending on the type and severity of symptoms.

12. **The correct answer is d.** The exact cause in unknown, but it is believed that diverticula develop in individuals with chronic constipation due to a lack of dietary fiber; hard stools require extra effort and higher intraluminal pressures for passage. This encourages a weak abdominal wall to pouch out, forming diverticula.

13. **The correct answer is d.** Any of these complications can happen depending on the size of the infection and whether or not it ruptures as a result of the inflammatory process.

14. **The correct answer is a.** Failure to move abdominal contents along results in vomiting and the inability of fluids to reach the colon, where fluid absorption occurs. Some fluids are lost through vomiting and more from inability of the body to absorb it.

15. **The correct answer is d.** Bacterial acute gastroenteritis is not contagious because it is an ingested toxin, and only those consuming contaminated food or water will become ill.

16. **The correct answer is a.** The other choices are real factors in the increased water content of diarrheal stools. Patients with diarrhea may ingest fluid, but this does not cause the problem. Eating and/or drinking often triggers additional bowel movements.

17. **The correct answer is d.** The rapid rise in esophageal cancer is due to Barrett's esophagus, which is a complication of chronic gastric esophagitis. The other choices are not associated with the development of adenocarcinoma of the esophagus.

18. **The correct answer is b.** Adenomatous polyps are considered to be the precursors of colorectal cancer. The association between the two is very strong, so screening examinations should be done routinely to excise any colonic polyps because they progress to a cancerous state within 10 years if left in place. The other choices are not generally associated with the development of colorectal cancers, although inflammatory bowel disease, particularly ulcerative colitis, is.

19. **The correct answer is a.** The liver is supplied with one-third of its blood from the hepatic artery delivered under high pressure and two-thirds from the portal vein delivered under low pressure. The mesenteric artery and vein are concerned with the blood supply for the intestines, not the liver.

20. **The correct answer is b.** These enzymes are contained in many types of tissue, including hepatic cells. They are released into the blood when hepatic tissue is injured.

21. **The correct answer is c.** Hepatitis B is the only one of the viral hepatitis viruses that has a vaccine to protect people from contracting it. Hepatitis D needs hepatitis B to exist, and if she cannot get hepatitis B, she will not get hepatitis D. Hepatitis A is transmitted by a fecal–oral route either from poor hand washing or from contaminated foods, often shellfish. The average incubation period for getting hepatitis A is 30 days, and for hepatitis C and E, it is longer. It is possible that hepatitis A is responsible for her friends' illnesses, and she may come down with it too. Symptoms may be so mild that she may not realize she is sick at all, just tired. She should go to her health care provider and be tested.

22. **The correct answer is b.** Hepatitis B is passed by sexual contact and contact with body fluid, especially blood, from infected people.

It is frequently passed at birth from mother to child, and that route produces most hepatitis B carriers. Both could have been infected as infants. Even though they are not experiencing symptoms, they can infect others, and there is a great risk they will infect children born to them.

23. **The correct answer is d.** Each of these conditions can produce cirrhosis, but by different mechanisms. Each results in the death of hepatocytes and changed liver architecture with the outcome being severely impaired liver function.

24. **The correct answer is b.** Esophageal varicosities are produced when the pressure increases within the gastrointestinal system. Collateral circulation develops to deal with blood flow. Esophageal varices are one type of collateral vessel.

25. **The correct answer is c.** Ammonia develops from the breakdown of urea and protein in the gut and the liver's inability to excrete them.

26. **The correct answer is b.** Alcohol forms plugs in the pancreatic ducts, causing edema, spasm, and the release of other enzymes. There is no association between pancreatitis and multiple sclerosis or rheumatoid arthritis. Diabetes does not cause pancreatitis, but repeated bouts of chronic pancreatitis can exacerbate diabetes.

27. **The correct answer is a.** Bile continues to be produced in the liver and flows directly into the duodenum in the presence of fats. Bile is not stored in the pancreatic ducts. Patients can eat fats in moderation. Neither dietary supplements nor bile enzymes are needed.

28. **The correct answer is d.** Nasogastric tube can increase risk of a stress-induced gastric ulcer due to continuous suctioning and presence of increased gastric acid.

29. **The correct answer is b.** Irritable bowel syndrome is characterized by periods of exacerbation and remission, and symptoms increase as a result of stress.

30. **The correct answer is a.** *H. pylori* produce urease that decomposes urea to produce ammonia. Ammonia neutralizes gastric acid, allowing the bacteria to thrive.

31. **The correct answer is d.** All answers are characteristic symptoms of diverticulitis.

32. **The correct answer is c.** Bloody diarrhea is a symptom of ulcerative colitis.

33. **The correct answer is b.** Celiac sprue is a gluten-sensitive enteropathy; therefore, all wheat products should be avoided.

Part IX

Renal System

Bernadette Madara, BC, APRN

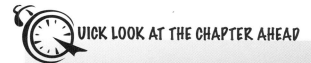

The regulation of fluid volume, blood pressure, and excretion of metabolic waste products and drug metabolites are the primary functions of the renal system. The kidneys are also responsible for conversion of vitamin D to its active form, serum pH regulation, and synthesis of hormones, such as **atrial natriuretic peptide,** erythropoietin, and renin.

58

Anatomy and Physiology of the Renal System

TERMS
- [ ] **angiotensin II**
- [ ] **atrial natriuretic peptide**
- [ ] **glomerulus**

Figure 58-1 Renal function tests.

Test	Related Physiology
BUN (blood urea nitrogen)	The end product of protein metabolism is urea, which is excreted entirely by the kidneys; therefore, the BUN is an indication of liver and kidney function
Serum creatinine	When creatinine phosphate is used in skeletal muscle contractions creatinine is formed, which is entirely excreted by the kidneys; therefore, the serum creatinine level is an indication of renal function. The creatinine level is not affected by hepatic function so it is a more precise indication of renal function than is the BUN. A 50% reduction in glomerular filtration rate (GRF) doubles the creatinine level
24-hour urine collection for creatinine clearance	Measures GFR and is dependent upon renal artery perfusion and glomerular filtration (GF)
Urinalysis	Cloudy, foul smelling, white blood cells (WBCs) ➡ urinary tract infection (UTI) Dark yellow ➡ dehydration Acetone odor ➡ diabetic ketoacidosis Presence of protein ➡ injured glomerular membrane Glucose ➡ diabetes mellitus Ketones ➡ fatty acid metabolism Crystals ➡ renal stone formation possible Many hyaline casts ➡ proteinuria Cellular casts ➡ nephrotic syndrome
Intravenous pyelogram (IVP)	IV-administered, radiopaque dye allows the visualization of the kidneys, renal pelvis, ureters, and bladder
PSA (prostatic specific antigen)	PSA is a glycoprotein found in all prostatic epithelial cells. An increase may be indicative of prostatic enlargement, thus this test is used to screen for prostatic cancer and as an indicator of treatment success/failure

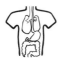

ANATOMY AND PHYSIOLOGY

Atrial natriuretic peptide, a hormone discovered in 1981, is released from muscle cells in the atria when the atrial walls are stretched. This hormone causes the vasodilation of afferent arterioles that lead into the glomerulus and efferent arterioles that lead

> ✓ The regulation of fluid volume, blood pressure, and excretion of metabolic waste products and drug metabolites are the primary functions of the renal system.

out of the glomerulus, resulting in an increased glomerular filtration rate (GFR). Atrial natriuretic peptide also inhibits aldosterone secretion and sodium reabsorption from the collecting tubules. All these actions result in increased urine production and reduced blood volume.

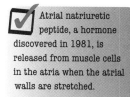
Atrial natriuretic peptide, a hormone discovered in 1981, is released from muscle cells in the atria when the atrial walls are stretched.

The hormone erythropoietin (released by the kidneys) stimulates the bone marrow to produce red blood cells in response to hypoxia from conditions such as anemia or from cardiac and/or pulmonary disease. If iron stores are adequate, an increase in red blood cells results in added oxygen-carrying capacity and reduced tissue hypoxia. As renal insufficiency progresses to renal failure, the kidneys' ability to produce erythropoietin declines, causing anemia.

 As renal insufficiency progresses to renal failure, the kidneys' ability to produce erythropoietin declines, causing anemia.

Blood pressure and blood volume are partially under the control of the renin-angiotensin-aldosterone regulatory cascade. A drop in renal blood flow stimulates the kidneys to release renin, which in turn converts angiotensinogen to angiotensin I. Angiotensin I enters the bloodstream and circulates through lung tissue, where the angiotensin-converting enzyme converts angiotensin I to **angiotensin II**, a powerful vasoconstrictor. Angiotensin II also causes the kidneys to reduce sodium and water excretion and stimulates aldosterone release, which increases sodium retention. These actions increase blood pressure, blood volume, and renal blood flow.

Vitamin D, in an inactive form, is either produced by the action of ultraviolet rays on cholesterol in the skin or is ingested. The inactive form of vitamin D is converted to the active form by the kidneys. Active vitamin D, necessary for calcium and phosphate absorption from the small intestine, helps maintain strong bone formation. People with renal disease cannot convert vitamin D to its active form.

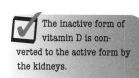
The inactive form of vitamin D is converted to the active form by the kidneys.

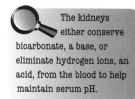
The kidneys either conserve bicarbonate, a base, or eliminate hydrogen ions, an acid, from the blood to help maintain serum pH.

The kidneys either conserve bicarbonate, a base, or eliminate hydrogen ions, an acid, from the blood to help maintain serum pH. Buffers in the urine, which combine with hydrogen ions so they can be eliminated, include bicarbonate, phosphate, and ammonia.

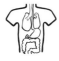

RENAL PERFUSION

The renal blood flow rate averages 20% to 25% of cardiac output or about 1,000 to 1,300 mL each minute, 600 to 700 cc of which is plasma, and the remainder of which is composed of cells. Adequate blood flow to the kidneys is required to produce a sufficient GFR and urine production. When the sympathetic nervous system is stimulated, such as occurs in a stress response, both the afferent and efferent renal arterioles constrict, producing a decrease in renal blood flow. Constriction of the afferent arteriole alone produces a reduction in renal blood flow, glomerular filtration pressure, and GFR, whereas constriction of the efferent arteriole produces an increased resistance to glomerular outflow and increases the glomerular pressure and filtration rate.

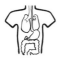

GLOMERULAR FILTRATION

The GFR is approximately 125 mL/min. The fluid that is not returned to the circulation becomes a component of urine. Daily urine production is approximately 1.5 L. Nephrons are the functional units of the kidneys, and each kidney has approximately 1.2 million nephrons. In each tubular-shaped nephron is a plasma-filtering capillary tuft created by the efferent and afferent arterioles called a **glomerulus,** which deposits its filtrate into a thin, double-walled capsule called *Bowman's capsule.* From Bowman's capsule the filtrate travels through the proximal convoluted tubule, the loop of Henle, the distal convoluted tubule, and finally the collecting tubule. The collecting tubules empty into the renal pelvis, which is drained by the ureters. The ureters then empty into the bladder.

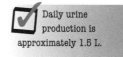

Daily urine production is approximately 1.5 L.

The role of the glomerulus is to filter plasma, and this filtering capability is controlled by capillary pressure, colloidal osmotic pressure, and capillary permeability. Approximately 125 mL of filtrate is processed each minute, although this GFR can vary from a few milliliters to a high of 200 mL/min. The proximal convoluted tubules are responsible for approximately 65% of the reabsorption and secretion functions of the tubular system. In the proximal tubules reabsorption of essential substances such as Na^+, Cl^-, HCO_3, phosphate, glucose, amino acids, and water and the secretion of H^+ ions and waste products, including drug metabolites, take place. The loop of Henle is primarily concerned with reabsorbing water, some Na and Cl, and calcium. The distal convoluted tubule reabsorbs Na^+, K^+, Cl^-, bicarbonate, urea, and water while secreting H^+ ions and K^+. The collecting duct either reabsorbs or secretes Na^+, K^+, H^+ ions, and ammonia depending on the body's requirements.

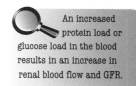

An increased protein load or glucose load in the blood results in an increase in renal blood flow and GFR.

In persons with uncontrolled diabetes mellitus, the increase in GFR results in polyuria and polydipsia.

An increased protein load or glucose load in the blood results in an increase in renal blood flow and GFR. This increased GFR allows urea, a waste product of protein metabolism, to be excreted in a timely manner. In persons with uncontrolled diabetes mellitus, the increase in GFR results in polyuria and polydipsia.

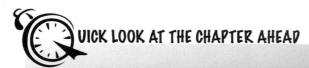
Urinary tract infections (UTIs) affect the renal system directly, whereas **hemolytic uremic syndrome (HUS)** affects the renal system indirectly. Pyelonephritis is classified as a tubulointerstitial disorder and is discussed in Chapter 64.

59

Urinary Tract Infections and Hemolytic Uremic Syndrome

TERMS
- [ ] cystitis
- [ ] hemolytic uremic syndrome (HUS)
- [ ] micturition
- [ ] pyuria
- [ ] thrombocytopenia
- [ ] urethritis

Figure 59-1 Urinary tract infection.

Urinary Tract Infection

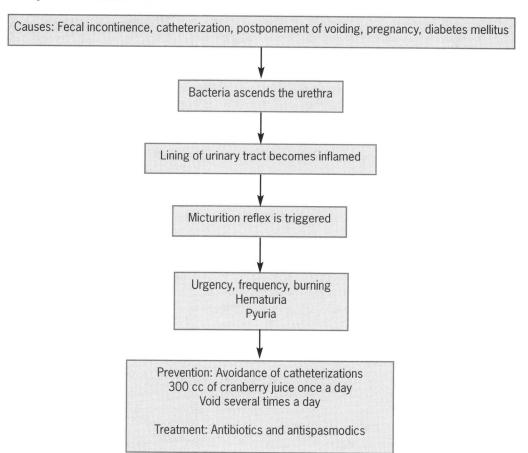

Causes: Fecal incontinence, catheterization, postponement of voiding, pregnancy, diabetes mellitus

Bacteria ascends the urethra

Lining of urinary tract becomes inflamed

Micturition reflex is triggered

Urgency, frequency, burning
Hematuria
Pyuria

Prevention: Avoidance of catheterizations
300 cc of cranberry juice once a day
Void several times a day

Treatment: Antibiotics and antispasmodics

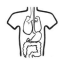

URINARY TRACT INFECTIONS

UTIs are classified as lower or upper tract infections. Upper UTIs involve the ureters and kidneys, whereas lower UTIs involve the urethra and bladder. **Urethritis** involves inflammation of the urethra, whereas **cystitis** indicates inflammation of the bladder. Lower UTIs are the second most common bacterial infections seen by doctors. It is estimated that 7 million people per year in the United States develop a UTI.

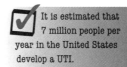

It is estimated that 7 million people per year in the United States develop a UTI.

Generally, acute UTIs are caused by a single pathogen common to the intestine (most commonly *Escherichia coli*) and are classified by the primary site affected, whereas chronic UTIs are caused by two or more pathogens. Although there are approximately 150 strains of *E. coli*, five subgroups are responsible for most UTIs. It has been estimated than 43% of women, 12% of men, 15% to 25% of the elderly living in a nursing home, and 5% to 20% of the elderly living at home will have a UTI sometime during their lifetime. Despite a long urethra, the incidence of UTI in men increases greatly with age as prostatic hypertrophy increases urinary retention and lessened bacteriostatic prostatic secretions (zinc) lower the body's defense mechanisms against infection.

Pathophysiology

Normally, a UTI is prevented by acidic urine, complete bladder emptying, a competent ureterovesical junction to prevent urine backflow, and bacteriostatic properties of the urethra and bladder. Ordinarily, the urinary tract above the urethra is sterile; therefore, if bacteria ascends the urethra and colonizes the bladder, an inflammatory process is initiated. The process of voiding routinely cleanses the bladder and urethra. Thus, anything that interferes with this process, such as outflow obstruction, postponement of voiding, pregnancy, or diabetes mellitus, increases the risk of a UTI. Use of a spermicide or diaphragms (both alter normal vaginal bacterial flora), fecal incontinence, and catheterization have also been implicated as UTI risk factors. Approximately 1% of adults who have a straight catheterization and almost 100% of patients who have an indwelling catheter develop a UTI within 3 to 4 days of catheter placement.

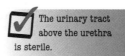

The urinary tract above the urethra is sterile.

Almost 100% of patients who have an indwelling catheter develop a UTI within 3 to 4 days of catheter placement.

Bacteria are introduced into the bladder during the catheterization procedure. The process of catheterization also causes irritation and minute scraping of the urethra, creating a portal for bacterial entry. Additionally, an indwelling catheter prevents normal flushing of the urethra by urine, and bacteria may travel to the bladder through the catheter itself or via the exudate that collects between the outside of the catheter and the urethral walls. As bacteria adhere to the catheter, they produce a protective film that covers the surface of the catheter and protects the bacteria against antibiotic action, making eradication of the infection difficult.

> As bacteria adhere to the catheter, they produce a protective film that covers the surface of the catheter and protects the bacteria against antibiotic action.

A UTI during pregnancy occurs for several reasons. During pregnancy the renal calices, pelves, and ureters dilate whereas peristaltic activity of the ureters decreases. These changes are thought to occur because of the muscle-relaxing effects of progesterone-like hormones. The enlarging uterus also causes ureteral and bladder displacement.

Signs and symptoms of a UTI commonly include lower abdominal pain, urgency, frequency, burning on urination, microscopic hematuria, offensive urine odor, and cloudy urine (i.e., **pyuria**). Frequency, urgency, and burning upon voiding occur because the inflamed lining of the urinary tract creates irritation, which triggers the **micturition** reflex.

Cystitis in the elderly may be manifested as confusion, malaise, incontinence, nocturia, lethargy, and anorexia instead of the classic signs of a UTI. Diagnostic tests that confirm a UTI include urinalysis and urine culture for bacteriuria. Over 100,000 bacterial organisms per 1 cc of blood was the former benchmark for a UTI; however, it is not essential for diagnosis. It is important to note that the degree of bacteriuria does not always correlate with the severity of the symptoms. White blood cells in the urine also signal an infection.

> Cystitis in the elderly may be manifested as confusion, malaise, incontinence, nocturia, lethargy, and anorexia instead of the classic signs of a UTI.

Management

Reduction of controllable risk factors is the primary way to prevent UTIs. Antibiotics, forcing fluids, and urinary antispasmodics are frequently used as treatments. Cranberry juice or blueberry juice has been used as a home remedy for UTIs for many years. The benefit of drinking cranberry juice lies in its ability to acidify urine, which decreases the bacteria's ability to adhere to bladder walls. Drinking 300 cc of cranberry juice daily has been shown to lessen the risk of incurring a UTI. Increasing fluid intake

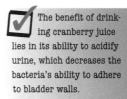

The benefit of drinking cranberry juice lies in its ability to acidify urine, which decreases the bacteria's ability to adhere to bladder walls.

before sexual activity can also lessen a UTI in a woman because voiding after intercourse removes bacteria from the bladder outlet. Screening for bacteriuria during the first prenatal visit allows for timely treatment of a UTI related to pregnancy. An untreated UTI may progress to pyelonephritis.

 An untreated UTI may progress to pyelonephritis.

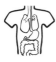

HEMOLYTIC UREMIC SYNDROME

HUS, which causes endothelial damage and coagulopathy of the kidneys, gastrointestinal system, and central nervous system, is the most common cause of acute renal failure (ARF) in children younger than 5 years. This disorder is characterized by microangiopathic hemolytic anemia, **thrombocytopenia,** and renal failure. In adults, HUS is associated with estrogen use, postpartum stage of pregnancy, delayed complication of high-dose steroid therapy, bone marrow or stem cell transplant, and nephrotoxic drugs or it may be inherited, although the exact cause is often unclear.

In contrast to noninfectious HUS, the epidemic form of HUS has an infectious etiology and is transmitted through food and person-to-person contact. Although *Salmonella typhimurium, Shigella dysenteriae,* and *Campylobacter* are associated with HUS, the most common causative organism related to HUS outbreaks is *E. coli* strain 0157:H7, which is usually transmitted via contaminated ground beef or unpasteurized milk or cheese.

 The epidemic form of HUS has an infectious etiology and is transmitted through food and person-to-person contact.

The toxin produced by the offending bacteria binds to cells on the renal, gastrointestinal, and central nervous systems. Once the toxin gains access to the inside of the cells, it prevents protein synthesis, leading to cellular death. Lipopolysaccharides produced by *E. coli* also activate the coagulation cascade, using up available platelets and putting down a fibrin network in the kidneys. As red blood cells pass through this fibrin network, they are hemolyzed. Signs and symptoms of HUS include diarrhea, which may be bloody; hemolytic anemia; renal failure; seizures; and fluid overload.

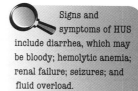 Signs and symptoms of HUS include diarrhea, which may be bloody; hemolytic anemia; renal failure; seizures; and fluid overload.

Management

Avoidance of undercooked beef and unpasteurized dairy products is the primary mode of prevention. Treatment includes blood transfusions, fluid and electrolytes, and dialysis, if needed. Antibiotics that cause *E. coli* cell death result in an additional release of toxins and therefore may not be used.

 Antibiotics that cause **E. coli** cell death result in an additional release of toxins and therefore may not be used.

Figure 59-2 Infectious hemolytic uremic syndrome.

Infectious Hemolytic Uremic Syndrome (HUS)

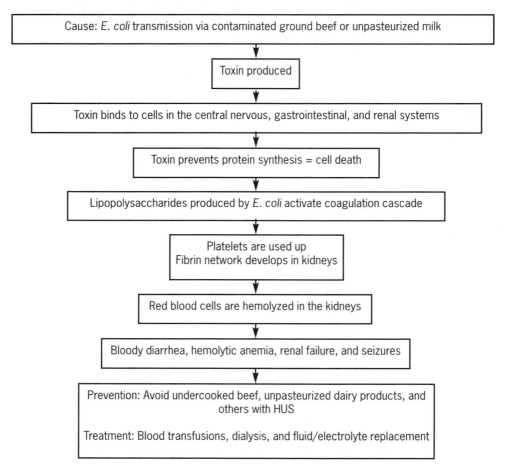

Cause: *E. coli* transmission via contaminated ground beef or unpasteurized milk

↓

Toxin produced

↓

Toxin binds to cells in the central nervous, gastrointestinal, and renal systems

↓

Toxin prevents protein synthesis = cell death

↓

Lipopolysaccharides produced by *E. coli* activate coagulation cascade

↓

Platelets are used up
Fibrin network develops in kidneys

↓

Red blood cells are hemolyzed in the kidneys

↓

Bloody diarrhea, hemolytic anemia, renal failure, and seizures

↓

Prevention: Avoid undercooked beef, unpasteurized dairy products, and others with HUS

Treatment: Blood transfusions, dialysis, and fluid/electrolyte replacement

Antibiotics = kill bacteria = release of more toxins; therefore, antibiotics are NOT generally used for HUS

Glomerulonephritis, classified as either nephritic syndrome or nephrotic syndrome, affects males more often than females and is the leading cause of chronic renal failure in the United States. Inflammatory injury to the glomeruli **(nephritic syndrome)** can occur as a result of antibodies interacting with normally occurring antigens in the glomeruli or as a result of antibody-antigen complexes that become lodged in the glomerular membrane **(nephrotic syndrome).** Chronic glomerulonephritis is the end stage of many types of glomerulonephritis, but it can also develop without a history of prior renal disease. In chronic glomerulonephritis, the kidneys are small and the glomeruli are sclerosed, leading to renal failure.

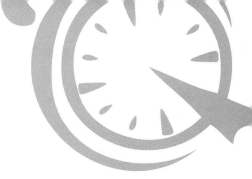

60

Glomerulonephritis

TERMS
- [ ] **azotemia**
- [ ] **glomerulus**
- [ ] **mesangial cells**
- [ ] **nephritic syndrome**
- [ ] **nephrotic syndrome**
- [ ] **plasmapheresis**
- [ ] **proteinuria**

Figure 60-1 Nephrotic syndrome and acute nephritic syndrome.

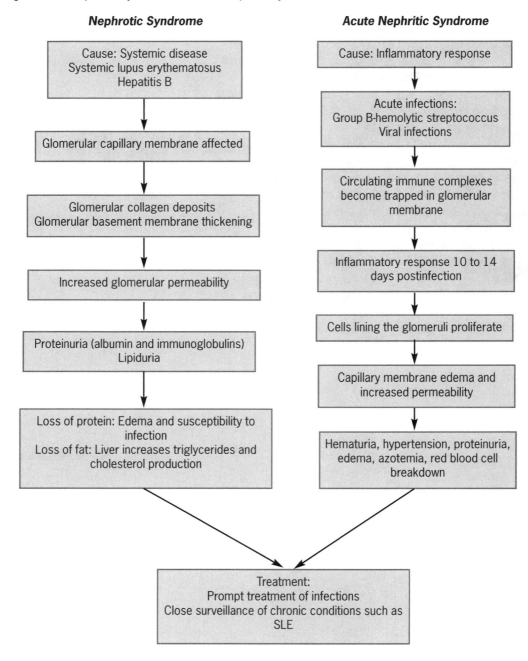

Chronic glomerulonephritis can develop without a history of prior renal disease.

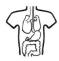

NEPHROTIC SYNDROME

Pathophysiology

Nephrotic syndrome is caused by systemic diseases such as systemic lupus erythematosus and hepatitis B, as a reaction to gold therapy, and idiopathically. This syndrome affects the glomerular capillary membrane, leading to increased glomerular permeability, secondary to collagen deposits in glomeruli and thickening of the glomerular basement membrane. **Proteinuria,** including loss of albumin and immunoglobulins, equal to or exceeding 3.5 g/day; lipiduria (i.e., fat in the urine); low serum albumin; generalized edema due to low serum colloidal osmotic pressure; and hyperlipidemia are characteristics of nephrotic syndrome. Loss of immunoglobulins increases the chance of developing infections. As a compensatory reaction to proteinuria, the body increases albumin production and the liver increases triglycerides and cholesterol production. This puts a person with nephrotic syndrome at risk for atherosclerosis. Hypercoagulability with resultant venous clot formation, especially in the renal veins, is thought to occur because of the loss of clot-inhibiting factors from the urine.

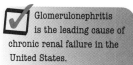 Glomerulonephritis is the leading cause of chronic renal failure in the United States.

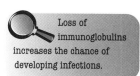 Loss of immunoglobulins increases the chance of developing infections.

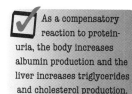 As a compensatory reaction to proteinuria, the body increases albumin production and the liver increases triglycerides and cholesterol production.

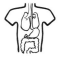

NEPHRITIC SYNDROME

Pathophysiology

Nephritic syndrome is caused by diseases such as infections that initiate an inflammatory response of the cells of the **glomerulus.** Signs and symptoms of nephritic syndrome include hematuria, urinary casts and leukocytes, low glomerular filtration rate, **azotemia,** oliguria (i.e., urine output less than 400 mL/day), and hypertension. Red blood cells spill into the urine as the glomerular capillary walls are damaged by the inflammatory process. A low glomerular filtration rate develops as a result of the change in hemodynamic pressure caused by the loss of red blood cells. As the glomerular filtration rate (GFR) drops, so does renal function, leading to azotemia, oliguria, and hypertension caused by water retention.

Acute glomerulonephritis (AG), a type of nephritic syndrome, may follow an infection caused by group B-hemolytic streptococci. Up to 8% of children who have a streptococcal infection, such as impetigo or pharyngitis, develop acute glomerulonephritis. Viral infectious agents, which cause chickenpox, mumps, and measles, may also cause acute glomerulonephritis. In acute glomerulonephritis, generalized infections result in circulating immune complexes that become trapped in the glomerular membrane and cause an inflammatory response 10 to 14 days after the initial infection. As the cells lining the glomeruli proliferate in response to the inflammatory process, the capillary membrane swells and becomes permeable. Signs and symptoms of acute glomerulonephritis include hematuria, hypertension, proteinuria, edema, azotemia,

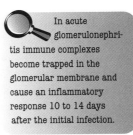

In acute glomerulonephritis immune complexes become trapped in the glomerular membrane and cause an inflammatory response 10 to 14 days after the initial infection.

and coffee-colored urine produced by red blood cell breakdown. Most children with acute glomerulonephritis recover completely, whereas 40% of adults with acute glomerulonephritis have permanent impaired renal function and possibly renal failure.

 Acute glomerulonephritis may follow an infection caused by group B-hemolytic streptococci.

 Forty percent of adults with acute glomerulonephritis have permanent impaired renal function and possibly renal failure.

The most common cause of primary nephritic syndrome in the United States is Buerger's disease, also called *IgA nephropathy.* In this type of acute glomerulonephritis, IgA and IgG immune complexes are deposited in the mesangial cells of the glomerulus. The **mesangial cells** are found between the capillary tufts and provide structural support for the glomerulus. IgA nephropathy presents as a single occurrence 50% of the time or may develop into a slowly progressing disease over several decades. Signs and symptoms of IgA nephropathy include hematuria lasting 2 to 6 days and mild proteinuria.

Rapidly progressive glomerular nephritis associated with systemic diseases such as systemic lupus erythematosus, vasculitis, and acute infections begins abruptly but rarely resolves spontaneously. In rapidly progressive glomerular nephritis, glomerular cells proliferate, macrophages are activated, and crescent-shaped structures are formed that block Bowman's capsule in the nephron. Approximately 70% of the glomeruli are affected, leading to a rapid decline in renal function. About half of the people with rapidly progressive glomerular nephritis require dialysis, and most of these people develop renal failure.

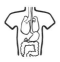

DIABETES-RELATED NEPHROTIC SYNDROME

Pathophysiology

Approximately 30% of people with type 1 diabetes mellitus develop diabetic nephropathy, which mainly affects the glomerulus, eventually producing non-nephrotic proteinuria, nephrotic syndrome, and renal failure. Diabetic nephropathy also affects people with type 2 diabetes. In diabetic nephropathy, the glomerular capillary membrane thickens, probably because of hypertension and hyperglycemia, and mesangial cells proliferate and block the capillary lumen, thereby reducing the area for glomerular filtration.

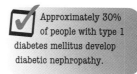

Approximately 30% of people with type 1 diabetes mellitus develop diabetic nephropathy.

Diabetic nephropathy occurs in five stages. Stage 1 is indicated by enlarged kidneys and increased intraglomerular pressure. Renal function begins to decline during stage 2. Hypertension develops and microalbuminuria is detected during stage 3. Stage 4 signals increased protein spilling into the urine and a further drop in renal function. Because the kidneys are failing, hypertension worsens. Dialysis and/or transplant is required in stage 5. Unfortunately, people with type 2 diabetes may already be in stage 3 by the time a diagnosis of diabetes is made.

> People with type 2 diabetes may already be in stage 3 by the time a
> diagnosis of diabetes is made.

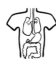

MANAGEMENT

Tight control of serum glucose and use of angiotensin-converting enzyme inhibitors can reverse early glomerular changes in diabetic nephropathy and prevent chronic renal failure. Prompt treatment of streptococcal infections with antibiotics can prevent acute glomerulonephritis.

Once glomerulonephritis has occurred, pharmacological interventions are used to manage the symptoms. Systemic steroids are given to reduce inflammation, angiotensin enzyme inhibitors prevent protein loss and slow the progression of renal failure, broad-spectrum antibiotics prevent a lingering infection, and antihypertensives maintain blood pressure at desired levels. Sodium is restricted until edema and hypertension resolve. **Plasmapheresis** has been used experimentally to remove serum immune complexes as a treatment for immune-mediated forms of glomerulonephritis.

QUICK LOOK AT THE CHAPTER AHEAD

Functional incontinence occurs in infants and young children when the bladder reaches a certain fullness. By the age of 2 or 3, a child learns to recognize the signals indicating the urge to void, and bladder training can begin. Enuresis, or bed-wetting, may last until late childhood. Children who sleep deeply may not notice the urge to void, and bed-wetting occurs. Elders with cognitive impairment may have functional incontinence.

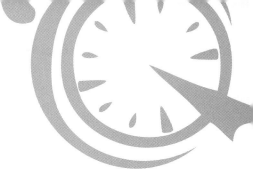

61

Micturition and Incontinence

TERMS
- ☐ chronic incontinence
- ☐ chronic overdistention
- ☐ reflex incontinence
- ☐ urge incontinence

Figure 61-1 Micturition.

Micturition

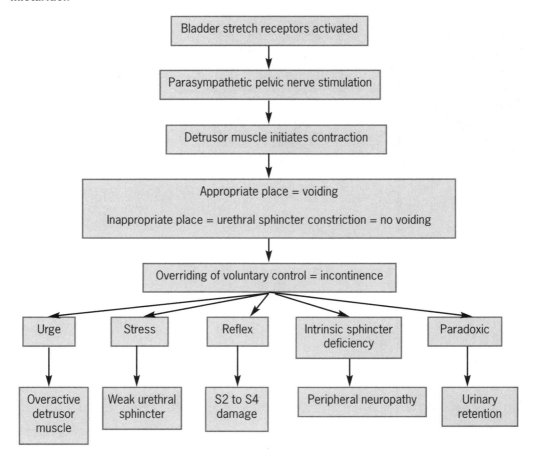

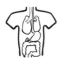

PATHOPHYSIOLOGY

As the bladder fills to between 150 and 300 cc, stretch receptors in the bladder walls are activated, creating the sensation of the need to void. Parasympathetic pelvic nerves transmit this signal to the detrusor muscle, initiating bladder contractions. The greater the amount of urine in the bladder, the stronger the impulse to micturate. Sympathetic nerve innervation of the detrusor muscle and internal sphincter prevents premature parasympathetic stimulation and maintains the muscle tone of the internal sphincter. Higher-level motor impulses inhibit the voiding reflex by constricting the urethral sphincter and delaying voiding. Generally, ignoring the urge to void prevents release of the external sphincter, and neuron fatigue delays further stimulation of the voiding reflex arc for a few minutes to 1 hour. If the urge to void continues to be ignored, bladder reflex contractions eventually take over and cause involuntary voiding. Although micturition is generally under voluntary control, an overfilled or irritated bladder causes incontinence or the involuntary passage of urine.

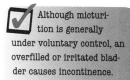

Although micturition is generally under voluntary control, an overfilled or irritated bladder causes incontinence.

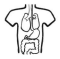

INCONTINENCE

The act of staying continent requires that a person have the motivation to do so, the ability to use toilet facilities, adequate mental functioning, and manual dexterity to manage clothing. Approximately 13 million adults over the age of 60 have either transient or chronic urinary incontinence. Complications of urinary incontinence include skin breakdown, depression, caregiver and personal stress, social isolation, and economic hardship caused by the cost of incontinence-related supplies. It is estimated that 50% of institutionalized elderly and 11% to 55% of community-dwelling elderly experience urinary incontinence. As a person ages, bladder capacity, sphincter tone, sensation, and the ability to inhibit detrusor contractions decrease, causing the involuntary passage of urine while the person is awake or, in some instances, asleep.

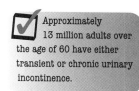

Approximately 13 million adults over the age of 60 have either transient or chronic urinary incontinence.

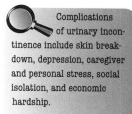

Complications of urinary incontinence include skin breakdown, depression, caregiver and personal stress, social isolation, and economic hardship.

Pathophysiology

Transient incontinence can be caused by many things, including delirium, infection, atrophic urethritis or vaginitis, medications, psychological factors, high urine output, restricted mobility, and fecal impaction.

Delirium prevents the patient from recognizing the urge to void and finding the nearest toilet. A symptomatic bladder infection leads to incontinence because the bladder and urethra are irritated. Medications such as beta-blockers, calcium channel blockers, alcohol, caffeine, and diuretics are the most common cause of transient incontinence. A severely depressed person may lack the motivation to stay continent.

Nocturia and a high nighttime urine output may occur in patients with congestive heart failure as peripheral edema is mobilized once they assume a recumbent position. The reason fecal impaction causes urinary incontinence is not known; however, once the impaction has been corrected, continence generally resumes. **Chronic incontinence** occurs when the bladder loses its ability to store urine or empty urine effectively.

> Transient incontinence can be caused by many things, including delirium, infection, atrophic urethritis or vaginitis, medications, psychological factors, high urine output, restricted mobility, and fecal impaction.

Urge incontinence, also called *instability incontinence* or *detrusor hyperreflexia,* is a type of chronic incontinence caused by inappropriate, repetitive, strong contraction of the detrusor muscle that eventually overcomes urethral sphincter control. This type of incontinence has numerous etiologies, such as central nervous system disease or damage from a brain attack (e.g., cerebrovascular accident), dementia, Parkinson's disease, and frontal lobe or cerebellum brain tumors. In urge incontinence, the detrusor muscle becomes overactive, the bladder contracts when the urge to void is felt, and the ability to postpone voiding is lost. A feeling of urgency precedes the passage of large amounts of urine, thus the name *urge incontinence.*

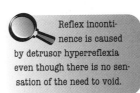

> Reflex incontinence is caused by detrusor hyperreflexia even though there is no sensation of the need to void.

Reflex incontinence is caused by trauma or damage to the nervous system as seen in spinal cord injury above S2-4, multiple sclerosis, and diabetes mellitus. Detrusor hyperreflexia occurs even though there is no sensation of the need to void. These conditions do not result in a feeling of urgency before the incontinence.

Urinary retention causes overflow incontinence (i.e., paradoxic incontinence) and involves a deficient detrusor muscle or bladder outlet obstruction. In this type of incontinence the bladder does not empty completely because of detrusor muscle malfunction, as occurs with polio and multiple sclerosis, or from blockage of the bladder outlet from conditions such as prostatic enlargement and urethral stricture. Pelvic surgery and diabetes mellitus may result in overflow incontinence because of damage to the parasympathetic innervation of the detrusor muscle. **Chronic overdistention,** also called *nurse's bladder* or *teacher's bladder,* occurs because of a perceived inability to interrupt work to void. This chronic avoidance to empty the bladder results in detrusor muscle areflexia and overflow incontinence. Symptoms associated with overflow incontinence may include urgency, frequency, nocturia, dribbling and an intermittent urinary stream, or a lack of urgency if nerve damage is present.

 Chronic overdistention, also called **nurse's bladder** or **teacher's bladder,** results in detrusor muscle areflexia and overflow incontinence.

Stress incontinence involves a weak urethral sphincter in contrast to urge incontinence and overflow incontinence, which involve the detrusor muscle. A person with stress incontinence experiences leakage of small amounts of urine with any activity that increases intraabdominal pressure, such as coughing, sneezing, or exercising. Pelvic floor relaxation, which results in the descent of pelvic organs and is associated with aging, vaginal childbirth, and obesity, has been implicated as a cause of stress incontinence. Pelvic floor relaxation causes the urethra to move out of its normal position. As a result the urethral sphincter does not sense the sudden increase in intraabdominal pressure; thus, when bladder pressure exceeds urethral closure pressure, the urethral sphincter does not close, and leaking of urine occurs.

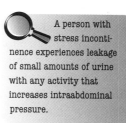 A person with stress incontinence experiences leakage of small amounts of urine with any activity that increases intraabdominal pressure.

Intrinsic sphincter deficiency (ISD) is another cause of stress incontinence. Intrinsic sphincter deficiency occurs when there is damage to the neuromuscular components of the proximal urethra or pelvic floor muscles. Conditions such as peripheral neuropathy associated with diabetes mellitus and nerve damage resulting from radical prostatectomy or transurethral resection of the prostate may result in intrinsic sphincter deficiency.

Diagnostic studies that identify the cause of incontinence include voiding cystourethrogram, urodynamic testing, cystoscopy, and urine culture.

Management

Prevention of incontinence is sometimes possible. Tight control of diabetes mellitus, for example, may prevent incontinence associated with diabetic neuropathy; not routinely delaying voiding may prevent some cases of overflow incontinence; and treatment of a urinary tract infection reverses incontinence associated with bladder wall and urethral irritation.

Other causes of incontinence cannot be avoided, but bladder retraining may be possible. Techniques used to correct incontinence include biofeedback to teach pelvic floor muscle exercises (e.g., Kegel exercises); timed voiding and habit training, which involve establishing a routine voiding schedule; and dietary modifications to reduce caffeine and alcohol, which act as diuretics.

Estrogen replacement in postmenopausal women may reduce stress incontinence. Anticholinergics and bladder smooth muscle relaxants, such as propantheline bromide and oxybutynin chloride, are used to reduce urge incontinence because they inhibit detrusor muscle contractions and increase bladder capacity. Drugs such as Sudafed (Pfizer, New York, NY) cause smooth muscle contractions of the bladder neck and help reduce stress incontinence. Urecholine (Odyssey Pharmaceuticals, East Hanover, NJ), a cholinergic receptor stimulator, increases detrusor muscle tone and is used to treat urinary retention and overflow incontinence. Doxazosin mesylate and finasteride are used to treat urinary retention caused by prostatic hypertrophy. Desmopressin acetate nasal spray, a form of vasopressin, is used to treat enuresis because it reduces urine volume by promoting water reabsorption.

Overflow incontinence can be relieved with intermittent self-catheterization. Surgical treatment of incontinence includes repairing of pelvic floor muscles, removing of the prostate gland to correct outflow obstruction (although this may result in incontinence if nerves are damaged), or implanting an artificial urethral sphincter.

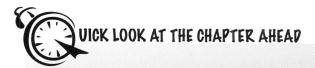

The presence of **renal calculi (urolithiasis)**, which can range in size from microscopic to several centimeters in diameter, is the most common cause of renal system obstruction. Calculi are more common in men than in women, are more likely in whites than in African Americans, and develop most frequently between the ages of 20 and 40. The most common sites for stone formation are the renal pelvis, ureters, and bladder.

Although the prostate is part of the male reproductive system rather than the renal system, some diseases of the prostate can cause prostate enlargement, with effects on the renal and urinary systems.

62

Renal Calculi and Benign Prostatic Hypertrophy

TERMS
- [ ] apoptosis
- [ ] benign prostatic hyperplasia (BPH)
- [ ] dihydrotestosterone
- [ ] extracorporeal shock wave lithotripsy
- [ ] hematuria
- [ ] hydronephrosis
- [ ] nidus
- [ ] renal calculi (urolithiasis)
- [ ] stromal cells
- [ ] struvite stones

Figure 62-1 Renal system obstruction.

Renal System Obstruction

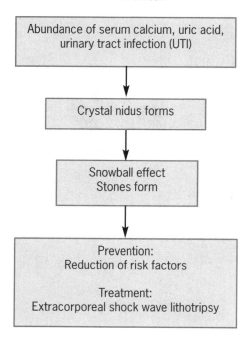

Renal Calculi

Abundance of serum calcium, uric acid, urinary tract infection (UTI)

↓

Crystal nidus forms

↓

Snowball effect
Stones form

↓

Prevention:
Reduction of risk factors

Treatment:
Extracorporeal shock wave lithotripsy

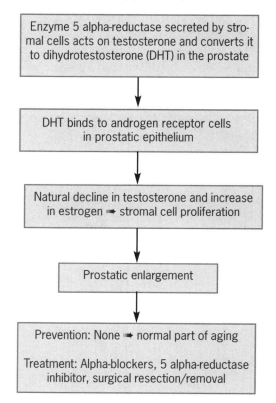

Prostatic Hypertrophy

Enzyme 5 alpha-reductase secreted by stromal cells acts on testosterone and converts it to dihydrotestosterone (DHT) in the prostate

↓

DHT binds to androgen receptor cells in prostatic epithelium

↓

Natural decline in testosterone and increase in estrogen ➡ stromal cell proliferation

↓

Prostatic enlargement

↓

Prevention: None ➡ normal part of aging

Treatment: Alpha-blockers, 5 alpha-reductase inhibitor, surgical resection/removal

Approximately 10% to 15% of individuals have renal calculi during their lifetime, with people living in the southern and midwestern United States at greatest risk for calculi development (thought to be related to high humidity levels and high temperature). Each year approximately 1 million people are hospitalized because of renal calculi and another 1 million are treated for this condition on an out patient basis.

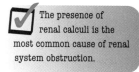 The presence of renal calculi is the most common cause of renal system obstruction.

It is estimated that over 50% of men over the age of 50 and 80% of men over the age of 70 will develop **benign prostatic hyperplasia (BPH)**, a nonmalignant enlargement of the prostate gland and a significant cause of urinary tract infection in men. This condition accounts for approximately 4 million office visits per year in the United States. The only identified risk factor thus far related to BPH is aging.

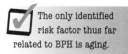

The only identified risk factor thus far related to BPH is aging.

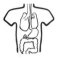

RENAL CALCULI

Pathophysiology

Renal calculi, polycrystalline aggregates of crystals, form either because of metabolic abnormalities, such as an urinary tract infection (UTI) or an aberrant urine pH. Normally, we are protected from calculi development by calculi inhibitors, including citrate, magnesium, and pyrophosphate, and endogenous compounds secreted by renal tubular cells, specifically nephrocalcin, uropontin, and Tamm-Horsfall protein.

When a nucleus (**nidus**) of crystals or organic material forms in the urinary tract and ions precipitate out of the urine and stick to the nucleus, a stone forms, much like a snowball that forms a larger and larger mass when rolled in the snow. Approximately 75% of renal calculi are calcium based, 10% are uric acid based, and 14% have a magnesium ammonium phosphate (i.e., struvite) base formed by urea-splitting bacteria associated with a UTI.

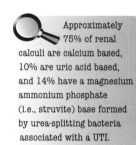

Approximately 75% of renal calculi are calcium based, 10% are uric acid based, and 14% have a magnesium ammonium phosphate (i.e., struvite) base formed by urea-splitting bacteria associated with a UTI.

Radiopaque calcium stones form because of an abundance of calcium in the blood as the result of excessive bone reabsorption secondary to immobility, bone disease, or renal tubular acidosis. Uric acid stones develop in acidic urine secondary to conditions such as gout, thiazide diuretic use, or a high-purine diet. Unlike calcium stones, they are not radiopaque and thus do not show up on x-ray.

 Uric acid stones are not radiopaque and thus do not show up on x-ray.

Struvite stones are composed of magnesium ammonium phosphate and form in alkaline urine when a UTI is present. Urease, an enzyme manufactured by bacteria, splits urea into ammonia and carbon dioxide. As the ammonia takes up a hydrogen ion, an ammonium ion is formed, which creates alkaline urine and results in an increase in urine phosphate levels. Phosphate, magnesium, and the ammonium ions then combine to form a stone, usually in the renal pelvis, often called *staghorn stones* because of their shape.

Small stones may not cause any signs and symptoms; however, large stones can block the renal pelvis or ureters. Ureteral spasms (renal colic) are intensely painful and occur when the body tries to move stones out of the ureters or urethra. Renal calculi in the renal pelvis may be asymptomatic or can cause **hydronephrosis** when the stone prevents the downward flow of urine into the bladder. Other signs and symptoms of renal calculi include **hematuria** as the result of trauma caused by sharp-edged stones, decreased urine output, and sediment or actual stones in the urine.

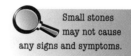

Small stones may not cause any signs and symptoms.

Management

General risk factors leading to calculi development are stasis of urine, high serum calcium or uric acid levels, vegetarian diet (changes urinary pH), high protein diet, UTI, abnormal urinary pH (urinary pH is normally around 5.85), deficiency of crystal-inhibiting factors, and low urine output. A urinary pH below 5.5 is a risk factor for uric acid stone formation, whereas a urinary pH above 7.5 is a risk factor for struvite stone formation. Dietary changes may be used to prevent the concentration of stone-forming crystals in the urine. A person with stones composed of calcium oxalate, for example, is encouraged to limit the intake of high oxalate foods such as spinach and chocolate. A person who has recurrent stone formation is encouraged to adopt a low-sodium low-protein diet. A high sodium intake increases the amounts of sodium and calcium excretion in the urine, increases the saturation of calcium phosphate, and decreases urinary citrate excretion. It also promotes increased monosodium urate saturation in the urine, which may act as a nidus for stone formation. A diet high in protein results in

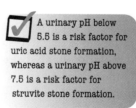

A urinary pH below 5.5 is a risk factor for uric acid stone formation, whereas a urinary pH above 7.5 is a risk factor for struvite stone formation.

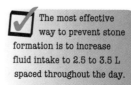

The most effective way to prevent stone formation is to increase fluid intake to 2.5 to 3.5 L spaced throughout the day.

Table 62-1 Types of Renal Stones

Type	Cause	Treatment
Calcium	Causes of renal stones include • Increased absorption of calcium from the small bowel • Hyperparathyroidism • Inability of renal tubules to reabsorb calcium • Dietary excess of calcium • Chronic bowel disease that results in steatorrhea; fat then combines with calcium and renders the calcium unable to bind to oxalate, causing stone formation	Treatment depends on the cause of the stone formation and includes • Cellulose phosphate or thiazide diuretics to decrease dietary absorption of calcium • Surgical resection of the parathyroid gland to reduce hyperparathyroidism • Thiazide diuretic therapy to correct renal tubular defects, resulting in the inability to reabsorb calcium • Purine dietary restrictions to reduce uric acid production • Increased fluid intake and treatment of chronic diarrhea
Struvite (magnesium-ammonium-phosphate)	Caused by urase-producing bacteria Urinary pH around 7.2 Usually large in size Texture is relatively soft Associated with frequent UTI More common in women	Prevention of UTI Percutaneous nephrolithotomy
Uric acid	Urine pH lower than 5.5 encourages insoluble urate salt formation Common causes of uric acid stone formation include rapid and dramatic weight loss, some malignancies	Large calculi can be dissolved by increasing the urine pH above 6.5 with potassium citrate (urate solubility salt is then increased)
Cystine	Abnormal excretion of cystine (amino acid), ornithine lysine, and arginine	Prevention: increase fluid intake and increase urine pH above 7.5

increased calcium, oxalate, and uric acid excretion, increasing the risk for stone formation. Regardless of the chemical composition of the calculi, the most effective way to prevent stone formation is to increase fluid intake to 2.5 to 3.5 L spaced throughout the day.

Small stones (under 5 mm) usually pass spontaneously, whereas larger stones may require **extracorporeal shock wave lithotripsy** in which high-frequency sound waves are directed at the stone to pulverize it. Occasionally, surgical removal may be necessary.

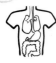

BENIGN PROSTATIC HYPERPLASIA

Pathophysiology

The exact cause of BPH is unknown, but two theories have emerged, both of which focus on the proliferation of prostatic **stromal cells** (composed of collagen and smooth muscle). One theory focuses on a hormonal cause associated with aging and the other on programmed cell death. As a man ages, the normal hormonal balance of androgens and estrogen changes as the testicular production of testosterone declines, leading to a relative increase of estrogen. In the prostate, circulating testosterone is converted to **dihydrotestosterone** (DHT) under the influence of an enzyme, 5α-reductase, secreted by stromal cells. Dihydrotestosterone then binds to androgen receptors in prostatic epithelium and promotes tissue growth. It is postulated that a naturally occurring decline in testosterone coupled with an increase in estrogen causes stromal cells proliferation, which in turn causes prostatic tissue growth. Before middle age, the balance between prostatic growth-inhibiting factors and growth-promoting factors is fairly constant. An imbalance in the factors may occur with aging, accounting for hyperplasia of the prostate gland. It is thought that stem cells in the prostate do not mature and die as programmed (**apoptosis**), resulting in an enlarged prostate gland. BPH produces a nodular growth pattern. These nodules compress the outer zones of the prostate and form a capsule. During a prostatectomy the capsule around the urethra is removed, leaving peripheral prostate tissue and capsule.

Regardless of the etiology, as the prostate enlarges it compresses the urethra, leading to outflow obstruction, stasis of urine, and UTI. Typically, a man with BPH complains of hesitancy, a weak urinary stream, frequency, dribbling, and a feeling of a full bladder. Because the bladder is constantly distended, overflow incontinence is common. Rectal examination reveals a large, palpable prostate with a rubbery surface. A uroflowmetry that records a urinary flow rate of less than 10 mL/s indicates outlet obstruction. Urinalysis shows white blood cells and microscopic white blood cells if inflammation and infection are present. Prostate size correlates poorly with symptoms. Some men with a seemingly normal-sized prostate gland have marked symptoms, whereas others with a very large prostate gland are asymptomatic.

Prostate size correlates poorly with symptoms.

Management

Prevention of BPH is not possible, although the risk for developing BPH increases if the man's father also had BPH in his fifties. Treatment is aimed at relieving bladder outlet obstruction and preserving renal function. Medications that can relieve the symptoms of BPH include alpha-blockers, such as terazosin and prazosin, which relax smooth muscle cells of the prostate and bladder neck (enhancing bladder emptying); and finasteride, a 5α-reductase inhibitor, which blocks the conversion of testosterone to dihydrotestosterone (reducing prostate size). Treatment with finasteride can reduce the size of a prostate gland by 20% to 50%.

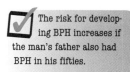 The risk for developing BPH increases if the man's father also had BPH in his fifties.

Surgical treatment includes newer, less invasive procedures, such as interstitial laser therapy, transurethral laser ablation, and balloon dilatation, and standard transurethral resection.

Table 62-2 Nonsurgical Treatment Options

Agent	Effect
Alpha-blockers	Reduces contraction of bladder neck
• Tamsulosin (Flomax)	
• Doxazosin (Cardura)	
• Prazosin (Minipress)	
• Terazosin (Hytrin)	
• Alfuzosin (Uroxatral)	
5α-Reductase inhibitors	Blocks conversion of testosterone to dihydrotestosterone—
• Finasteride (Proscar)	reduces gland size approximately 20%
• Dutasteride (Avodart)	
Phytotherapy (use of plants or	How phytotherapy acts is unknown
plant extracts)	To date, prospective, randomized, double-blind studies
• Saw palmetto berry	have failed to demonstrate the effectiveness of phytotherapy
• Bark of *Pygeum africanum*	for BPH
• Roots of *Echinacea purpurea*	
and *Hypoxis rooperi*	
• Leaves of the trembling poplar	

Table 62-3 Minimally Invasive Therapy

Technique	
Laser therapy	Two main energy sources used
Advantages	• Neodymium:yttrium aluminum garnet (Nd:YAG)
• Minimal blood loss	• holmium-YAG
• Rare occurrence of transurethral resection syndrome	• TULIP → transurethral laser-induced prostatectomy—ultrasound-guided procedure
• Outpatient treatment	• Visually directed → coagulation → requires up to 12 weeks for tissue sloughing to complete
Disadvantages	
• Lack of tissue for pathological exam	
• Longer post-op catheterization	
• Irritation when voiding	
• Equipment expense	
TUNA (transurethral needle ablation)	Urethral approach Tissue heated and necrosis results
Transurethral electrovaporization of the prostate	Tissue vaporized in response to heat
Hyperthermia	Microwave hyperthermia technique destroys tissue
HIFU (high-density forced ultrasound)	Short bursts of high-energy ultrasound delivered to the tissue—heats tissue and results in coagulative necrosis
Intraurethral stents	Placed in the prostatic fossa to keep it patent
Transurethral balloon dilation	Most effective if the enlargement is small—rarely used

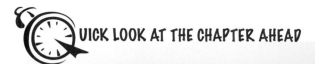
Renal failure is classified as acute or chronic. **Acute renal failure (ARF)** (now frequently called "acute kidney injury") has a mortality rate of 10% to 60%, begins abruptly, and is characterized as a sudden decline in renal function resulting in the inability to maintain fluid and electrolyte balance and excretion of waste products. ARF is generally reversible, whereas **chronic renal failure (CRF)** has an eventual mortality rate of 100% (without dialysis and/or renal transplantation), is irreversible, and results in a slow, steady decline of renal function. This chapter discusses the pathophysiology and treatment for acute and chronic renal failure.

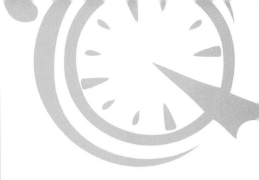

63

Renal Failure

TERMS
- [ ] acute renal failure (ARF)
- [ ] acute tubular necrosis (ATN)
- [ ] chronic renal failure (CRF)
- [ ] glomerulosclerosis
- [ ] intrarenal ARF
- [ ] postrenal ARF
- [ ] prerenal ARF
- [ ] renal insufficiency
- [ ] renal osteodystrophy
- [ ] uremic frost

Figure 63-1 Renal failure.

Renal Failure

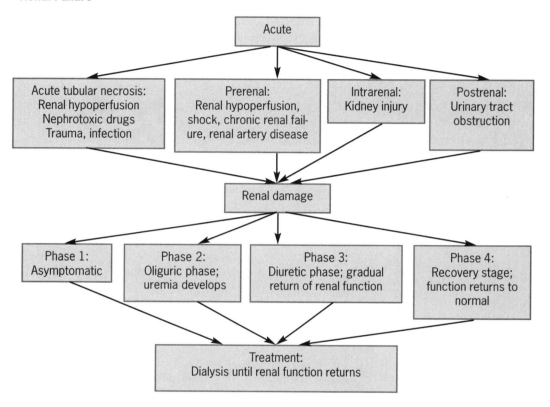

Prevention of ARF depends in part on limiting one's exposure to nephrotoxic agents and prevention and prompt treatment of shock, especially in the elderly and people with renal insufficiency. CRF can be avoided with tight control of hypertension and diabetes; genetic counseling for persons with polycystic renal disease, which is an inheritable cause of renal failure; and prompt treatment of ARF.

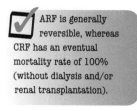
ARF is generally reversible, whereas CRF has an eventual mortality rate of 100% (without dialysis and/or renal transplantation).

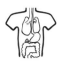

ACUTE RENAL FAILURE

Pathophysiology

Approximately 10,000 people develop ARF each year. It has been estimated that 5% of hospital admissions, 30% of clients in critical care units, and 25% of all hospitalized patients develop ARF.

> It has been estimated that 5% of hospital admissions, 30% of clients in critical care units, and 25% of all hospitalized patients develop ARF.

Acute tubular necrosis (ATN), one cause of ARF, occurs because of renal hypoperfusion or in response to nephrotoxic drugs, such as aminoglycosides, and chemicals, such as radiological dyes, which set up an inflammatory process leading to tubular edema, obstruction, and ischemia. Up to 12% of patients exposed to radiocontrast agents develop ATN. Other causes of ATN are major trauma, systemic infections, and muscle breakdown, which produces myoglobin, a substance that clogs renal tubules. Damaged tubules result in a decreased ability to maintain homeostasis. ATN usually resolves in about 8 weeks.

 Up to 12% of patients exposed to radiocontrast agents develop ATN.

The factors that instigate **prerenal ARF** (i.e., factors that occur before blood being filtered by the kidneys) are caused by renal hypoperfusion and account for approximately 40–80% of ARF cases per year. Prerenal factors include those that cause decreased cardiac output such as shock and congestive heart failure, volume depletion from vomiting, or increased renal vascular resistance as occurs in renal artery stenosis. If perfusion can be restored in a short amount of time, permanent renal damage can be averted. In prerenal ARF, urine osmolality is high and urine sodium is low, because although renal perfusion is greatly decreased, renal tubular function is normal.

Intrarenal ARF results from injury to the kidney itself from emboli or ATN. Sodium cannot be conserved and urine cannot be concentrated because of glomerular damage. **Postrenal** or obstructive **ARF** results from urinary tract obstruction by renal calculi or prostatic enlargement; thus urine osmolarity and sodium levels are usually unaffected.

ARF has four phases. In the initial phase the patient may be asymptomatic, although renal damage is occurring. During the oliguric phase,

which lasts a few days to a few weeks, impaired glomerular filtration causes solute and water reabsorption, urine output declines to 400 cc or less per day, and serum waste products cannot be removed. As the patient becomes symptomatic, a condition known as uremia (i.e., urine in the blood) develops. Neurotoxicity from uremia causes an altered mental status and altered peripheral sensation. Electrolyte imbalance causes dysrhyth-
mias, water retention may lead to congestive heart failure and hypertension, and meta-
bolic acidosis may develop because of the kidney's inability to excrete hydrogen ions. In addition to anemia caused by decreased

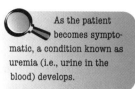

As the patient becomes sympto-
matic, a condition known as uremia (i.e., urine in the blood) develops.

erythropoietin production, blood loss may be caused by gastrointestinal bleeding secondary to platelet and protein anticoagulant dysfunction.

 In the initial phase, the patient may be asymptomatic although renal damage is occurring.

During the third phase, or the diuretic phase, which lasts days to weeks, there is a gradual return of renal function because of cellular regeneration and healing. Excessive urine output leading to dehydration and electrolyte imbalance may occur during this stage because of incompetent tubular transport of water and solutes. The fourth and final stage is the recovery stage during which glomerular function gradually returns to normal. The recovery stage may take 3 to 12 months.

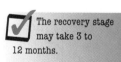

The recovery stage may take 3 to 12 months.

Table 63-1 Signs and Symptoms of ARF

Nausea	Vomiting
Malaise	Anemia
Pericardial effusion	Pericardial friction rub
Cardiac tamponade	Dysrhythmias → peaked T waves, QRS widening, prolonged PR interval
Hyperkalemia	Abdominal pain and ileus
Platelet dysfunction → bleeding	Asterixis and confusion, possible seizures
Elevated blood urea nitrogen and creatinine	High serum phosphorus, low serum calcium

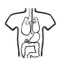

CHRONIC RENAL FAILURE

Pathophysiology

In CRF, renal function steadily declines as nephrons are replaced with scar tissue. **Renal insufficiency** denotes a 20% to 50% reduction in the glomerular filtration rate. When renal function in each kidney is reduced by 50%, signs and symptoms of mild azotemia (i.e., buildup of nitrogenous waste products in the blood), polyuria, nocturia, hypertension, and anemia become apparent. The term *renal failure* is used when the glomerular filtration rate drops to 20% to 25% of normal. During renal failure uremia (symptom complex indicating multiple organ system dysfunction) is apparent along with fluid and electrolyte imbalances. When the glomerular filtration rate drops from a normal level of 125 mL/min to less than 10 mL/min, the kidney's loss of ability to maintain its homeostatic functions occurs, denoting the destruction of 90% of the nephrons and the onset of end-stage renal disease (ESRD).

Approximately 20 million Americans (one in nine adults) have chronic renal disease, including 500,000 people in ESRD, with men, African Americans, and Native Americans affected more often than women and whites. Diabetes and hypertension cause 70% of ESRD cases. Other major causes of ESRD include sickle-cell disease, glomerulonephritis, and polycystic kidney disease.

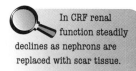

In CRF renal function steadily declines as nephrons are replaced with scar tissue.

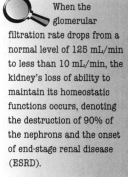

When renal function in each kidney is reduced by 50%, signs and symptoms of mild azotemia, polyuria, nocturia, hypertension, and anemia become apparent.

When the glomerular filtration rate drops from a normal level of 125 mL/min to less than 10 mL/min, the kidney's loss of ability to maintain its homeostatic functions occurs, denoting the destruction of 90% of the nephrons and the onset of end-stage renal disease (ESRD).

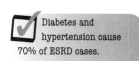

Diabetes and hypertension cause 70% of ESRD cases.

ESRD is the result of glomerulosclerosis, tubulointerstitial injury, and/or vascular injury. **Glomerulosclerosis** is the progressive hardening of the glomerular capillaries. This process of epithelial and endothelial injury results in protein spilling into the urine. Tubulointerstitial injury causes the loss of tubular transport functions as the tubules become inflamed, edematous, and necrotic. Vascular injury to renal blood vessels causes ischemia and damage to renal tissue.

Clinical signs and symptoms of CRF develop slowly and are similar to those of ARF but include additional effects of long-term uremia such as renal osteodystrophy, malnutrition, pruritus, peripheral neuropathy, and altered reproductive functioning. **Renal osteodystrophy**, or demineralization of bone, has three major causes. First, the kidneys lose their ability to activate vitamin D, which results in decreased absorption of calcium from food. Second, there is a decreased excretion of parathyroid hormone, which leads to demineralization of bones and teeth. Third, there is retention of phosphate, which leads to increased renal excretion of calcium.

Malnutrition occurs because of anorexia, malaise, dietary protein restriction, and proteinuria. Dietary protein is restricted in an attempt to reduce the protein load on the kidneys. Hypoalbuminemia causes fragile capillaries, poor wound healing, and decreased immune system function, which increases susceptibility to infections.

Retained serum toxins cause a dermal inflammatory process and pruritus. The skin may have a grayish-yellowish cast because of the buildup of urinary pigments. **Uremic frost** occurs when the body attempts to rid itself of uric acid and other toxins through sweat.

Restless leg syndrome (i.e., spontaneous movement of the feet and legs), altered sensation, weakness, and diminished deep tendon reflexes occur because of neurotoxicity caused by uremia. An alteration in hormone levels causes a lack of ovulation and menstruation, the inability to carry a fetus to term, impotence, and decreased sperm counts.

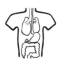

MANAGEMENT

ARF is treated by dialysis until renal function returns. CRF is treated by conservative management of renal insufficiency and then by dialysis or renal transplantation as needed. Conservative management aimed at retaining as much renal function as possible includes a protein-restricted diet and control of hypertension. Anemia has been successfully treated with recombinant human erythropoietin (i.e., Epogen®, Amgen Inc., Thousand Oaks, CA). Dietary restriction of phosphates and the administration of phosphate-binding antacids and activated vitamin D and calcium have been shown to reduce osteodystrophy. Metabolic acidosis is treated with sodium bicarbonate. Salt and water restriction, along with antihypertensives, may be necessary to control hypertension.

Table 63-2 Complications of CRF

System	Etiology	Treatment
General appearance	Tired, weak, sallow skin color due to anemia, toxins	Dialysis, Epogen®
Integumentary	Itching (uremic frost) occurs in an attempt to remove toxins from the body	Dialysis and palliative care
Sensory	Metallic taste in mouth, fishy breath odor (uremic fetor) due to toxins	Dialysis
Cardiopulmonary	Hypertension • Related to salt and water retention, erythropoietin (20% of patients on this therapy), or increased renin production • Accelerated renal damage if not controlled • Congestive heart failure develops	• Limiting salt and fluids • Angiotensin-converting enzyme inhibitors (ACE), angiotensin II receptor blockers, calcium channel blockers, beta-blockers • Blood pressure goal is 130/80 mm Hg
	Pericarditis • Result of metabolic toxins • Chest pain, fever, friction rub, decreased cardiac output	• Hemodialysis
	Congestive heart failure (75% of patients needing dialysis) • Result of increased workload of the heart (left ventricular hypertrophy) secondary to anemia, dialysis (shunting of blood), fluid overload, hypertension, atherosclerosis	• Salt and fluid restriction • Diuretics (Loop) • Angiotensin-converting enzyme inhibitors, angiotensin II receptor blockers
Hematological	Coagulopathy • Platelet dysfunction due to abnormal aggregation and "stickiness" • Bleeding time increases • Platelet count slightly decreased • May have petechiae or purpura	• Desmopressin (causes release of factor VIII from endothelial cells)—used before surgery
	Anemia • Related to decreased erythropoietin production (occurs when glomerular filtration rate falls below 20–25 mL/min) and iron deficiency • Hemodialysis causes some red blood cell destruction	• Epogen® if hematocrit is below 33% (hemoglobin levels should increase no more than 1 g/dL every 3–4 weeks so hypertension does not develop) • Intravenous iron for patients on dialysis (PO absorption poor)
Gastrointestinal	Anorexia, nausea, vomiting, hiccups—related to metabolic toxins	Dialysis
Endocrine	Decreased libido, impotence, and infertility • Decreased estrogen levels in women—do not ovulate • Decreased testosterone levels in men	• Dialysis and a healthy diet may restore fertility
	Glucose intolerance • Peripheral insulin resistance Serum insulin high • Kidneys cannot clear insulin from bloodstream	• Patients with diabetes may require lower doses of hypoglycemic agents

(continued)

Table 63-2 *Continued.*

Mineral metabolism	Renal osteodystrophy (disorder of calcium, phosphorus, and bone) leading to bone pain, fractures, muscle weakness, calcium deposits in blood vessels, soft tissue, heart and lungs	
	• Low glomerular filtration rate = phosphorus excretion slowed so calcium excretion increases → parathyroid hormone secretion rises and causes a high bone turnover • In ESRD, excess hydrogen ions are buffered by leeching large stores of calcium phosphate and calcium carbonate from the bones = bone demineralization	• Restrict dietary phosphorus • Administer phosphorus-binding drugs such as calcium carbonate • Vitamin D (suppresses parathyroid hormone)
Neurological	Uremic encephalopathy • Appears when glomerular filtration rate falls below 10–15 mL/min or by hyperparathyroidism • Symptoms: poor concentration (first sign) and progresses to confusion, asterixis, weakness, nystagmus, hyperreflexia • Peripheral neuropathy (restless leg syndrome, distal pain, loss of deep tendon reflexes) • Impotence and autonomic dysfunction	• Dialysis
Metabolic	Hyperkalemia • Glomerular filtration rate falling below 10–20 mL/min • Hemolysis, trauma, acidosis • Diet high in citrus fruits/juices • Medications such as angiotensin-converting enzyme inhibitors, NSAIDs	• Monitor cardiac status • Administer calcium chlorides, insulin, and glucose (insulin moves K into cells), bicarbonate or an exchange resin • Dietary K restriction
Acid–base disorders	Damaged kidneys • Cannot produce enough ammonia or buffer hydrogen ions • Arterial pH generally between 7.33 and 7.37 • Excess hydrogen ions are buffered by large stores of calcium phosphate and calcium carbonate from the bones	• Maintain serum bicarbonate above 21 mEq/L by giving alkali supplements such as sodium bicarbonate, calcium bicarbonate, or sodium citrate

NSAIDs, nonsteroidal antiinflammatory drugs.

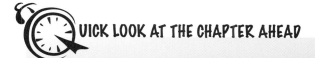

Renal disorders that affect the proximal and distal tubules and sometimes the tissue surrounding the tubules are termed **tubulointerstitial disorders.** These disorders, which include **renal tubular acidosis**, pyelonephritis, and drug-related nephropathies, may be acute or chronic in nature. Acute disease produces an abrupt onset of signs and symptoms, whereas chronic disorders result in fibrosis and atrophy of nephrons. Early signs of tubulointerstitial disorders include signs and symptoms of fluid and electrolyte imbalance such as nocturia, polyuria, and metabolic acidosis.

64

Tubulointerstitial Disorders

TERMS
- [ ] **casts**
- [ ] **pyelonephritis**
- [ ] **renal tubular acidosis**
- [ ] **tubulointerstitial disorders**

Figure 64-1 Renal tubular acidosis.

Renal Tubular Acidosis

Proximal tubule defects:
Loss of bicarbonate and sodium
Hypovolemia
Increased aldosterone secretion
Hypokalemia

Distal tubule defects:
Inability to excrete hydrogen ions
Loss of sodium and bicarbonate
Hypovolemia
Increased aldosterone secretion
Hypokalemia
Increased parathyroid production
Osteomalacia
Renal calculi
Growth retardation

Prevention: Prompt diagnosis of urinary
tract infection (UTI)

Treatment: Replacement of bicarbonate
reverses the other electrolyte losses

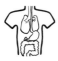

RENAL TUBULAR ACIDOSIS

Pathophysiology

Proximal tubular defects hinder bicarbonate reabsorption, whereas distal tubular defects result in a reduction of the secretion of metabolic acids. Both lead to metabolic acidosis, bone disease, renal calculi, and growth retardation in children.

 Early signs of tubulointerstitial disorders include signs and symptoms of fluid and electrolyte imbalance such as nocturia, polyuria, and metabolic acidosis.

Because the proximal tubules are where 90% to 95% of filtered bicarbonate is reabsorbed, defects affecting this area result in a loss of bicarbonate and sodium into the urine. Associated with the loss of bicarbonate and sodium is a reduction of serum bicarbonate levels, hypovolemia, increased aldosterone secretion, and hypokalemia. The distal tubules

Table 64-1 Types of Renal Tubular Acidosis

Type	Characteristics	Etiology
Type I (classic distal renal tubular acidosis)	• Hypokalemic hyperchloremic metabolic acidosis • Alkaline urine • Hypercalciuria • K excretion • Hyperaldosteronism • Renal calculi formation	• Selective deficiency in hydrogen ion secretion of cells in the collecting tubules • Autoimmune disease • Drugs/toxins, i.e., amphotericin B
Type II (proximal renal tubular acidosis)	• Hypokalemic hyperchloremic metabolic acidosis • Bicarbonate is not reabsorbed by the proximal tubule • Distal nephron tries to reabsorb some bicarbonate but becomes overwhelmed by the bicarbonate load and does not function adequately • As bicarbonate is lost in the urine, the serum bicarbonate level falls and the distal nephron can again reabsorb some bicarbonate	• Selective defects in the proximal tubule inhibit reabsorption of bicarbonate • May be caused by carbonic anhydrase inhibitors • Multiple myeloma • Nephrotoxic drugs
Type IV* (hyporeninemic [low levels of renin in plasma] hypoaldosteronemic renal tubular acidosis)	• Most common form of renal tubular acidosis • Hyperkalemic, hyperchloremic acidosis	• Aldosterone deficiency—impairs distal nephron sodium reabsorption and potassium and hydrogen ion excretion • Diabetic nephropathy • Hypertensive nephrosclerosis • Acquired immunodeficiency syndrome

*A type III does not exist.

continue to function and excrete metabolic acids. Eventually, the proximal tubules regain enough function to reabsorb a small amount of bicarbonate.

Distal tubular defects, in contrast, result in a decreased ability to excrete hydrogen ions into the urine with a concomitant loss of sodium and bicarbonate. As in proximal tubular defects, hypovolemia results, leading to increased aldosterone secretion and hypokalemia. In an attempt to buffer the rising serum hydrogen ions, calcium is leeched from the

> Because the proximal tubules are where 90% to 95% of filtered bicarbonate is reabsorbed, defects affecting this area result in a loss of bicarbonate and sodium into the urine.

bones. As calcium is excreted in the urine, the production of parathyroid hormone occurs, leading to osteomalacia, bone pain, renal calculi, and impaired growth in children.

Management

Prompt treatment of a urinary tract infection may help prevent tubular defects. Treatment of proximal and distal tubular defects is focused on replacement of bicarbonate, which then leads to a return of Na^+ and K^+ balance.

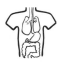

PYELONEPHRITIS

Pathophysiology

Pyelonephritis, an upper urinary tract infection and inflammatory disorder of the renal pelvis and parenchyma classified as a tubulointerstitial disorder, can be acute or chronic. Females over the age of 50 are more likely to develop pyelonephritis than females under the age of 50. Risk factors include renal calculi; presence of an indwelling urinary catheter; diabetes mellitus, which lowers resistance to infection; and catheterization. In children, a condition called vesicoureteral reflux, which moves urine from the bladder back to the kidneys, is associated with pyelonephritis. In adults, a risk factor for developing pyelonephritis is bladder outflow obstruction resulting from calculi, tumors, or prostatic hypertrophy.

> Risk factors include renal calculi; presence of an indwelling urinary catheter; diabetes mellitus, which lowers resistance to infection; and catheterization.

Acute pyelonephritis is caused by a bacterial infection that travels from the urethra to the kidney or from bloodborne bacteria. It generally involves patchy foci of infection and sometimes small areas of localized abscess formation; however, the glomeruli are spared from major damage. Gram-

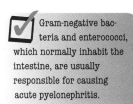

Gram-negative bacteria and enterococci, which normally inhabit the intestine, are usually responsible for causing acute pyelonephritis.

negative bacteria and enterococci, which normally inhabit the intestine, are usually responsible for causing acute pyelonephritis.

Signs and symptoms of acute pyelonephritis include abrupt onset of dull, constant flank pain or back pain, fever and chills, and other signs of infection, such as malaise and headache. Symptoms of bladder irritation such as urgency, frequency, and burning are common. Urinalysis may reveal **casts**, which are clumps of cells that form in the collecting tubules and are shed in the urine because they are indicative of an inflammatory process. Bacteria in the urine above 100,000/mL and elevated serum neutrophil count indicate infection. Untreated acute pyelonephritis can lead to septic shock, abscess formation, and/or chronic pyelonephritis.

In contrast to acute pyelonephritis, chronic pyelonephritis is a progressive process. Chronic pyelonephritis is associated with recurring acute bacterial or nonbacterial infections or, most commonly, an autoimmune process involving the kidneys. Inflammation, fibrosis, and scarring of the tubules occur, which results in renal tissue destruction. Approximately 11% to 20% of end-stage renal disease is caused by chronic pyelonephritis.

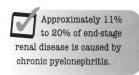
Approximately 11% to 20% of end-stage renal disease is caused by chronic pyelonephritis.

A person with chronic pyelonephritis may be asymptomatic or have some of the signs and symptoms associated with acute pyelonephritis. Polyuria and nocturia occur as the kidneys lose their ability to concen-

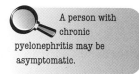
A person with chronic pyelonephritis may be asymptomatic.

trate urine. Hypertension may develop as the disease progresses. An intravenous pyelogram detects a change in kidney size and function.

Management

Prevention of acute pyelonephritis can be accomplished by avoiding the risk factors associated with its development. Of primary importance is prevention of lower urinary tract infections. In women, wiping from front to back after a bowel movement prevents spread of fecal bacteria to the urinary tract. Therapy for acute pyelonephritis includes antibiotics, hydration, and urinary analgesics. The treatment of chronic pyelonephritis is aimed at removing the underlying cause to prevent renal damage. Surgery to correct structural defects associated with outflow problems is indicated.

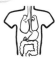

DRUG-RELATED NEPHROPATHIES

Pathophysiology

Several classes of drugs can cause functional and structural changes in the kidneys, especially in the elderly. Tubulointerstitial nephritis is caused by a hypersensitivity reaction to commonly prescribed drugs such as sulfonamides, methicillin, and other synthetic antibiotics, Lasix, and thiazide diuretics. It takes from 2 to 40 days after exposure to the offending drug for signs and symptoms of nephritis, including fever, hematuria, mild proteinuria, rash, and eosinophilia, to appear. Half of those with tubulointerstitial nephritis develop acute renal failure. Most people fully recover once the drug is stopped.

 Several classes of drugs can cause functional and structural changes in the kidneys, especially in the elderly.

 It takes from 2 to 40 days after exposure to the offending drug for signs and symptoms to appear.

Prostaglandins help to regulate tubular blood flow. Nonsteroidal antiinflammatory drugs (NSAIDs) inhibit prostaglandin synthesis and thereby cause renal damage in some individuals. The elderly, people with renal insufficiency and/or disease, and those who are dehydrated are at greatest risk from developing NSAID-related renal damage.

The elderly, people with renal insufficiency and/or disease, and those who are dehydrated are at greatest risk from developing NSAID-related renal damage.

Management

Avoidance of drugs known to cause renal damage, especially in the elderly and those with renal insufficiency, and adequate hydration are ways to prevent drug-induced renal pathology.

Figure 64-2 Pyelonephritis.

Pyelonephritis

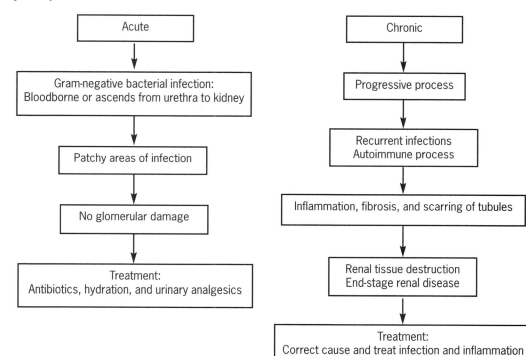

PART IX · QUESTIONS

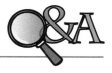

1. Which of the following is a major function of the kidneys?
   a. Converting vitamin D to the active form
   b. The proliferation of leukocytes
   c. Converting angiotensin I to angiotensin II
   d. Producing antibodies

2. Which of the following laboratory results would give the nurse the best information concerning a patient's renal function?
   a. Blood urea nitrogen
   b. Serum creatinine
   c. Urinalysis
   d. Red blood cell count

3. Which of the following statements about urinary tract infections (UTIs) is *true?*
   a. UTIs are more common in men than in women.
   b. UTIs frequently result from highly acidic urine.
   c. UTIs are prevented by voiding.
   d. UTIs occur in 70% of patients with an indwelling catheter.

4. A nurse explains hemolytic uremic syndrome (HUS) to the parents of a child with the disorder. Which of the following statements is *true?*
   a. Antibiotics are the treatment of choice for HUS.
   b. Seizure activity is a symptom of HUS.
   c. HUS is spread by dairy products.
   d. HUS is caused by *S. alternans.*

5. The pathology of the nephrotic syndrome includes which of the following?
   a. Thickening of the basement membrane and glomeruli collagen deposits
   b. Glomeruli damage by group B hemolytic streptococci
   c. IgA hyperactivity
   d. Glomerular proliferation

6. The treatment plan for a patient with glomerulonephritis includes which of the following?

   a. Blood transfusions to correct anemia

   b. A high protein diet to restore albumin levels

   c. Potassium restriction to correct electrolyte imbalance

   d. Systemic steroids to reduce inflammation

7. Stretch receptors in the bladder are initially stimulated when the bladder fills to

   a. 150 cc

   b. 400 cc

   c. 550 cc

   d. 600 cc

8. Which of the following causes urge incontinence?

   a. Damage to the spinal cord at the level of S2-4

   b. Urinary retention

   c. An overactive detrusor muscle

   d. A weak urethral sphincter

9. Which of the following statements about struvite renal calculi is *true?*

   a. Struvite calculi are caused by an abundance of calcium in the blood.

   b. Struvite calculi may result from a UTI.

   c. Struvite calculi are more common when the urine is acidic.

   d. Struvite calculi are frequently composed of uric acid.

10. When explaining finasteride to a patient, the nurse stresses which of the following?

   a. It can reduce the size of the prostate gland by 50% to 75%.

   b. It is an estrogen supplement associated with reduction in prostate size.

   c. It causes the proliferation of stromal cells in the prostate.

   d. It blocks the conversion of testosterone to dihydrotestosterone, thereby reducing prostate size.

11. Which of the following is *true* about acute renal failure (ARF)?

   a. ARF usually progresses to chronic renal failure.

   b. ARF initially produces profuse urine with a low specific gravity.

   c. ARF may take 1 year to resolve.

   d. ARF is commonly caused by radiological dyes.

12. Renal insufficiency develops when the glomerular filtration rates drop by which of the following percentages?
a. 10%
b. 30%
c. 60%
d. 90%

13. A patient with renal tubular acidosis exhibits
a. An imbalance of bicarbonate levels
b. Hyperglycemia
c. Fluid retention
d. Hypernatremia

14. Signs and symptoms of drug-related nephropathy include which of the following?
a. Cardiac dysrhythmia
b. Subnormal body temperature
c. Bradycardia
d. Rash

15. ANP has several functions including (select all that apply)
a. Vasoconstriction of arteries
b. Slowing the glomerular filtration rate
c. Inhibition of aldosterone secretion
d. Inhibition of Na^+ reabsorption

16. Angiotensin I is converted to angiotensin II in the
a. Kidneys
b. Lungs
c. Gastrointestinal tract
d. Atria

17. The nurse teaching a class on renal function stresses that a high protein diet
a. Results in a high urine output
b. Decreases renal blood flow
c. Causes polydipsia
d. Decreases the glomerular filtration rate

18. The nurse conducting a community education program in an adult health clinic is asked how someone can develop a urinary tract infection. The nurse correctly responds (select all that apply)
    a. "Pregnant women may develop a UTI because their bladder does not empty completely as the baby grows."
    b. "Ignoring the urge to void and 'holding' urine for a long time can cause a UTI."
    c. "Drinking large amounts of an acidic juice like cranberry juice can cause a UTI."
    d. "Using spermicides may cause a UTI."

19. The new graduate asks the nurse why patients who are incontinent of urine do not have a Foley catheter inserted on a routine basis. The nurse explains that a Foley catheter (select all that apply)
    a. Introduces bacteria into the bladder during catheterization
    b. Prevents normal flushing of the urethra
    c. Allows bacteria to ascend into the bladder
    d. Causes minute cuts to the urethra upon insertion

20. The nurse explains to a patient with a Foley catheter who has developed a UTI that antibiotic therapy may be prolonged because
    a. Many different kinds of bacteria are present
    b. It is hard for the antibiotic to reach the bladder
    c. The bacteria protect themselves from antibiotics by developing a protective "coat"
    d. Antibiotic therapy is very safe and inexpensive, so it is customary to administer the antibiotic for several weeks

21. Which of the following patients is at risk for developing HUS? (Select all that apply.)
    a. Marie, a 26-year-old who delivered a baby 6 hours ago
    b. Scott, a 56-year-old with acute respiratory distress syndrome who is on prednisone 80 mg IV every 6 hours
    c. Timmy, a 4-year-old who lives on a dairy farm and routinely drinks unpasteurized milk
    d. Maureen, a 72-year-old who had a bone marrow transplant 24 hours ago

22. The nurse is caring for Mr. Tuzik, a patient with nephrotic syndrome. Which of the following laboratory values is consistent with Mt. Tuzik's diagnosis? (Select all that apply.)
   a. Fat in the urine
   b. Serum albumin of 3.8 mg/dL
   c. Total cholesterol of 256
   d. Protein in the urine

23. Mark, a 22-year-old, has just developed chickenpox. The nurse practitioner will monitor Mark for acute glomerulonephritis for
   a. 3 days
   b. 7 days
   c. 2 weeks
   d. 2 months

24. Ms. Paliwal, a 46-year-old newly diagnosed with type 2 diabetes, is told by the nurse to return to the clinic in 1 week for renal function tests. The nurse realizes that patients with type 2 diabetes
   a. Generally develop diabetic nephropathy 5–10 years after diagnosis
   b. Have a 30% or greater chance of developing diabetic neuropathy
   c. Develop a very thin glomerular capillary membrane
   d. Increase their glomerular filtration rate by 30%

25. The nurse is explaining incontinence to new graduates. Which of the following statements is *correct?* (Select all that apply.)
   a. "Transient urinary incontinence may be caused by fecal impaction."
   b. "Nurses are at risk for developing overflow incontinence."
   c. "Stress incontinence is caused by a weak detrusor muscle."
   d. "Reflex incontinence occurs during high anxiety situations."

26. The nurse is explaining renal calculi to a patient who has had several calculi over the past 5 years. Which of the following statements made by the nurse is *correct?*
   a. "Most kidney stones are formed from uric acid."
   b. "All kidney stones show up on x-ray."
   c. "Even small stones cause pain."
   d. "A diet low in sodium and protein helps prevent more stone formation."

27. The nurse conducting a community education program about benign prostatic hypertrophy was asked to explain the condition. The nurse should respond that BPH is

a. Associated with multiple risk factors, including frequent UTIs

b. Thought to occur because of declining testosterone levels

c. Rare until the seventh decade of life

d. Responsible for symptoms such as a weak urinary stream, and the size of the prostate gland directly correlates to the severity of the symptoms.

28. While discussing BPH at a urology clinic, the nurse is asked to explain some treatment options available. The nurse correctly responds that

a. "Herbal products such as saw palmetto berry have been shown to safely reduce prostate gland size."

b. "Laser therapy produces an immediate reduction in prostate mass."

c. "Although effective, laser therapy does not allow for tissue sampling."

d. "Transurethral balloon dilation is one of the most frequently used methods to treat BPH."

29. The nurse explaining the complications of chronic renal failure to a new graduate should state (select all that apply)

a. "Uremic frost is an early indication of renal failure."

b. "Epogen® causes hypertension in one in five patients on this therapy."

c. "The amount of hypoglycemic medication is usually increased."

d. "Bleeding time is increased in a patient with CRF, although the platelet count may be near normal."

PART IX · ANSWERS

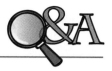

1. **The correct answer is a.** Inactive vitamin D is converted to the active form by the kidneys.

2. **The correct answer is b.** Creatinine is cleared from the blood by the kidneys. Unlike the blood urea nitrogen, it does not rise or fall in response to fluid balance.

3. **The correct answer is c.** Voiding removes bacteria from the bladder and urethra.

4. **The correct answer is b.** Seizure activity, bloody diarrhea, anemia, and renal failure are symptoms of HUS.

5. **The correct answer is a.** The nephrotic syndrome causes increased glomerular capillary membrane permeability and basement membrane thickening as a result of collagen deposits in the glomeruli.

6. **The correct answer is d.** Systemic steroids help reduce inflammation, whereas a low protein diet slows the progression to renal failure.

7. **The correct answer is a.** Parasympathetic pelvic nerves are stimulated when the bladder fills to between 150 and 300 cc.

8. **The correct answer is c.** An overactive detrusor muscle causes repetitive strong contractions of the muscle, which overcomes urethral sphincter control.

9. **The correct answer is b.** The bacteria that causes a UTI produces an enzyme that splits urea into ammonia and carbon dioxide, creating an alkaline urine and increased phosphate, which combines with magnesium and ammonium to form a calculus.

10. **The correct answer is d.** Lowering the level of dihydrotestosterone results in less prostatic tissue growth. The prostate normally converts testosterone to dihydrotestosterone.

11. **The correct answer is c.** The resolution stage of acute renal failure may take 3 to 12 months.

12. **The correct answer is b.** The term renal insufficiency is used when the glomerular filtration rate drops to between 20% and 50%.

13. **The correct answer is a.** When either the distal or proximal tubules are damaged, bicarbonate is excreted.

14. **The correct answer is d.** Signs and symptoms of drug-related nephropathy include fever, hematuria, proteinuria, rash, and an elevated eosinophil count.

15. **The correct answers are c and d.** ANP is produced by the atria in response to fluid overload. It helps to produce diuresis.

16. **The correct answer is b.**

17. **The correct answer is a.** A high-protein diet produces a large amount of urea that must be excreted by the kidneys; therefore, the renal blood flow increases, as does the glomerular filtration rate.

18. **The correct answers are a, b, and d.** Drinking cranberry juice helps to prevent a UTI.

19. **All of the answers are correct.**

20. **The correct answer is c.** As bacteria adhere to the catheter, they produce a protective film that covers the surface of the catheter and protects the bacteria against antibiotic action.

21. **All of the answers are correct.**

22. **The correct answers are a, c, and d.** A serum albumin level of 3.8 mg/dL is within the normal range. Patients with nephritic syndrome spill fat and protein in the urine and have a high serum cholesterol level because the liver increases triglycerides and cholesterol production in an attempt to replace what is lost in the urine.

23. **The correct answer is c.** Circulating immune complexes may become trapped in the glomerular membrane and cause an inflammatory response 10 to 14 days after the initial infection.

24. **The correct answer is b.** Approximately 30% of people with type 2 diabetes mellitus develop diabetic nephropathy. In diabetic nephropathy, the glomerular capillary membrane thickens, probably due to hypertension and hyperglycemia, and mesangial cells proliferate and block the capillary lumen, thereby reducing the area for glomerular filtration.

25. **The correct answers are a and b.** Reflex incontinence is caused by trauma or damage to the nervous system. Stress incontinence involves a weak urethral sphincter.

26. **The correct answer is d.** Most stones have a calcium base. Those without a calcium base do not show up on x-ray. Small stones may not cause pain.

27. **The correct answer is b.** The only known risk factor for BPH is aging. It is estimated that over 50% of men over the age of 50 will develop BPH, with the incidence increasing with age. Prostate size correlates poorly with symptoms.

28. **The correct answer is c.** To date, prospective, randomized, double-blind studies have failed to demonstrate the effectiveness of phytotherapy for BPH. Transurethral balloon dilation is rarely used.

29. **The correct answers are b and d.** Uremic frost is a late sign of renal failure, and the amount of hypoglycemic medication may need to be decreased as insulin cannot be cleared from the bloodstream normally.

Part X

Orthopedics

Vanessa Pomarico-Denino, MSN, APRN

The human body is made up of 206 bones, which provide support and protection for soft tissue and body organs. Bones work interdependently with muscles and ligaments that allow for movement. There are four categories of bones, all of which provide specific functioning to the particular part of the body that makes up the framework. Any impairment of the bone due to disease or trauma affects its ability to properly function.

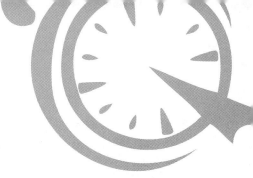

65
Bone Physiology

TERMS
- [ ] compact bone
- [ ] compartment syndrome
- [ ] fibroblasts
- [ ] glycosaminoglycans
- [ ] Haversian system
- [ ] matrix
- [ ] medullary canal
- [ ] osteogenesis
- [ ] osteomyelitis
- [ ] remodeling
- [ ] resorption
- [ ] trabecular bone

Figure 65-1 Age-related changes in bone.

Age-Related Changes in Bone

- Decreased bone mass
- Decreased bone strength
- Decreased calcium absorption
- Increased demineralization

Types of Fractures

- Simple (closed)—Skin intact
- Compound—Skin broken, bone exposed
- Displaced—Bone continuity disrupted
- Nondisplaced—Fractured bone remains in alignment
- Incomplete—Portion of the bone remains intact
- Comminuted—Three or more bone fragments
- Impacted—One fragment imbedded in another
- Depressed—Fractured bone driven inward (skull)
- Pathological—Associated with disease/disorder
- Avulsion—Fragment torn off due to twisting/pulling
- Compression—Crushed
- Stress—Minute fracture related to repetitive stressd

Table 65-1 Structural Elements of Bone

Bone Cells	Function
Osteoblasts	Builds bone through collagen
Osteoclasts	Cells of the bone that enable matrix to be absorbed and assists with release of calcium and phosphate
Osteocytes	Mature bone cells that help maintain bone matrix; also play a major role in release of calcium into blood

The main function of bone is to protect and support internal organs of the body. Bones also function as an attachment site for muscles and skeletal tissue that allow for movement. Bone consists of an organic **matrix** upon which mineral salts are deposited. Protein, vitamin A, and vitamin C are needed for its formation by **fibroblasts.** Calcium, phosphorus, and vitamin D are needed to form the inorganic compounds. Bone serves as a reservoir for calcium, phosphorus, and other minerals. Cancellous or **trabecular bone** is made up of thin plates, is spongy, and contains marrow. It is formed in response to stress and is found in bones such as vertebrae and skull as well as the ends of long bones. The interlacing structure of these plates provides tensile strength and structural support for compact bone. Compact or cortical bone is found primarily in the long bones (upper and lower extremities) and in the outer layers of all bones. It is firm, dense, and resistant to compression and shearing.

Collagen is the basic building block of bone matrix. It provides resilience or tensile strength. Without the collagen matrix, bone would be too hard and brittle. Calcium and other minerals lend strength and rigidity and provide compressive strength to bone. Ground substance consisting of protein polysaccharides or **glycosaminoglycans** serves as an adhesive between the layers of collagen matrix. It serves as a medium for diffusion of nutrients, oxygen, waste products, electrolytes, and minerals between bone tissue and blood vessels and influences calcium deposition and calcification. Vitamins A and C are also needed for its formation.

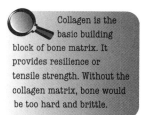

Collagen is the basic building block of bone matrix. It provides resilience or tensile strength. Without the collagen matrix, bone would be too hard and brittle.

Osteoblasts and osteoclasts work synergistically to form and maintain bone. Osteoblasts synthesize osteoid, which forms the organic protein of the matrix. Osteocytes are calcified osteoblasts. Osteoblasts lay down bone, and osteoclasts cause its **resorption** and removal. It is this constant process of breakdown and buildup of bone, termed **remodeling,** that repairs damage and keeps bones strong in response to environmental stressors. Bone is laid down where it is needed and reabsorbed where it is not needed. A small percentage of bone is undergoing remodeling at any given time. The remodeling process takes approximately 4 months to complete one cycle. Bone turnover depends on many factors, such as the influence from various hormones, amount of stress on the bones, nutritional status, adequacy of circulation, age, and overall health. Physical stress on bone leads to deposition of additional bone at the site of increased stress. This is the principle underlying weight-bearing exercise for menopausal women and ambulation in the latter stages of bone healing after fractures.

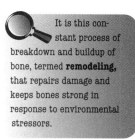

It is this constant process of breakdown and buildup of bone, termed **remodeling,** that repairs damage and keeps bones strong in response to environmental stressors.

The basic unit of cortical bone is the **Haversian system.** It is the channels within this system that allow nutrients from the blood to reach

Figure 65-2 Haversian system.

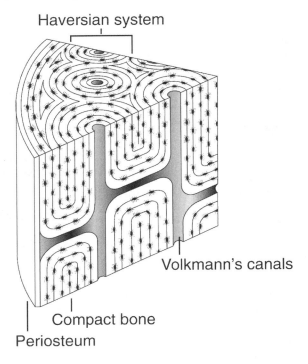

the osteocytes. Circulation within compact bone is supplied by one or more arteries and veins, which pierce the bone and enter the marrow. Blood then enters the Haversian system to nourish the bone. Necrosis of the bone can occur if this blood supply is obstructed or obliterated. Cancellous bone lacks the Haversian system. Circulation in cancellous bone takes place within the trabeculae, which are filled with red marrow.

Periosteum is a tough connective tissue or fibrous membrane that covers the outermost aspect of bone. It is very vascular, contains pain receptors, and is responsible for **osteogenesis.** It supplies blood to the bones via Volkmann's canals. The inner portion of the long bones is referred to as the **medullary canal.** The medullary canal and trabecular spaces (mesh-type layers) are lined by the endosteum that contains osteogenic cells and the bone marrow. Intact periosteum is necessary for healthy bone; if disrupted by mechanical stress due to trauma or disease, it leads to the death of the bone because of interference with the blood supply.

Other factors also play a critical role in bone metabolism. Vitamin D is a fat-soluble vitamin that controls the absorption of calcium from the intestine and increases calcium reabsorption in the kidneys. Parathyroid hormone regulates blood levels of calcium and phosphate while promoting formation of osteoclasts. Parathyroid hormone is regulated by the negative feedback system in response to ionized calcium in the blood and initiates the release of calcium from bone via activation of vitamin D and increased intestinal absorption of calcium. Calcitonin, a thyroid hormone, decreases osteoclastic activity and increases osteoblastic activity, thereby reducing bone breakdown and enhancing its formation. It achieves this activity by inhibiting secretion or release of stored calcium in bone into the blood in response to increased serum calcium. Estrogen inhibits formation of osteoclasts in women, whereas testosterone increases bone length and density in men.

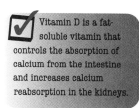

Vitamin D is a fat-soluble vitamin that controls the absorption of calcium from the intestine and increases calcium reabsorption in the kidneys.

Longitudinal and circumferential bone growth occurs via growth of cartilaginous tissue, which gradually ossifies into bone. This ossification process is accelerated during puberty. Longitudinal growth of long bones takes place at the growth plate at the ends of long bones. Good nutrition, physical activity, and exercise from childhood onward are essential for the development and maintenance of healthy bones. Calcium and/or vitamin D should be supplemented during periods of increased need (such as rapid growth spurts or during pregnancy) through dietary means, if at all possible. Oral calcium supplements are available. Calcium carbonate contains the highest amount of elemental calcium, whereas calcium citrate is best absorbed. Vitamin D enhances calcium absorption.

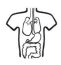

FRACTURES AND BONE HEALING

A local inflammatory process is necessary for bone healing to occur, as with healing of any other tissue. The edges of the fracture site become necrotic, are reabsorbed, and are eventually replaced by new bone. Bone healing begins with formation of a hematoma and granulation tissue, which gradually transforms into callus. It takes 2 to 6 weeks for callus formation. Callus, which is osteoid tissue, binds the bone but is initially neither stable nor strong. As calcium deposits within the callus, it is transformed into bone tissue. This process of ossification can take from 3 weeks to several months; however, bone healing ordinarily takes 4 to 6 weeks. Healing time depends on a variety of factors, such as age, nutrition, blood supply and type and location of the fracture. Compact or cortical bone develops callus both externally and internally. The external callus often forms a palpable lump at the site of the fracture, which gradually decreases in size as ossification occurs, although it may not disappear entirely.

Cancellous or trabecular bone develops internal callus, and healing is ordinarily faster in this type of bone. The remodeling phase of bone healing may take as long as a year depending on the degree and type of fracture, as well as other factors. It is during this phase that the bone reshapes to meet the mechanical requirements placed

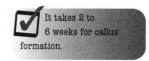 It takes 2 to 6 weeks for callus formation.

on it. Delayed union, malunion, or nonunion may occur due to poor nutrition, poor circulation, malalignment, premature weight bearing, and/or other factors. Ossification occurs more quickly in children and more slowly in the elderly.

> The external callus often forms a palpable lump at the site of the fracture, which gradually decreases in size as ossification occurs, although it may not disappear entirely.

The growth plate is a site of common fracture in children and has the potential to lead to limb length discrepancies. These fractures may not always be visible on x-ray. Cancellous bone is more susceptible to compression fractures and is a common site of postmenopausal fractures and other osteoporotic fractures.

Fractures are often accompanied by extensive soft tissue damage, depending on the site, the cause, and the degree of injury. **Compartment syndrome** is a serious complication that results from an increase in pressure in the given compartment. The pressure impinges on the nerves and blood vessels contained within it and can compromise the distal extremity if not identified and treated promptly. Infection is also a serious complication that can lead to **osteomyelitis.**

Figure 65-3 Long bone structures.

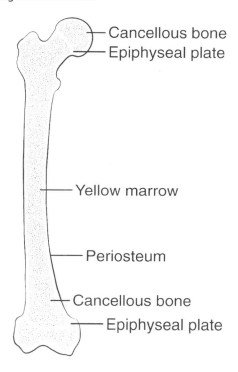

Cancellous bone
Epiphyseal plate

Yellow marrow

Periosteum

Cancellous bone
Epiphyseal plate

Management

Rest, immobilization, compression, and elevation, or RICE, is the mainstay of initial treatment of orthopedic injuries. Immobilization of fractures until callus forms and ossification begins is critical. Partial weight bearing is prescribed once ossification has begun as determined by x-ray. Full weight bearing without external support is prescribed once ossification is complete.

Bleeding, inflammation, and possible contamination need to be considered in management. Pain management with pharmacological and nonpharmacological measures and prevention of complications of immobility are also critical.

Osteoporosis is a disease of decreased bone mass and occurs when the rate of bone **resorption** exceeds the rate of bone formation. Approximately 10 million people have osteoporosis, but it is more common among the older adult female population, affecting one in three women and one in eight men. **Osteopenia** is a condition of bone thinning that leads to osteoporosis if not diagnosed.

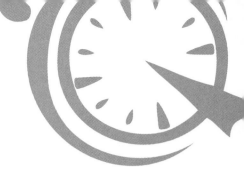

66
Osteoporosis

TERMS
- ☐ **iatrogenic**
- ☐ **osteopenia**
- ☐ **Paget's disease**
- ☐ **resorption**

Figure 66-1 Bone remodeling and types of osteoporosis.

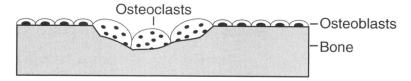

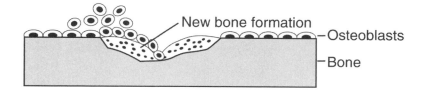

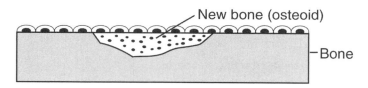

Postmenopausal	**Senile**	**Secondary**
55 to 70 years	75 to 90 years	Variable
F 20:1	F 2:1	F 1:1
Vertebrae	Vertebrae, hip, pelvis, and humerus	Vertebrae and hip

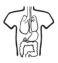

PATHOPHYSIOLOGY

There are two types of osteoporosis: Type I or primary osteoporosis is associated with postmenopausal estrogen loss but can also be contributed to as a result of not building necessary bone mass during the formative years. Secondary, or Type II, osteoporosis is due to some underlying disease or pathology or from certain medications. Osteoporosis can be due to either a decrease in activity of the osteoblasts, which are responsible for bone

> ✓ Osteoporosis is more common among the older adult female population, affecting one in three women and one in eight men.

Figure 66-2 Risk factors for osteoporosis.

Risk Factors for Osteoporosis

Caucasian or Asian	Female	Early menopause
Scandinavian	Fair, blonde	Late menarche
Small frame	Physical inactivity	Postmenopausal
Excessive nicotine	Excessive alcohol intake	Family history
Internal fixation with metal implant		

Red Flags for Osteoporosis

- Presence of risk factors
- Kyphosis
- Fracture with slight or nontrauma
- Hip fracture preceding a fall
- Loss of height >2 inches of adult height

Common Diagnostic Tests

- MRI, CT, bone scan
- Bone density tests—DEXA (safest and most reliable)
- Blood work—Ca, PO_4, vitamin D, parathyroid, alkaline phosphatase

Drugs and Health Problems Associated with Osteoporosis

Drugs	Health Problems
Thyroid replacement	Thyrotoxicosis
Glucocorticoids	Cushing's disease
Heparin	Type 1 diabetes
Lithium	Malabsorption
Chemotherapy	Rheumatoid arthritis
Anticonvulsants	Hemolytic anemia
Tetracyclines	Anorexia nervosa
Selected diuretics	Hepatobiliary dysfunction
Phenothiazines	
Cyclosporine	
Selected antacids	

formation, or an increase in activity of the osteoclasts, which are responsible for bone breakdown. It can be either regional or generalized. Early osteoporosis is asymptomatic, and considerable bone loss (30–50%) can occur before it is detectable on x-ray.

Osteoporosis is more common in women than in men, with the peak incidence

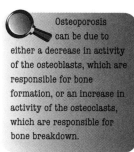

Osteoporosis can be due to either a decrease in activity of the osteoblasts, which are responsible for bone formation, or an increase in activity of the osteoclasts, which are responsible for bone breakdown.

in women beginning within 5 years of menopause. Estrogen influences bone density. When that source is decreased, cytokinins increase and stimulate osteoclast (bone break-down) activity. In men, demineralization begins around the age of 65 to 70 due to a decrease in testosterone and other factors.

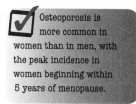

Osteoporosis is more common in women than in men, with the peak incidence in women beginning within 5 years of menopause.

Osteoporosis in males has less clinical significance because their bones are larger and denser than those of women. Men also do not have the influence of estrogen on their bones. The bone loss during menopause is due to an increase in osteoclastic activity, whereas that occurring with aging is mediated by a decrease in osteoblastic activity.

Cancellous or trabecular bone such as vertebrae or distal wrist is more susceptible to osteoporosis associated with the decrease in estrogen with menopause. Osteoporosis associated with aging occurs in both genders and involves both cancellous and cortical bone. The cortical bone becomes thinner, and there is a reduction in the number and size of trabeculae in cancellous bone. Fractures in type II osteoporosis frequently occur in the femoral neck, proximal humerus, and proximal tibia. The effect of osteoporosis is most significant in cancellous bone, which results in a decrease in the resilience or tensile strength of the bone and a decrease in the amount of internal support it affords surrounding compact or cortical bone.

The bone remodeling cycle in persons with osteoporosis may take up to 2 years versus the normal time of 4 months. If circulation to the bone is impaired, the remodeling process is hindered, further contributing to the development of osteoporosis and likelihood of fractures. There is a very high morbidity and mortality rate after hip fracture in the elderly, so every effort should be made to prevent osteoporosis and reduce fall risk in this population. Fifty percent die within 1 year of presentation. Most of those who survive have a significant reduction in independence and functional ability that contributes to other illnesses and risk of infection and possibly death.

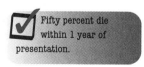

Fifty percent die within 1 year of presentation.

Factors that contribute to bone loss include genetic predisposition; hormonal imbalance; nutritional deficits, especially protein, calcium, and vitamins C and D; age; use of certain medications; and certain diseases. Excessive coffee, tobacco, and alcohol use can also contribute.

Osteoporosis due to the use of certain medications is termed **iatrogenic** osteoporosis. Steroids interfere with glucose utilization and cause breakdown of protein, which forms the matrix of bone. They also depress osteoblastic activity. Long-term heparin use increases collagen breakdown. Other medications that can contribute to osteoporosis include anticonvulsants, barbiturates, thyroid hormones, and, possibly, loop diuretics.

Disuse osteoporosis is due to lack of stress on long bones caused by physical inactivity. This results in a decrease in osteoblastic activity and an increase in osteoclastic activity, with an overall decrease in bone mass. It is thought that muscular activity plays a role in enhancing circulation to the bone and in stimulating osteoblastic activity. In addition, stress on bones alters electrical charges on the surface of the bone, which stimulates new bone formation.

Metastatic bone tumors result in osteoporotic changes in bone tissue, particularly in older adults. This can be particularly painful because of the pressure exerted upon the periosteum from the proliferating cell mass. If the tumor causes elevation of the periosteum, new bone formation becomes erratic or impaired. Pathological fractures can occur as a consequence of osteoporosis, bone metastasis, or other causes.

Paget's disease is a disease of chronic bone inflammation that results in softening and bowing of the long bones. It has no known cause, but viral involvement has been studied. In widespread disease, it can involve most bones. There is an increase in osteoclastic activity with a compensatory increase in osteoblastic activity. The newly formed bone exceeds that broken down; however, it is structurally abnormal, resulting in bone that is porous and soft. The long bones are bowed and other bones are often misshapen. Fractures are common. This may be a very painful condition if accompanied by fractures and/or compression of nerves. Other more common causes of secondary osteoporosis include hyperthyroidism, hyperparathyroidism, Cushing's disease, diabetes mellitus, and chronic renal failure.

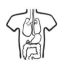

MANAGEMENT

Prevention of risk factors and early detection is critical with osteoporosis. Good nutrition in women is particularly important from childhood through the age of 30, because those are the years when maximum bone formation takes place. The recommended intake of calcium in children and adolescents is 1,500 mg/day. Premenopausal and postmenopausal women on hormone replacement therapy as well as adult men require 1,000 mg of elemental calcium daily; postmenopausal women without hormone replacement therapy require 1,500 mg of elemental calcium daily. Calcium carbonate contains the highest amount of elemental calcium; however, calcium citrate is better absorbed. In addition to calcium, phosphorus and vitamin D are needed for adequate mineralization, and protein and vitamins A and C are needed for formation of bone matrix. Weight-bearing exercise and calcium and vitamin D supplementation have an important role in long-term management.

Once osteoporosis is present, the goal of management is to slow the rate of calcium and bone loss and stop progression of the disease. Medications are available to either increase bone formation or osteoblastic activity or to decrease osteoclastic activity or bone loss. Current therapies available for the treatment of osteoporosis include bisphosphonates, calcitonin, selective estrogen receptor modulators, and teriparatide (a parathyroid hormone). Treatment in postmenopausal women also includes estrogen or hormone replacement therapy, but these do not increase bone mass but rather halt further progression of disease. Estrogen or hormone replacement therapy is recommended unless contraindicated, especially in those women with a history of breast cancer or strong family history of breast cancer. Weight-bearing exercise combined with calcium and vitamin D supplementation is essential in long-term management. Management of secondary osteoporosis lies in correcting or ameliorating the underlying cause when possible.

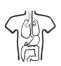

OSTEOMYELITIS

Osteomyelitis is an infection of the bone and bone marrow that results in some of the same structural abnormalities as osteoporosis, such as destruction of cortical and cancellous bone and propensity to fracture. Osteomyelitis can be severe and is a very serious problem because of the difficulty of eradicating the infection once it is present. It can occur when there is an open wound, which serves as a portal of entry for bacteria, or in the

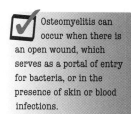

Osteomyelitis can occur when there is an open wound, which serves as a portal of entry for bacteria, or in the presence of skin or blood infections.

presence of skin or blood infections. Therefore, meticulous attention is paid to prevention.

Pathogenic gram-positive or gram-negative organisms can reach the body via the blood adjacent to soft tissue or can be introduced directly with trauma or during or after surgery. The nature of circulation to and within bone makes it difficult for antibiotics to reach involved tissue in sufficient concentrations to eradicate the organisms. It also contributes to the difficulty of removal of waste products of the inflammation/immune response and necrotic tissue. Organisms can remain sequestered within the bony tissue, and infection can reactivate at a later time if the person becomes immunosuppressed or after trauma. Osteomyelitis can also become chronic, especially if initial treatment was insufficient. Aggressive antibiotic therapy is the mainstay of treatment. Sometimes surgical debridement and/or replacement of orthopedic appliances (such as artificial joints) are necessary.

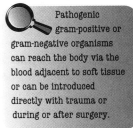

Pathogenic gram-positive or gram-negative organisms can reach the body via the blood adjacent to soft tissue or can be introduced directly with trauma or during or after surgery.

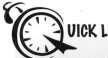

Arthritis, a term applied to many different conditions, is the second leading cause of disability in the United States. Arthritis is the inflammation of a joint that can manifest as many different forms. Some forms are due to disease or trauma, whereas others are related to infections and metabolic or autoimmune disorders. Three major forms of arthritis include osteoarthritis, rheumatoid arthritis (RA), and gout. All three of these diseases involve the entire joint structure, including the synovial membrane, articular cartilage, tendons, ligaments, adjacent bone, and joint spaces. X-ray is used to confirm diagnosis and monitor progression. Specific laboratory tests are available for rheumatoid or autoimmune forms.

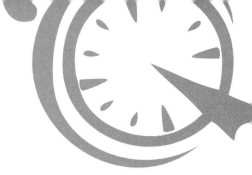

67

Arthritis

TERMS
- [ ] chondrocytes
- [ ] hyperuricemia
- [ ] pannus
- [ ] synovitis

Figure 67-1 Types of joints.

Types of Joints

- Synarthrosis—Immovable (e.g., cranial sutures)
- Fibrous—Rigid surface (e.g., cranial)
- Amphiarthrosis—Partially moveable (e.g., symphysis)
- Cartilaginous—Slightly moveable (e.g., ribs, sternum)
- Diarthrosis—Freely moveable (e.g., hip, knee)
- Synovial—Considerable movement (e.g., fingers, elbow)

Types of Cartilage

- Elastic—Most flexible (e.g., ear, epiglottis)
- Hyaline—Most common (e.g., most joints, nose)
- Fibrous—Most rigid (e.g, pelvis, intervertebral discs)

Definitions

- Tendons—Attach muscle to bone
- Ligaments—Attach bone to bone

Common Diagnostic Tests with Gout

- Joint aspiration
- Serum uric acid
- ESR
- WBC

Common Diagnostic Tests with Rheumatoid Arthritis

Rh factor titer	Urinalysis
Complete blood count with differential	FOBT
Sedimentation rate	Joint aspiration
Chemistry	X-ray
LFT	ANA if indicated

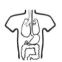

OSTEOARTHRITIS

Osteoarthritis is a progressive degenerative joint disease affecting primarily peripheral and central weight-bearing joints and fingers and is the most common form of arthritis in adults and elderly. The hallmark of this disease is progressive loss of articulating cartilage. Primary or idiopathic osteoarthritis is associated with aging, whereas secondary osteoarthritis is related to some other condition or

> ✓ Arthritis, a term applied to many different conditions, is the second leading cause of disability in the United States.

process and is often a result of repeated or severe joint stress or trauma. Osteoarthritis has an asymmetrical distribution and is a local disease. Degenerative changes often begin between the ages of 40 and 50. Early symptoms are often mild and frequently ignored or compensated for by those who have them. The incidence is higher in males.

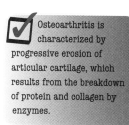

Primary or idiopathic osteoarthritis is associated with aging, whereas secondary osteoarthritis is related to some other condition or process and is often a result of repeated or severe joint stress or trauma.

Collagen is the primary building block of cartilage. It is continuously being renewed and remodeled by **chondrocytes.** Cartilage does not possess a blood supply or nerve endings; therefore, it requires long periods of time to heal. It is nourished by diffusion of nutrients from surrounding capillaries. Its function is to absorb shock, reduce friction, and distribute weight bearing. Tendons have pain receptors but a limited blood supply, so they also take a long time to heal. Joint spaces are filled with synovial fluid, which lubricates, nourishes, cushions, and facilitates movement.

Pathophysiology

Osteoarthritis is characterized by progressive erosion of articular cartilage, which results from the breakdown of protein and collagen by enzymes. Increased water is absorbed because of disruption in pumping action, so the cartilage becomes less able to tolerate weight bearing and loses some of its tensile strength. As osteoarthritis progresses, bits of articular cartilage flake off and longitudinal fissures develop. The cartilage becomes thin or absent, leaving the bone unprotected. Subchondral bone thickens and becomes sclerotic with potential of cyst formation. Osteophytes (bone spurs) develop at the joint margin, which can also break off, causing **synovitis** and joint effusion. The joint capsule becomes thickened and may adhere to underlying structures. Knees, hips, vertebrae, and fingers are the most common sites. Pain associated with osteoarthritis arises from a combination of articular distension, inflammation, and fibrosis.

Osteoarthritis is characterized by progressive erosion of articular cartilage, which results from the breakdown of protein and collagen by enzymes.

 Pain associated with osteoarthritis arises from a combination of articular distension, inflammation, and fibrosis.

Management

Osteoarthritis is managed by a combination of rest and exercise, including range of motion exercises to maintain joint mobility. Weight reduction is important if indicated. Ambulation aids may be necessary to reduce stress on weight-bearing joints. Pain management with acetaminophen and other nonsteroidal antiinflammatory drugs (NSAIDs) is the mainstay of therapy. Cyclooxygenase-2 inhibitors are used sparingly and in those patients without risk of vessel disease or bleeding abnormalities. Patient education is important in the management of this chronic condition. Surgery and joint replacement is sometimes indicated.

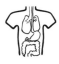

RHEUMATOID ARTHRITIS

RA is a systemic inflammatory disease of connective tissue with an onset of disease between ages 20 and 50. For many, there is a strong autoimmune component, although a genetic predisposition is also a possibility. The joints most commonly involved are the hands, wrists, knees, feet, and upper cervical spine. In adults, joint involvement is symmetrical.

Rheumatoid arthritis is characterized by inflammatory damage or destruction of the synovial membrane and articular cartilage. It eventually involves the joint capsule, ligaments, and tendons, resulting in pain, joint deformity, and loss of function. RA is accompanied by systemic inflammatory symptoms, leading to nonarticular pathological manifestations in other body systems such as cardiac, pulmonary, or ophthalmic.

RA is more common in women. It is characterized by remissions and exacerbations and can progress to severe debilitation with significant loss of functional ability.

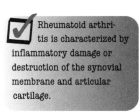

Rheumatoid arthritis is characterized by inflammatory damage or destruction of the synovial membrane and articular cartilage.

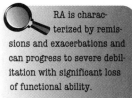

RA is characterized by remissions and exacerbations and can progress to severe debilitation with significant loss of functional ability.

Pathophysiology

Rheumatoid factor has been found in most people with RA, and 60% to 80% have the B lymphocyte alloantigen HLA-DR4. The stimulus for the abnormal immune reaction is not known, but several theories have been postulated, including injury, stress, autonomic changes, and physical activity.

The immune complexes formed between rheumatoid factor and IgG activate the complement system and leukocyte release of lysosomal enzymes. These initiate and enhance the inflammatory response. Immune complexes are deposited on synovial membranes and phagocytized by macrophages. The enzymes that are released degrade synovial tissue and articular cartilage. This continued inflammatory response results in hypertrophy, which impairs local circulation and invades local joint structures. Granulation tissue forms, which covers the articular cartilage, leading to pannus formation.

> The enzymes that are released degrade synovial tissue and articular cartilage. This continued inflammatory response results in hypertrophy, which impairs local circulation and invades local joint structures.

Pannus is vascularized scar tissue that erodes and destroys articular cartilage, leading to bone erosion, cysts, fissures, and bone spurs. As the pannus becomes more fibrotic, it causes tendons and ligaments to shorten. Secondary muscle atrophy, fibrosis, and the inflammatory destruction that follows it contribute to laxity of ligaments and tendons, causing joint instability, subluxation, and contractures. The characteristic ulnar deviation and swan-neck deformity of the hands are easily recognized. Subcutaneous nodules composed of inflammatory cells and cellular debris may present over extensor surfaces of elbows and fingers as well as other areas.

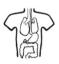

CLINICAL MANIFESTATIONS

The onset of RA is usually insidious, with a small percentage of acute onset of symptoms. It may initially present with inflammation or acute arthralgias accompanied by fever, fatigue, malaise, and weakness. Symmetrical joint pain and swelling occurs as an inflammatory response within the synovial membrane mainly involving the metacarpophalangeal and metatarsophalangeal joints. The joint may appear boggy with an overlying ruddy discoloration and may feel

Figure 67-2 Synovial joint.

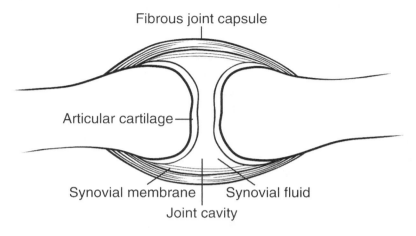

Figure 67-3 Cross-section of the knee joint.

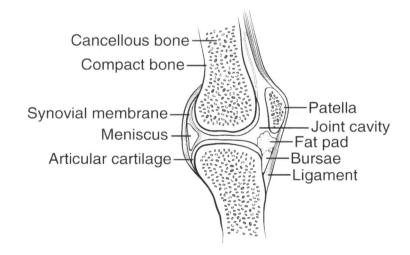

warm to the touch. Limited range of motion can progress to permanent deformities of the hand. Rheumatoid nodules over areas of infection are characteristic of RA.

Diagnosis is based on symptomatology, x-rays and serum rheumatological factors.

Figure 67-4 Osteoarthritis.

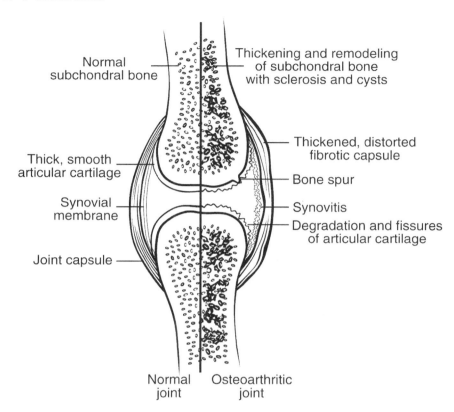

Normal subchondral bone

Thickening and remodeling of subchondral bone with sclerosis and cysts

Thick, smooth articular cartilage

Thickened, distorted fibrotic capsule

Bone spur

Synovial membrane

Synovitis

Degradation and fissures of articular cartilage

Joint capsule

Normal joint

Osteoarthritic joint

Management

The goals of management are to decrease pain, prevent deformity, and maintain functional ability. Local joint rest and periodic daily systemic rest, as well as exercise, are mainstays of management. Physical measures include use of heat, cold, and other physical therapy techniques. Pain management is a priority. Acetylsalicylic acid and NSAIDs are used; disease-modifying antirheumatic drugs and biological response modifiers are used for those with more advanced disease.

Many patients benefit from oral or injectable corticosteroids but must be surveyed for osteoporosis with prolonged use. Surgery may be done to correct deformity, improve function, and decrease pain.

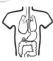

GOUT

Gout, which is asymptomatic in the early phase, is a disorder characterized by disturbances of uric acid metabolism. This leads to **hyperuricemia** and deposition of urate salts in articular, periarticular, and subcutaneous tissue, which initiates an inflammatory response. Renal stones are common sequelae. Gout is most frequently found in middle-aged men and postmenopausal women. Those taking diuretics are at an increased risk, as are uncontrolled diabetics and postmenopausal women. It involves weight-bearing joints of the lower extremities, particularly the great toe.

Pathophysiology

Uric acid is a breakdown product of purines, a byproduct of metabolism. An increase in uric acid can result from either an increased breakdown or production of purine. Two other mechanisms are an increased turnover of nucleic acids, which are necessary for various intracellular processes, and a lack of uricase, an enzyme that oxidizes uric acid to a soluble compound such as plasma and urine. The resultant hyperuricemia and deposition of urate crystals are accompanied by an acute local inflammatory response and severe pain. An acute attack, which lasts 3 to 10 days, is often triggered by trauma, stress, high-fat diet, or use of alcohol or drugs. Periods between attacks are asymptomatic and are termed intercritical periods.

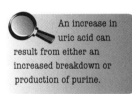

An increase in uric acid can result from either an increased breakdown or production of purine.

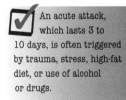

An acute attack, which lasts 3 to 10 days, is often triggered by trauma, stress, high-fat diet, or use of alcohol or drugs.

As the disease progresses, urate crystals in subcutaneous tissue and joints cause the formation of nodules, called tophi. The most common site for tophi is the helix of the ear. This is the chronic phase of the disease. The tophi can erode and drain through the skin. The chronic inflammation caused by the tophi can lead to deforming arthritis. Uric acid is excreted by the kidneys. If its excretion is impaired or its reabsorption is increased, uric acid levels become elevated.

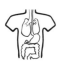

CLINICAL MANIFESTATIONS

Patients typically present with a sudden onset of monarticular pain in the absence of trauma. Over 50% occur in the great toe, but it can also occur in knees, ankles, or elbows. The joint becomes reddened with exquisite tenderness. Diagnosis is based on symptomatology and serum uric acid levels.

Management

The goals of management are to control pain, prevent acute attacks, prevent or reverse complications, and prevent renal calculi. NSAIDs are used for pain management. Medications are also used to reduce hyperuricemia by either increasing the excretion of uric acid or decreasing its formation. Additional measures during an acute attack include decreased weight bearing, elevation, and ice. Dietary measures include a low-purine diet and increased fluid intake. Intraarticular steroid injections may be indicated.

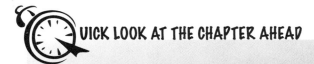

Low back pain of musculoskeletal origin is one of the most common causes of pain in adults and results in significant loss of work hours. Although it is sometimes caused by acute injury, it is commonly chronic and often caused by soft tissue strain, sprain, or overuse due to muscle weakness, deconditioning, obesity, poor body mechanics, or poor posture. It may be accompanied by sciatica in which pain occurs along the distribution of one or both sciatic nerves. Other musculoskeletal or neurological conditions can also cause low back pain, such as degenerative disc disease, arthritis, herniated nucleus pulposus (herniated disk), fibromyalgia, bursitis, radiculitis, fibrosis, stenosis, and vertebral fracture. Ninety percent of acute low back problems resolve spontaneously within 4 weeks, regardless of treatment.

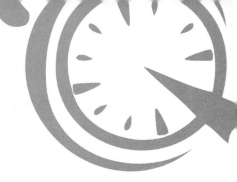

68

Low Back Pain

TERMS
- ☐ **amphiarthroses**
- ☐ **ligaments**
- ☐ **nucleus pulposus**
- ☐ **radicular pain**

Figure 68-1 Changes with aging.

Changes with Aging

- Dehydration of intervertebral discs
- Narrowing of disc spaces
- Decreased height, kyphosis
- Decreased flexibility of lumbar curve and flattening of lumbar curve

Definitions

- Tendons—Attach muscle to bone
- Ligaments—Attach bone to bone

Grades of Strains/Sprains

Grade 1

- Minimal tearing and edema
- Local tenderness
- No change in muscle mass
- Moderate tearing
- Moderate pain, edema
- Muscular defect may be palpable

Grade 3

- Severe or complete tear
- Severe pain and edema
- Large palpable defect

Common Diagnostic Tests and PE Maneuvers

- Lumbosacral x-ray
- Magnetic resonance imaging (MRI)/computed tomography (CT)
- Electromyogram (EMG)
- Neurological exam
- Straight leg raise test

The vertebral column is supported by a complex group of strong serially arranged muscles, fascia, and **ligaments** that extend from the skull to the pelvis. Functionally, these serve as a single muscle and maintain extension of the vertebral column. These structures work in conjunction with those of the abdomen, thorax, pelvis, neck, and head

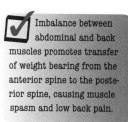
Imbalance between abdominal and back muscles promotes transfer of weight bearing from the anterior spine to the posterior spine, causing muscle spasm and low back pain.

to afford the trunk full range of motion. The muscles of the abdomen are particularly important in providing additional support to the back. Imbalance between abdominal and back muscles promotes transfer of weight bearing from the anterior spine to the posterior spine, causing muscle spasm and low back pain.

Vertebral joints are classified as **amphiarthroses**, or partially moveable joints. The intervertebral discs are pad-like structures between the vertebrae that help stabilize them and act as shock absorbers between them. They also help to maintain the normal spinal curvatures. The outer layer of the disc is a tough, fibrous layer referred to as the annular layer. The inner portion is more viscid and is called the **nucleus pulposus**. It lies close to the posterior portion of the disc. The nucleus pulposus changes shape with spinal movement, causing bulging of the annulus. The discs are strongly attached to adjacent vertebral bodies. They are a common cause of back pain. Because of their high water content, the discs are subject to dehydration as people age, resulting in thinning of the discs, a decrease in shock absorbency, less spinal stability, and less ability to tolerate stress and strain.

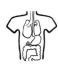

PATHOPHYSIOLOGY

The pain associated with low back pain may be due to a variety of mechanisms, and consideration of the underlying causes directs the selection of the most appropriate treatment options. Direct tissue injury and inflammation and spasm all contribute to the degree of pain experienced. Vertebral malalignment and disc degeneration can likewise result in low back pain. Pain from other sites, such as renal and aortic, may also be referred to the low back. Inflammation commonly accompanies low back pain, regardless of the cause. Compression, inflammation, and edema of nerve roots can also contribute to back pain of musculoskeletal origin. Muscle spasm, which is a compensatory or protective mechanism associated with trauma, can be exceedingly painful.

Muscular changes with aging that can predispose to or exacerbate low back pain include a decrease in size and number of muscle cells and capillaries, a decrease in muscle fiber diameter, and a decrease in muscle mass. There is also increased fat deposition, decreased elastic tissue, and increased collagen. Inactivity as one ages contributes to the development of muscle atrophy and chronic back problems. Muscle cells are less responsive to neurotransmitters, which contributes to a decrease in response to stimulation by the nervous system. These cellular changes result in decreased muscle tone, strength, endurance, and elastic tissue. Over time, these changes result in a functional decrease in muscle strength of 30% to 50%. However, this process can be slowed by good nutrition and regular active exercise as one ages.

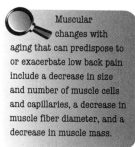

Muscular changes with aging that can predispose to or exacerbate low back pain include a decrease in size and number of muscle cells and capillaries, a decrease in muscle fiber diameter, and a decrease in muscle mass.

Herniated nucleus pulposus, referred to by lay persons as a "slipped" disc, is a protrusion of the posterior portion of the nucleus pulposus through the fibrous annular capsule. The nucleus pulposus may also protrude into the annulus and cause bulging of the disc without an actual herniation. Both protrusion of the nucleus pulposus and bulging of the annulus can cause compression of adjacent nerve roots and pain. Actual rupture of the disc is relatively uncommon.

Disc problems are most common between L3–4 and L5 to S1, which is the most flexible portion of the vertebral column. The precise location of the defect or injury can be assessed by examination of the distribution of the lumbosacral nerves and appropriate reflexes. Herniations at C5–7 also occur but are less frequent. Ligamentous injury frequently occurs in conjunction with a herniated nucleus pulposus, and significant muscle spasm is often present.

Pain caused by pressure of a protruding disc on adjacent nerve roots or spinal nerves is referred to as **radicular pain.** In addition to pain, paresthesias, weakness, and decreased reflexes may also accompany nerve root compression or irritation. With

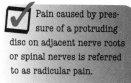

Pain caused by pressure of a protruding disc on adjacent nerve roots or spinal nerves is referred to as radicular pain.

appropriate management and self-care, these often resolve fairly rapidly.

Degenerative disc disease results from a fibrosis and thinning of the nucleus pulposus, which is associated with aging. This narrowing can result in vertebral instability, spinal stenosis, or rupture of the disc.

Spinal stenosis, which occurs primarily in middle-aged and older adults, is the narrowing of the spinal canal by soft tissue such as fibrosis or bony tissue. Pressure on nerve roots results in pain and neurogenic claudication, which is relieved by sitting or flexion of the lumbar spine.

Figure 68-2 Dermatomes (lumbar/sacral nerve root innervation).

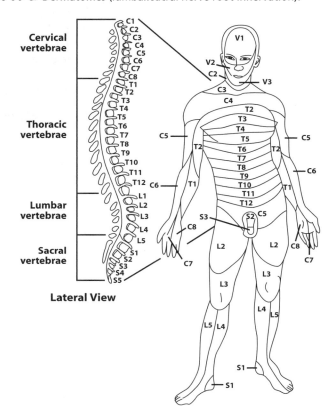

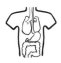

MANAGEMENT

It is important that management be tailored to the pathophysiology involved such as muscle relaxants for muscle spasm and nonsteroidal antiinflammatory drugs (NSAIDs) for pain and inflammation. Bed rest reduces pressure on the discs, allowing water, which was forced out by compression, to reenter and reestablish compressibility. Intermittent rest for 2 to 3 days is recommended if the injury is severe. Otherwise, normal activity may be maintained as tolerated. Prolonged bed rest is avoided because of the muscle weakness that accompanies immobility.

Figure 68-3 Vertebral segment.

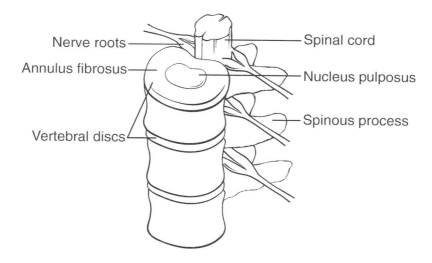

Nerve roots

Annulus fibrosus

Vertebral discs

Spinal cord

Nucleus pulposus

Spinous process

Figure 68-4 Herniated nucleus pulposus.

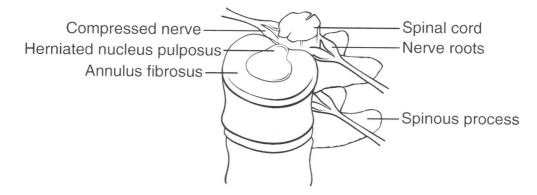

Compressed nerve

Herniated nucleus pulposus

Annulus fibrosus

Spinal cord

Nerve roots

Spinous process

Physical measures such as support, heat, ice, and other physical therapy techniques are an important part of treatment.

It is important to make pain management a priority. Non-narcotic analgesics are the mainstay of pain management. NSAIDs, including acetaminophen, are the initial drugs of choice. Mild muscle relaxants are used for brief periods during acute attack combined with NSAIDS, but only if NSAIDs are ineffective or contraindicated. Narcotics are avoided unless all other pharmacological and nonpharmacological measures have been exhausted and are a last resort for intractable pain due to the potential for addiction. Care must be taken to avoid or compensate for side effects and avoid toxic effects of analgesic medications because some of these medications may be used for long periods of time, depending on the particular disorder.

Patient education regarding body mechanics, stretching, and strengthening exercises (once the acute phase has passed) and techniques to reduce strain to back muscles is very important. Weight loss is advised if indicated. Increasing flexibility and strength of the lower extremities and strength of the abdominal muscles is important, as is regular exercise for overall musculoskeletal health. Occupational factors need to be considered and modified if indicated. Occasionally, surgery is necessary with certain conditions, such as spinal stenosis and herniated nucleus pulposus, if there is severe compression or if more conservative management is unsuccessful.

PART X · QUESTIONS

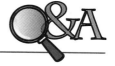

1. Changes associated with aging that can contribute to low back pain include all the following *except*
   a. Muscle spasm
   b. Narrowing of disc spaces
   c. Decreased water content of intervertebral discs
   d. Decreased flexibility of lumbar curve

2. Mrs. L., your neighbor, is 62 years old, 5′ 3″ tall, and weighs approximately 160 lbs. She is complaining of low back pain. She cannot identify any precipitating factor but she reports having had "back problems" off and on for years. It ordinarily goes away on its own if she "takes it easy." She reports sometimes taking acetaminophen or ibuprofen, which helps. This time, however, she says her back has been bothering her for the last 2 months and is present most of the time, although it gets worse when she's been more active. She mentions that she just took a week off and "stayed in bed the entire time." When she returned to her normal activity yesterday, her back pain came right back and may even be a little worse. What is the most appropriate response?
   a. "You probably have a slipped disc. You should make an appointment to be seen by your primary care provider to have some tests done."
   b. "Back pain is commonly associated with aging. You could try one of the nutritional supplements from the health food store."
   c. "Lots of times exercises and weight loss help back problems. I'd recommend that you join a gym and try to lose 25 to 30 lbs."
   d. "Staying in bed for a week may have caused your muscles to become weaker. You should see your primary care provider to check your back and suggest some exercises and other things that can help you."

3. Most low back pain is due to which of the following?
   a. Vertebral fractures
   b. Herniated intervertebral discs
   c. Muscle sprain/strain
   d. Obesity

4. Degenerative disc disease commonly occurs in whom?
   a. Those with a poor dietary calcium intake
   b. Those with a narrowing of the spinal canal
   c. People as they age
   d. In athletes, particularly African-American males

5. What is the basic pathophysiology underlying osteoporosis?
   a. An imbalance between osteoclastic and osteoblastic activity
   b. An increase in osteoblastic activity
   c. A decrease in osteoclastic activity
   d. Impaired calcium absorption that leads to a decrease in osteoclastic activity

6. Which of the following is an appropriate response for you to make to a 40-year-old woman who is interested in learning what she can do to decrease her risk for osteoporosis?
   a. "You should take hormones to replace estrogen once you reach menopause."
   b. "If you do not have risk factors in your history, you probably don't need to do anything special."
   c. "Weight-bearing exercises and an adequate intake of calcium and vitamin D are important factors in preventing osteoporosis."
   d. "Osteoporosis is inevitable, so there's nothing much you can do to prevent it."

7. Which of the following medications may contribute to iatrogenic osteoporosis?
   a. Steroids
   b. Thyroid hormones
   c. Heparin
   d. NSAIDs

8. Which of the following statements about osteoporosis in men is *true?*
   a. Osteoporosis is less significant in men because their bones are more dense.
   b. Demineralization in men begins in the late 70s or early 80s.
   c. Men do not get osteoporosis because it is an estrogen-dependent disorder.
   d. Men have fewer vertebral compression fractures than women because they have less trabecular bone.

9. What provides tensile strength?
   a. Compact bone
   b. Trabecular bone
   c. Periosteum
   d. Haversian system

10. What portion of the bone contains pain receptors?
   a. Endosteum
   b. Marrow
   c. Haversian system
   d. Periosteum

11. The matrix of bone is made of which of the following?
   a. Bone marrow
   b. Collagen
   c. Calcium
   d. Cartilage

12. Callus formation at the site of a fracture takes 2 to 6 weeks. Which of the following statements about bone healing is true?
   a. The most important vitamin in bone healing is vitamin B.
   b. Callus is strong and stable.
   c. The palpable bump at the site of a fracture gradually disappears as ossification takes place.
   d. Bone remodeling takes 6 to 8 weeks, during which time it is important for the patient to avoid stress to the fracture site.

13. Which of the following statements *best* reflects the pathophysiology of osteoarthritis?
   a. It is characterized by thinning of the articular cartilage, commonly affects weight-bearing joints, and has an asymmetrical distribution.
   b. It is a systemic inflammatory disease that affects many joint structures in a symmetrical fashion and can also involve other body systems.
   c. It is a systemic disease with several phases and is accompanied by hyperuricemia with deposition of urate crystals in joints and other tissues.
   d. It is a disease of aging that ultimately results in profound disability. It commonly contributes to pathological fractures due to increased excretion of calcium and protein by the kidneys.

14. Mrs. T. has rheumatoid arthritis and has been told that she needs to exercise regularly and that a plan will be worked out with her the next day. Which of the following statements indicates that she understands the rationale for exercise with this disease?

a. "I know I have to do lots of exercises now so the inflammation in my joints will go away."

b. "I understand that exercise of my joints is important to help prevent loss of motion."

c. "Because exercise is so important, I plan to do as much as I can, regardless of whether it hurts or not—'no pain, no gain'."

d. "They told me I needed to do regular exercise. I think they mean just for my hips and shoulders, because my knees and hands hurt too much."

15. Which of the following classifications of medications is commonly used with osteoarthritis, rheumatoid arthritis, and gout?

a. Narcotics

b. Steroids

c. Uricosurics

d. NSAIDs

16. What is involved in the pathophysiology of gout?

a. A reduction of uric acid, which allows calcium to precipitate

b. Inflammation resulting from intraarticular deposition of urate crystals

c. Thinning of the articular cartilage, leading to splitting and fragmentation

d. Formation of tophi in the kidneys, which impairs excretion of uric acid

17. _____ initiates the release of serum calcium.

a. Phosphate

b. Vitamin D

c. Calcitonin

d. Parathyroid hormone (PTH)

18. The most common fracture site of type II osteoporosis is

a. Ankle

b. Proximal humerus

c. Wrist

d. Vertebrae

19. Monoarticular joint pain is a common finding of
a. Gouty arthritis
b. Rheumatoid arthritis
c. Osteoarthritis
d. None of the above

PART X · ANSWERS

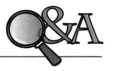

1. **The correct answer is a.** Muscle spasm is usually a consequence of strain, overuse, or injury.
2. **The correct answer is d.** Postural muscles lose strength at approximately 3% per day with bed rest. A referral is indicated for appropriate diagnosis and treatment. The other options contain inappropriate suggestions or incorrect information.
3. **The correct answer is c.** This is the most common cause, usually due to deconditioning or overuse. Answers a and b are less common sources of back pain; d is sometimes a contributing factor.
4. **The correct answer is c.** Degenerative disc disease results from fibrosis and thinning of the nucleus pulposus associated with aging.
5. **The correct answer is a.** It is a disturbance in the balance between osteoclastic and osteoblastic activity, from a variety of causes, and results in osteoporosis. The other choices are incorrect or incomplete.
6. **The correct answer is c.** Weight bearing helps increase osteoblastic activity. Vitamin D is needed for calcium absorption, which is necessary for new bone formation. The other choices are incorrect because estrogen replacement is not recommended for all women, and all older women are at some degree of risk and should modify their lifestyle and/or diet as indicated.
7. **The correct answer is a.** Long-term use of glucocorticoid hormones can commonly cause osteoporosis; the others do not.
8. **The correct answer is a.** Bones in men are denser and thicker than those of women. The other choices are incorrect because demineralization in men begins in the late 60s, and men do get osteoporosis and vertebral compression fractures.
9. **The correct answer is b.** The mesh-like network provides tensile strength. The other options include parts of bone structure but do not provide tensile strength.
10. **The correct answer is d.** Because this is the only bone tissue that contains pain receptors, any process that disrupts or results in pressure on the periosteum causes pain.
11. **The correct answer is b.** The matrix is collagen tissue. Minerals deposit on this tissue.

12. **The correct answer is c.** Vitamins D and C are the most important for bone healing. The callus is unstable and not as strong as bone tissue, and bone remodeling can take as much as a year, depending on a number of factors.

13. **The correct answer is a.** Osteoarthritis is caused by wear and tear and trauma and can occur in middle age and in the elderly. The other options describe other forms of arthritis.

14. **The correct answer is b.** Individualized exercise plans are important to maintain as much joint function as possible, while at the same time preventing additional joint damage. (This is the rationale for why choice d is incorrect.) Choices a and c are incorrect because arthritis does not go away and exercise should not be done to the point of pain.

15. **The correct answer is c.** These are antiinflammatory medications used with all these conditions. The other choices are incorrect because narcotics are not used for long-term treatment of arthritis; under certain circumstances, steroids are sometimes used with rheumatoid arthritis; and NSAIDs are used with gout.

16. **The correct answer is b.** This is the only option that describes the pathology of gout.

17. **The correct answer is d.** PTH regulates blood calcium levels and phosphate while promoting formation of osteoclasts.

18. **The correct answer is b.** The proximal humerus is among the most common sites for type II osteoporotic fractures. The other sites include the femoral neck and proximal tibia.

19. **The correct answer is a.** Monoarticular joint pain, especially of the great toe, is a hallmark of gout.

Glossary

Accessory muscles   muscles used during dyspnea to assist in ventilation and include the sternocleidomastoid and scalenus muscles in the neck and possibly facial muscles

Achlorhydria   the absence of hydrochloric acid in gastric juice

Acid   a substance containing more than one H⁺ ion

Acidosis   decreased base or excess acid

Acquired active immunity   immunity provided because the body makes its own antibodies

Acquired immunodeficiency syndrome (AIDS)   T-cell immune system failure

Active transport   movement of molecules by a protein transporter across a membrane against a concentration gradient and requiring an expenditure of energy.

Acute renal failure (ARF)   renal failure that begins abruptly and is generally reversible

Acute respiratory distress syndrome (ARDS)   acute hypoxemia as the result of a systemic or pulmonary event that is not cardiac in origin

Acute tubular necrosis (ATN)   inflammatory process leading to tubular edema, obstruction, and ischemia

Addison's disease   adrenal insufficiency caused by deficient adrenal cortical hormones and elevated adrenocorticotropic hormone (ACTH) levels

Adenocarcinoma   a form of cancer that begins in glandular tissue

Adenosine triphosphate   a nucleic acid that powers cellular activity

Aerobes   pathogens that require oxygen for growth and metabolism

Affinity   ability of the receptor sites to bind with the hormone

Afterload   resistance to ejection of blood from the left ventricle during systole

Agranulocytes leukocytes without cytoplasmic granules

Akinesia inability to initiate movement

Alkalosis excess base or loss of acid

Allogenic non-self donor

α Thalassemia caused by a short α chain on chromosome 16

α₁-Antitrypsin (AAT) enzyme an enzyme that inactivates proteolytic enzymes such as trypsin involved in tissue remodeling in response to infection so that tissue damage is controlled

Alveolar macrophages macrophages in the lungs

Amphiarthroses slightly moveable joint such as the symphysis pubis, vertebrae, or ribs

Anaerobes bacteria that die when exposed to oxygen

Anastomosis removal of diseased portion of the colon and reattaching to healthier aspects of the colon

Anemia decrease in hemoglobin level

Aneurysm a localized dilation of a blood vessel or cardiac chamber wall due to congenital or acquired weakness of the muscle

Angina chest pain that occurs due to hypoxia or ischemia

Angiotensin II powerful vasoconstrictor

Antibody (also called immunoglobulins) proteins formed by B cells in response to antigens. Antibodies bind to antigens and destroy the antigen.

Antigen any substance recognized as foreign by the immune system

Antinuclear antibody (ANA) test that detects autoantibodies which are a marker for systemic lupus erythematosus

Apoptosis programmed cell death

Asbestos a mineral fiber that is carcinogenic

Ascites the accumulation of fluid in the peritoneal cavity

Aseptic meningitis viral infection limited to the meninges

Asterixis flapping tremor of the hand

Asthma a respiratory disease characterized by acute airway inflammation, bronchoconstriction, bronchospasm, edema of the bronchioles, and increased production of mucus

Ataxia impaired gait or staggering

Atelectasis incomplete alveolar expansion

Atherosclerosis a chronic disease characterized by thickening and hardening of the arterial wall

Atrial natriuretic peptide hormone released from muscle cells in the atria

Atypia cell abnormality that may or may not be a precursor to cancer

Aura a manifestation of symptoms or prodrome that occurs before the onset of a seizure

Automaticity ability of specialized tissue cells in the sinoatrial node to spontaneously initiate impulses

Autonomic hyperreflexia an acute episode of a syndrome consisting of hypertension, vasospasm, and skin pallor; considered a clinical emergency

Autonomic nervous system (ANS) regulation of the internal environment and involuntary control of organs

Autoregulation the brain's ability to regulate or maintain blood volume under a constant change in arterial pressure

Azotemia a condition in which abnormal levels of urea, creatinine, and other waste products are in the blood because they cannot be filtered out into the urine

Bacille Calmette-Guérin vaccine (BCG) made from a live weakened strain of *Mycobacterium bovis* (similar to *M. tuberculosis*); only preventative tuberculosis vaccine available

Bacteria organism that contains both RNA and DNA; they have a rigid cell wall and reproduce by cell division

Bacterial meningitis infection of the pia mater, arachnoid, and subarachnoid, the ventricular system, and cerebrospinal fluid

Bands immature neutrophils

Barrett's esophagus abnormal changes or metaplasia in the lower esophagus

Base a substance with the ability to combine with H$^+$ ions from a solution

Basophils type of white blood cell involved in an allergic response or stress, although their function is unclear

B cells lymphocytes that produce antibodies

Benign prostatic hyperplasia (BPH) enlargement of the prostate gland not caused by a malignancy

Blebs *see* bullae

β Thalassemia caused by a mutation on chromosome 11

Bone remodeling when existing bone is resorbed and new bone is formed to replace it

Borborygmi bowel sounds caused by movement of intestinal gas

Bronchopneumonia patchy pneumonia in several lobes

Brudzinski's sign a neurological sign causing hip flexion when neck is flexed

Bullae large ineffective air spaces

Ca 50 (carbohydrate antigen) Tumor marker used to plot progression of many types of tumors; especially useful for tumors of the gastrointestinal tract

Calcitonin hormone produced by the parafollicular cells of the thyroid

Carbonic acid carbon dioxide plus water

Carbonic anhydrase enzyme in red blood cells that causes 60% of the carbon dioxide produced by cell metabolism to rapidly combine with water and create carbonic acid

Carcinoembryonic antigen (CEA) antigen released during rapid proliferation of epithelial cells, particularly of the gastrointestinal tract; not diagnostic, but frequent measurement helps to guide management and evaluate success of treatment measures

Cardiac output the amount of blood in liters, pumped out by the ventricles in a minute

Caseous necrosis central section of a tubercle that becomes necrotic and forms a yellow "cheesy" mass

Casts clumps of cells that form in the collecting tubules and are shed in the urine

CD antigen enables cells to be identified

Celiac disease malabsorption of nutrients found predominantly in whites

Cell-mediated immunity immunity provided by T cells and macrophages

Central nervous system (CNS) brain and spinal cord

Centrilobular emphysema associated with both smoking and chronic bronchitis, primarily affecting the respiratory bronchioles

Chain of infection process by which infection moves from host to host

Chelating agent binds with a substance such as iron so it can be eliminated from the body

Chemical mediators   responsible for initiating and sustaining the inflammatory response (i.e., histamine)

Cholecystitis   inflammation of the gallbladder usually caused by an obstruction, either gallstone or tumor

Cholescintigraphy (HIDA scan)   evaluates gallbladder and common bile duct function

Chondrocytes   cartilage cells

Chronic airflow limitation   three common respiratory diseases—asthma, chronic bronchitis, and emphysema—that limit ventilation

Chronic bronchitis   inflammation of the bronchi, a productive cough, and increased mucous production for at least 3 months of the year for 2 consecutive years

Chronic incontinence   bladder loses its ability to store urine or empty urine effectively

Chronic obstructive pulmonary disease (COPD)   chronic, often progressive, airflow limitation related to chronic bronchitis or emphysema

Chronic overdistention   occurs when urine is held in the bladder for prolonged periods of time rather than voiding

Chronic renal failure (CRF)   renal failure that progresses to end-stage renal disease

Chvostek's sign   Ipsilateral contraction of facial muscles elicited by tapping facial nerve anterior to the ear

Chylomicrons   large lipoproteins that serve as a transport system of exogenous or dietary lipids to the liver and adipose, cardiac, and skeletal tissues

Chyme   partially digested food

Cirrhosis   condition of chronic, progressive, irreversible damage to the liver resulting in compromised hepatic functioning due to a variety of causes

Colonization   presence of microorganisms without cellular injury

Colorectal cancer allelotyping for chromosomes 17p and 18q   Blood and tissue samples are used to determine the presence of cellular *p53* and *DCC* genes located on chromosomes 17p and 18q, respectively

Community-acquired pneumonia   pneumonia acquired outside of a hospital/health care setting

Compact bone   cortical bone that forms the outermost aspect of bone

Compartment syndrome   compromised vascular perfusion caused by increased pressure within the limited space of bone

Complement system   plasma proteins that aid in the inflammatory process

Concussion   temporary loss of brain function with or without loss of consciousness

Conductivity   ability to transmit impulses from one fiber to another

Constipation   abnormally delayed or decreased number of hard, dry feces

Contractility   ability of the myocardial fibers to shorten

Contusion   injury to the brain causing small hemorrhages and swelling

Cor pulmonale   development of right-sided heart failure in response to chronic pulmonary artery resistance

Cortex   outermost part of the adrenal that secretes glucocorticoids, mineralocorticoids, and adrenal sex hormones

Coup-countrecoup injury   when an external force strikes the head, forcing the brain to move and hit the opposite side of the skull, causing a contusion on both sides

Cretinism   lack of thyroid hormone at birth or within the first several months of life; also referred to as "congenital hypothyroidism"

Crohn's disease   insidious, slow-developing, chronic, progressive disorder that involves the full thickness of the bowel wall

Crypt abscesses   ulcerative hemorrhages in the mucosal layer of the rectum that cause abscess

Cushing's reflex   decreased pulse, elevated systolic pressure, and widened pulse pressure

Cushing's syndrome   excess glucocorticoids causing "moon face," hirsutism, buffalo hump, and truncal obesity

Cushing's triad   elevated systolic pressure, bradycardia, and widening pulse pressure that is accompanied by respiratory changes

Cyclooxygenase   enzyme necessary for prostaglandin production

Cystitis   inflammation of the bladder

Cytoxic T cells   destroy infected cells

Decerebrate posturing   rigid extension of all extremities with hyperpronation of forearms and plantar extension

Decorticate posturing   arm, wrist, and finger flexion with upper extremity flexion at elbows and external rotation and extension of lower extremities

Defecation   the act of passing stool or feces from the bowels through the rectum

Dendritic cells   macrophages in lymphoid tissue

Diarrhea   increased number of watery or loose stools

Diastole   ventricular relaxation

Diastolic dysfunction   classic findings of congestive heart failure with abnormal diastolic but normal systolic function/normal ejection fraction

Diffuse axonal injury (DAI)   characteristic injury occurring when the head strikes an inanimate object or a moving object strikes the head, causing a rotational movement of the head

Diffusion   movement of solutes across a semipermeable membrane

Dihydrotestosterone   androgen created from the hormone testosterone by the enzyme 5α-reductase secreted by stromal cells

Dilated cardiomyopathy   cardiomegaly due to ventricular dilation and by impaired myocardial contractility and mixed systolic and diastolic dysfunction

Dissecting aneurysm   tear in the inner layer of an arterial wall that allows blood to collect between layers of the wall

Diurnal rhythm   cyclic secretion of hormones that begins with onset of sleep and decreases as the day progresses

Diverticulitis   acute inflammation of diverticula

Diverticulosis   asymptomatic presence of diverticula, or outpouching of the sigmoid colon

Down-regulation   a higher concentration of hormones causing a decrease in the number of receptor sites

Dressler's syndrome   pain, fever, and arthralgias occurring after a myocardial infarction as an inflammatory response or hypersensitivity reaction to necrotic heart tissue

Dysarthria   difficulty forming words

Dyslipidemia   increased level of plasma lipid concentration made up of cholesterol and/or triglycerides

Dysphagia   difficulty swallowing

Dysplasia   abnormality of cell that is a precursor to cancer

Edema   accumulation of fluid within the interstitial spaces

Effector cells   killer T cells

Emphysema   anatomical term that denotes loss of lung elasticity as a result of the breakdown of connective tissue support of the lower airways, abnormal dilatation of air spaces distal to the terminal bronchioles, and abnormal enlargement and eventual destruction of the alveoli

Empyema   a collection of pus within the pleural space surrounding the lungs

Endocardium   innermost lining of the heart and blood vessels

Endocrine glands   ductless glands that secrete hormone directly into the circulation (such as the adrenal or thyroid glands)

Endotoxins   bacteria found in gram-negative bacteria cell walls

Eosinophils   type of white blood cell found mainly in the gastrointestinal and respiratory tracts where they protect the body from parasitic infections by secreting toxic enzymes that destroy the invader

Epilepsy   recurrent seizures with no known underlying or correctable cause

Erythema chronicum migrans   characteristic "bull's eye" rash of Lyme disease

Erythropoietin   hormone that stimulates the bone marrow to produce red blood cells in response to hypoxia

Essential hypertension   *see* primary hypertension

Excitability   response to stimulation

Exertional dyspnea   shortness of breath with exercise or exertion

Exocrine glands   secrete hormones to epithelial surface either directly or through a duct (such as sweat or salivary glands).

Exophthalmus   anterior bulging of the eye from its orbit

Exsanguinations   an abdominal aortic aneurysm that bleeds into the peritoneal cavity, causing death

Extracorporeal shock wave lithotripsy   procedure during which renal calculi are broken apart by sound waves

Extrinsic asthma   "allergic" asthma; the result of increased IgE synthesis and hypersensitivity of the airways

Extrinsic pathway   clotting cascade begins as a reaction to chemical mediators released from damaged endothelial cells

Facilitated diffusion   movement of molecules by a protein transporter across a membrane without an expenditure of energy

Fecal antigen assay   one test of choice to verify eradication of the *Helicobacter pylori* bacteria after treatment for the disease

Fecal fat   used to diagnose conditions associated with poor fat absorption (i.e., pancreatic disorders, Crohn's disease, hepatobiliary diseases)

Festinating gait   short accelerating steps in attempt to maintain upright position

Fibrinous exudate   thick and clotted exudate

Fibroblasts   connective tissue cell that synthesizes and secretes collagen

Filtration   movement of water and dissolved substances from an area of high pressure to one of lower pressure

Flagella a whip-like projection on a bacterium that allows movement

Flatus gas generated in the intestines that is expelled through the rectum

Frank-Starling law of the heart the greater the stretch of the ventricle during diastole, the greater the volume of blood ejected during systole

Fungi organism that digests food externally and then absorbs nutrients into their cells (i.e., yeast)

Fusiform aneurysm a circumferential and relatively uniformly shaped malformation of the artery

Gastroscopy used to visualize mucosal irregularities, varices, ulcers, perforations, or tears or to obtain brushings of gastric mucosa to identify the presence of *Helicobacter pylori*

Ghon's focus *see* granulomatous lesions

Glomerulosclerosis progressive hardening of the glomerular capillaries

Glomerulus plasma-filtering capillary tuft created by the efferent and afferent arterioles and surrounded by Bowman's capsule in nephrons

Gluconeogenesis release of glucose from stored glycogen

Glycosaminoglycans long-chain polysaccharides derived from carbohydrates

Goiter diffuse thyroid enlargement

Granulocytes leukocytes that contain cytoplasmic granules

Granuloma small nodule that results in area of inflammation

Granulomatous lesions tubercles composed of fused elongated macrophages that have engulfed the bacilli and are surrounded by lymphocytes

Greenfield filter inferior vena cava filter used to prevent deep vein thrombosis from traveling to right atria and then to the lungs via the pulmonary artery

Haversian system internal structure of compact bone

Helminths worm-like parasites

Helper T cells stimulate the production of other T cells, activate macrophages, help killer T cells, and activate B cells to produce antibodies

Hematemesis blood in vomitus typically with a "coffee-ground" appearance

Hematochezia rectal bleeding

Hematocrit the percent of whole blood that is composed of red blood cells

Hematuria blood in the urine

Hemiparesis contralateral weakness

Hemiplegia loss of mobility

Hemoglobin the oxygen-carrying component of red blood cells

Hemoglobin F fetal hemoglobin

Hemolytic uremic syndrome (HUS) disorder characterized by microangiopathic hemolytic anemia, thrombocytopenia, and renal failure

Hemoptysis coughing up blood

High-density lipoprotein (HDL) contains the largest proportion of apoprotein; "good" cholesterol

Hila areas where the bronchus splits into the right and left bronchi

Histiocytes macrophages in connective tissue

Horner's syndrome   a syndrome caused by injury to the sympathetic nerves of the face; signs and symptoms include sinking of the eyeball into the face, constricted pupil, drooping eyelid (ptosis), and a lack of face sweating, all occurring on the same side of the body

Human immunodeficiency virus (HIV) virus that causes T-cell failure

Human leukocyte antigens (HLA)   part of our individual genetic makeup; recognizes self from non-self

Humoral immunity   antibody-mediated immunity controlled by B lymphocytes

Hydronephrosis   condition in which the kidney is distended with urine that cannot pass through the ureters

Hydrostatic pressure   mechanical force of water against cellular membranes.

Hyperaldosteronism   excessive production of mineralocorticoids

Hypercalcemia   increased calcium

Hypercapnia   excess carbon dioxide in the blood

Hyperglycemic hypertonic nonketotic syndrome   severe hyperglycemia, osmotic diuresis, hypovolemia, and dehydration accompanied by decreased urine output, lactic acidosis, presence of ketosis, and neurological abnormalities

Hyperinsulinemia   excess levels of circulating insulin in blood

Hyperkalemia   increased potassium

Hypermagnesemia   increased magnesium

Hypernatremia   increased sodium

Hyperparathyroidism   increased secretion of parathyroid hormone

Hypersensitivity reaction   excessive immune response

Hypertensive emergency   life-threatening hypertension requiring immediate medical intervention

Hypertonic   higher concentration of solute than body fluid

Hyperuricemia   increased levels of uric acid in blood

Hypocalcemia   decreased calcium

Hypocapnia   low carbon dioxide in the blood

Hypokalemia   decreased potassium

Hypokinesia/bradykinesia   slowed or diminished movements characterized by difficulty initiating, continuing, and synchronizing movements

Hypomagnesemia   decreased magnesium

Hyponatremia   decreased sodium

Hypoparathyroidism   decreased secretion of parathyroid hormone

Hypotonic   lower concentration of solute than body fluid

Iatrogenic   state or condition that occurs as a result of medical or therapeutic intervention

Icteric phase   symptomatic with presence of jaundice

IgA   One of the five classes of immunoglobulins (antibodies), it is found in saliva; tears; and gastrointestinal (gastrointestinal), bronchial, prostatic, and vaginal secretions

IgD   One of the five classes of immunoglobulins (antibodies), it may be responsible for binding the antigen to the surface of the B cell

IgE   One of the five classes of immunoglobulins (antibodies), it binds to mast cells and causes the release of histamine etc.

IgG   One of the five classes of immunoglobulins (antibodies), it is the most common of the immunoglobulins and the only one to cross the placenta

IgM One of the five classes of immunoglobulins (antibodies), it activates complement and is the first antibody formed when B cells initially encounter an antigen

Immune complex dissociated p24 assay detects the p24 antigen, which is an indication of active human immunodeficiency virus replication

Incontinence involuntary passage of urine

Indirect bilirubin insoluble form of bilirubin

Inflammatory response general response to any cell injury

Insensible losses loss of fluids through vaporization from skin or lungs

Interleukin-1 substance produced by neutrophils and macrophages primarily responsible for fever production

Intestinal villi finger-like projections lining the intestinal tract that assist with digestion

Intrarenal ARF acute renal failure caused by injury to the kidney itself

Intrinsic asthma nonallergic asthma triggered by events such as a upper respiratory tract infection

Intrinsic factor glycoprotein secreted by the parietal cells of the stomach necessary for vitamin B_{12} absorption from the intestines

Intrinsic pathway clotting cascade begins as a reaction to vascular injury

Intussusception telescoping of the bowel onto an adjacent part of the bowel

Isotonic same concentration (osmolality) of solute as body fluid

Jaundice condition in which the skin, tissues, and conjunctiva become yellow because of the excess bilirubin in the blood

Kernig's sign neurological sign that causes resistance to leg extension when the hip is flexed at a right angle

Ketosis release of fatty acids from adipose tissue and converted to ketones by the liver

Ki-67 proliferation marker determines prognosis and outcomes in patients with specific types of cancers, including colorectal cancer

Killer T cells effector cells

Kupffer cells macrophages in the liver sinusoids

Kussmaul's respiration deep rapid respiration

Langerhans' cells macrophages in the skin

Large-volume diarrhea increased volume of feces

Left ventricular dysfunction elevation of pressure in the left ventricle

Leukocytes white blood cells

Leukocytosis increase in number of circulating white blood cells

Leukotrienes acidic sulfur-containing lipids released from the mast cell membrane that produce a slower and more prolonged inflammatory response

Ligaments attach bone to bone

Lipogenesis mobilization and redistribution of fatty acids for energy use

Lobar pneumonia confined to a single lobe of the lung

Low-density lipoprotein (LDL) the highest concentration of cholesterol and are the major transporter of cholesterol; "bad" cholesterol

Lyme disease caused by the spirochete *Borrelia burgdorferi*, it is the most common tick-borne illness in the United States

Lymphocytes type of white blood cell involved in the immune response

Macrophages largest of the white blood cells

Major histocompatibility complex (MHC) large cluster of genes located on chromosome 6 enabling the body to code its own antigens

Mantoux test intradermal method of injecting purified protein derivative

Mast cells activate the initial inflammatory response

Matrix extracellular connective tissue made up of collagen, proteins, and minerals that stores mineral salts or calcium

Medulla innermost portion of the adrenal glands that secretes epinephrine, norepinephrine, and dopamine

Medullary canal innermost part of the bone containing bone marrow

Mesangial cells found between the capillary tufts and provide structural support for the glomerulus; macrophages in the kidney

Mesenteric angiography used with conscious sedation to localize and possibly perform therapeutic embolization of a bleeding site that does not respond to conservative therapy and cannot be visualized by endoscopy

Mesothelioma primary tumor arising from the surface of the pleura (80%) or the peritoneum (20%)

Metabolic acidosis a decrease in pH due to a decrease in HCO_3

Metabolic alkalosis increase in HCO_3 concentration due to an increase in pH

Metaplasia replacement of one cell type with a differentiated cell type affecting the linings of various organs

Microglia macrophages in the nervous system

Micturition act of voiding

Mitral valve regurgitation backward or retrograde flow of blood during ventricular systole due to the incomplete closing of the mitral valve

Mitral valve stenosis valve in which the leaflets have become thickened and restrict the forward flow

Monocytes mature macrophages

Mononuclear phagocyte system monocytes and macrophages

Monro-Kellie hypothesis volume and pressure relationship between intracranial pressure, cerebrospinal fluid volume, blood and brain tissue, and cardiopulmonary pressure

Motility diarrhea diarrhea caused by surgical intervention or pathological process that alters motility of intestines

Mycoplasmata organisms one-third smaller in size than bacteria that can reproduce independently but do not have a rigid cell wall

Myocarditis inflammation of the middle layer of the heart as a result of infection, medications, or viruses

Myocardium middle layer of the heart consisting of cardiac muscle; the thickest of all the layers

Myxedema adult onset of hypothyroidism

Natriuretic hormones peptides that promote excretion of sodium and water through urination

Natural killer cells cytoxic cells that act as surveillance agents

Negative feedback mechanism inhibition or release of a target gland hormone to maintain hormone levels

Nephritic syndrome inflammatory injury to the glomeruli

Nephrotic syndrome injury to the glomerular membrane resulting in proteinuria

Neurotransmitters chemicals (acetylcholine, norepinephrine, epinephrine, dopamine, and serotonin) released from the neuron causing inhibitory or excitatory actions

Neutrophils type of white blood cell with a short lifespan (48 hours) and is responsible for the phagocytosis of bacteria and small particles of debris

Nidus nucleus or center of a stone

Norwalk virus severe gastroenteritis spread by infected food or shellfish or through aerosolization

Nosocomial pneumonia pneumonia that develops 48 hours after admission to the hospital

Nucleus pulposus elastic fibers found at the center of the intervertebral disc

Obstipation severe constipation caused by intestinal obstruction

Oncogenes a modified gene that increases the malignancy of a tumor cell

OraSure HIV-1 test for human immunodeficiency virus infection that uses an oral fluid specimen

Orthopnea difficulty breathing while lying down

Osmolality concentration of molecules by weight of water

Osmosis movement of water across a semipermeable membrane from low solute concentration to higher solute concentration

Osmotic diarrhea large-volume diarrhea produced by increase in stool weight and volume due to osmotic effect

Osmotic (oncotic) pressure overall osmotic effect of colloids (protein molecules)

Osteoblasts bone-forming cells that produce collagen

Osteoclasts macrophages in the bone that remove or resorb bone

Osteogenesis the process of laying down of new bone

Osteomyelitis serious bone infection that requires extensive and prolonged antibiotic therapy

Osteopenia bone thinning

Overflow the bladder does not empty completely because of detrusor muscle malfunction or from blockage of the bladder outlet from conditions such as prostatic enlargement and urethral stricture; may also occur because of a chronic avoidance of bladder emptying

Paget's disease a progressive skeletal disorder causing bone deterioration

Pancreatitis self-limiting inflammation of the pancreas with spontaneous regression in 3–7 days

Panlobular emphysema associated with α_1-antitrypsin deficiency and senile emphysema, which affects the terminal and respiratory bronchioles and alveoli

Pannus granulation tissue

Paraneoplastic characteristics symptoms that develop when substances released by some cancer cells mimic the normal function of other cells, such as the parathyroid gland

Parasympathetic nervous system (ANS-P) maintains organ function antagonist to sympathetic nervous system

Parathyroid hormone (PTH) regulates calcium metabolism

Parietal pleura a double-layered membrane that lines the inside of the thoracic cavity

Paroxysmal nocturnal dyspnea difficulty breathing unless the person stands or sits up

Passive immunity obtained when a person receives antibodies made outside the body by another person, animal, or recombinant DNA

Pericarditis inflammation of the pericardium, a thin, double-layered, fibrous covering of the heart

Pericardium outermost double-walled layer of the heart

Peripheral nervous system (PNS) composed of cranial nerves and spinal nerves

Peristalsis contraction and relaxation of the muscular layer of gastrointestinal tract allowing forward passage of food

Pernicious anemia B_{12} deficiency caused by lack of intrinsic factor

Peroral pneumogram evaluates the terminal ileum; can be performed concurrently with an upper gastrointestinal series

Petechiae minor hemorrhages caused by injured capillary blood vessels

Phagocytosis process whereby pathogens and foreign material are engulfed by white blood cells

Plasma viral load number of viral particles per millimeter of blood

Plasmapheresis removing and filtering of the blood to eliminate waste products and then returning the blood to the body.

Pleural effusion accumulation of excess pleural fluid

Pneumonia an inflammatory process of lung tissue

Polycythemia overproduction of red blood cells

Polydipsia excessive thirst caused by cellular dehydration due to osmotic effect of hyperglycemic state

Polyneuropathies a condition where many peripheral nerves throughout the body malfunction all at once; malfunction is often symmetrical and involves the distal extremities

Polyphagia depletion of stored carbohydrates, fats, and proteins, which causes hunger

Polyuria increased urination due to hyperglycemic state acting as osmotic diuretic

Positive feedback mechanism release of one hormone in response to an elevated level of another stimulating hormone

Postrenal ARF acute renal failure caused by urinary tract obstruction

Preicteric period also known as the prodromal phase; symptomatic but without jaundice

Preload degree of stretch in muscle length before contraction or at the end of diastole

Prerenal ARF acute renal failure caused by renal hypoperfusion

Primary or essential hypertension also known as idiopathic; high blood pressure, for which there is no known cause

Primary lymphoid organs thymus gland and the bone marrow

Prinzmetal's angina also known as variant angina; form of angina caused by coronary artery spasm, with or without atherosclerotic plaque, that occurs unpredictably and almost exclusively at rest

Proctitis inflammation of the rectum

Projectile vomiting spontaneous, forceful vomiting not preceded by any symptoms

Proprioception the ability to sense where the body and body parts are in relation to position, location, and orientation

Prostaglandins cause actions similar to histamine, inhibit the inflammatory response, produce fever and pain, or promote platelet aggregation

Proteinuria leaking of protein into the urine

Protozoa minute unicellular animals

Pruritus sensation of itching caused by release of histamines or accumulation of bile salts depositing in skin

Pulmonary capillary wedge pressure indirect measure of left atrial pressure

Pulmonary embolism any bolus of blood-borne material that travels to the lungs

Pulmonary hypertension reflexive pulmonary vascular narrowing

Purified protein derivative (PPD) an antigen derived from dead tuberculosis bacteria, which stimulates the immune system to produce an inflammatory response

Purulent exudate exudates composed of leukocytes, pus, and dead cells

Pyelonephritis upper urinary tract infection and inflammatory disorder of the renal pelvis and parenchyma

Pyuria pus in urine

Radicular pain caused by lumber nerve root compression

RBC sickling development of a crescent shape

Reentry generalized mechanism underlying many dysrhythmias, such as premature beats, supraventricular tachycardias, and atrial flutter

Reflex incontinence caused by trauma or damage to the nervous system as seen in spinal cord injury above S2–4, multiple sclerosis, and diabetes mellitus; detrusor hyperreflexia occurs even though there is no sensation of the need to void

Refractory period time during the cardiac cycle that follows depolarization

Regulator cells includes helper T cells, which activate B-cell antibody production, and suppressor T cells, which turn off antibody production

Regurgitation backward flow of blood into a chamber

Remodeling process mediated by the renin-angiotensin-aldosterone system that results in hypertrophy and abnormal contractile function both leading to ventricular failure

Remodeling process by which old bone is broken down and resorbed and new bone is manufactured

Renal calculi (urolithiasis) polycrystalline aggregates of crystals that form stones in the renal system

Renal failure inability of the kidneys to regulate fluid volume and filter waste products from the blood

Renal insufficiency denotes a 20% to 50% reduction in the glomerular filtration rate

Renal osteodystrophy demineralization of bone caused by renal failure

Renal tubular acidosis metabolic acidosis that develops because the proximal or distal tubules malfunction and either do not reabsorb bicarbonate or retain hydrogen ions

Resorption ability of a cell to dissolve itself

Respiration exchange of oxygen and carbon dioxide between cells, the alveoli, and the environment

Respiratory acidosis increase in Pa_{CO_2} due to a decrease in pH

Respiratory alkalosis decrease in Pa_{CO_2} resulting in an increase in pH

Reticulocyte immature red blood cell

Reticuloendothelial system older term used to describe the mononuclear phagocyte system

Reverse transcriptase enzyme that converts viral RNA to DNA

Rhythmicity regulates the generation of impulses

Rotaviruses the most common cause of infectious diarrhea found in infants and young children

Saccular aneurysm bulge with a narrow neck or spherical in shape connecting it to one side of the artery

Schilling test a 24-hour urine test used to diagnose pernicious anemia

Secondary hyperparathyroidism increased secretion of parathyroid hormone

Secondary hypertension hypertension caused by an altered hemodynamic state associated with a specific disease

Secondary lymphoid organs spleen, lymph nodes, tonsils, and Peyer's patches in the small intestine

Secretory diarrhea large-volume diarrhea caused by excessive secretion of fluid from intestines

Segs mature neutrophils

Seroconversion human immunodeficiency virus antibody production at a level detectable in blood samples

Serous exudate watery fluid made of plasma

Sigmoidoscopy test used to visualize the mucosa of the sigmoid colon; can detect obstruction, carcinoma, inflammatory disease, and other irregularities

Small-volume diarrhea excessive intestinal motility that produces small amounts of feces

Somatic nervous system (SNS) regulates voluntary control such as skeletal muscle

Spinal shock complete loss of all reflex function that occurs in all areas below the area of trauma immediately after a spinal cord injury

Spirochetes anaerobic bacteria capable of movement by filaments that cover the entire cell wall

Splenic pulp lymphoid tissue in the spleen

Squamous cell carcinoma cancer that arises from epithelial cells

Stabs immature neutrophils

Status asthmaticus severe, prolonged asthma attack that does not respond to usual treatment

Status epilepticus persistent seizure that does not allow restoration of consciousness

Stenosis narrowing of a valve causing decreased blood flow

Stress incontinence related to a weak urethral sphincter so urine leaks out when intraabdominal pressure increases

Stromal cells make up the support structure of the prostate gland

Struvite stones stones with a magnesium ammonium phosphate base created by urease, an enzyme made by bacteria

Superinfection infection that follows or coincides with a previous infection due to resistance or overgrowth of bacteria

Superior vena cava syndrome syndrome that occurs when a tumor compresses blood vessels and impairs blood return to the right atrium

Suppressor T cells turn off the immune response

Surfactant fluid that coats the inner surface of each alveoli and allows it to remain partially opened during exhalation.

Sympathetic nervous system (ANS-S) maintains body temperature and adjusts blood pressure and blood flow; "fight-or-flight" response

Syncope brief loss of consciousness (fainting) due to reduction in blood flow to the brain

Synovitis inflammation of the inner lining of the joint capsule

Systemic lupus erythematosus (SLE) chronic, multisystem, inflammatory disease of unknown cause

Systemic vascular resistance (SVR) decreased or resistive blood flow by the systemic arteries and determines diastolic blood pressure

Systole ventricular contraction

Systolic dysfunction diminished CO (ejection fraction < 40%) due to decreased contractility

Tachypnea rapid respirations

T cells lymphocytes responsible for cell-mediated immunity

Tendons attach muscle to bone

Tenesmus feeling of incomplete evacuation

Thalassemia hereditary disorders of hemoglobin synthesis

Thalassemia major (Cooley's anemia) anemia resulting from the inheritance of a defective gene from each parent leading to the production of excess α chains that attach to the RBC membrane, damaging RBCs and forming toxic substances

Thalassemia minor mutation in one β globin allele (β thalassemia trait)

Third spacing movement of transcellular fluid from one compartment to another

Thrombocytopenia decreased platelet count

Thyroid-stimulating hormone (TSH) hormone released from the anterior pituitary that causes stimulation of the thyroid gland

Thyroid storm life-threatening form of thyrotoxicosis

Thyrotoxicosis state of excessive thyroid hormone

Thyrotropin-releasing hormone (TRH) hormone secreted by the hypothalamus that influences release of TSH

Thyroxine (T_4) hormone stored in the thyroid that is composed of active iodine compound

Tine test multiple-puncture test method of injecting purified protein derivative

Trabecular bone cancellous or spongy bone found on the inside aspect of bone

Transient incontinence temporary incontinence caused by irritation to the bladder and urethra

Triglycerides highly concentrated energy source found in fats and oils absorbed from the diet

Triiodothyronine (T₃) hormone stored in the thyroid that contains three iodine molecules and has a faster release into the bloodstream than T4

Trousseau's sign carpal spasm related to ischemia of nerves in upper arm during inflation of blood pressure cuff (for 3–5 minutes) above systolic pressure

True aneurysms occur as a result of atrophy of the medial layer of the artery

Tuberculosis (TB) chronic recurrent infection caused by *Mycobacterium tuberculosis* that involves the lung and, less commonly, other tissues

Tubulointerstitial disorders disorders that affect the proximal and distal tubules and sometimes the tissue surrounding the tubules

Up-regulation lower concentration of hormone causing an increase in the number of receptor sites

Upper gastrointestinal series fluoroscopic study used to evaluate the upper gastrointestinal tract

Urea breath test/C-Urea noninvasive study of choice to verify eradication of *Helicobacter pylori* after treatment

Urease enzymatic byproduct of urea that produces ammonia

Uremic frost uric acid and other toxins deposited on the skin during the final stage of renal failure

Urethritis inflammation of the urethra

Urge incontinence a type of chronic incontinence caused by inappropriate, repetitive, strong contraction of the detrusor muscle that eventually overcomes urethral sphincter control

Variant angina *see* Prinzmetal's angina

Ventilation movement of air denoting inhalation and exhalation

Ventilation-perfusion scan used to evaluate both ventilation and perfusion of lungs

Virchow's triad venous stasis, vessel wall injury, and hypercoagulability

Viruses smallest pathogens that can reproduce outside of a living cell and are composed of a protein coat that surrounds a nucleic acid core of either RNA or DNA

Visceral pleura a double-layered membrane that lines the outside of the lungs

Vitamin B₁₂ absorption test (Schilling test) 24-hour urine test that detects ileal disease or resection, Crohn's disease, pancreatitis, postgastrectomy, and cystic fibrosis

Volvulus torsion or twisting of the bowel

Vomiting sudden, forceful emptying of stomach contents

References

PART I

Bullock, B., & Henze, R. (2000). *Focus on pathophysiology*. Philadelphia: Lippincott, Williams & Wilkins.

Huether, S., & McCance, K. (2004). *Understanding pathophysiology* (3rd ed.). St. Louis, MO: Mosby.

Porth, C. (2005). *Pathophysiology: Concepts of altered health states* (7th ed.). Philadelphia: Lippincott, Williams & Wilkins.

Price, S., & Wilson, L. (2003). *Pathophysiology: Clinical concepts of disease processes*. St. Louis, MO: Mosby.

PART II

Dambro, M. R. (Ed.). (2001). *Griffith's 5-minute clinical consultant*. Philadelphia: Lippincott, Williams & Wilkins.

Groer, M. W. (2001). *Advanced pathophysiology: Application to clinical practice*. Philadelphia: Lippincott, Williams & Wilkins.

Hansen, M. (1998). *Pathophysiology: Foundations of disease and clinical interventions*. Philadelphia: W. B. Saunders.

Huether, S. E., & McCance, K. L. (2004). *Understanding pathophysiology* (3rd ed.). St. Louis, MO: Mosby.

Langford, R. W., & Thompson, J. D. (2000). *Mosby's handbook of diseases* (2nd ed.). St. Louis, MO: C. V. Mosby Co.

LeMone, P., & Burke, K. M. (2004). *Medical surgical nursing: Critical thinking in client care* (3rd ed.). Upper Saddle River, NJ: Prentice Hall Health.

McPhee, S., Papadakis, M., & Tierney, L. Jr. (Eds). (2007). *Current medical diagnosis and treatment* (46th ed.). New York: McGraw-Hill.

Pagana, K. D., & Pagana, T. J. (2006). *Mosby's diagnostic and laboratory test* (3rd ed.). St. Louis: Mosby.

Porth, C. M. (2005). *Pathophysiology: Concepts of altered health* (7th ed.). Philadelphia: Lippincott, Williams & Wilkins.

Zollo, A. J. (2004). *Medical secrets* (4th ed.). Philadelphia: Hanley & Belfus.

PART III

Blackwell, S., & Hendrix, P. (2001). Common anemias. *Clinician Reviews, 11*, 3.

Crowley, L. V. (2007). *An introduction to human disease: Pathology and pathophysiology correlations* (7th ed.). Sudbury, MA: Jones and Bartlett Publishers.

Dambro, M. R. (Ed.). (1999). *Griffith's 5-minute clinical consult.* Philadelphia: Lippincott, Williams & Wilkins.

Fischbach, F. (2000). *A manual of laboratory and diagnostic tests* (6th ed.). Philadelphia: Lippincott, Williams & Wilkins.

Groer, M. W. (2001). *Advanced pathophysiology: Application to clinical practice.* Philadelphia: Lippincott, Williams & Wilkins.

Huether, S. E., & McCance, K. L. (2004). *Understanding pathophysiology* (3rd ed.). St. Louis, MO: Mosby.

Kumar, V., Cotran, R. S., & Robbins, S. L. (1997). *Basic pathophysiology* (6th ed.). Philadelphia: W. B. Saunders.

McPhee, S., Papadakis, M., & Tierney, L. Jr. (Eds.). (2007). *Current medical diagnosis and treatment* (46th ed.). New York: McGraw-Hill.

Mulvihill, M. L., Zenman, M., Holdaway, P., Tompary, E., & Turchany, J. (2001). *Human diseases: A systemic approach* (5th ed.). Upper Saddle River, NJ: Prentice Hall Health.

Nicoll, D., McPhee, S. J., Pignone, M., Detmer, W. M., & Chou, T. (2001). *Pocket guide to diagnostic tests* (3rd ed.). New York: Lange Medical Books/McGraw-Hill.

Porth, C. M. (2005). *Pathophysiology: Concepts of altered health* (7th ed.). Philadelphia: Lippincott, Williams & Wilkins.

Tierney, L. M. Jr., McPhee, S. J., & Papadakis, M. A. (2001). *Current medical diagnosis and treatment* (40th ed.). New York: Lange Medical Books/McGraw-Hill.

PART IV

Beers, M., Porter, R., & Jones, T. (2006). *The Merck manual of diagnosis and therapy* (18th ed.). Whitehouse Station, NJ: Merck Publishers.

Bullock, B., & Henze, R. (2000). *Focus on pathophysiology*. Philadelphia: Lippincott, Williams & Wilkins.

Huether, S., & McCance, K. (2004). *Understanding pathophysiology* (3rd ed.). St. Louis, MO: Mosby.

Porth, C. (2005). *Pathophysiology: Concepts of altered health states* (7th ed.). Philadelphia: Lippincott, Williams & Wilkins.

Price, S., & Wilson, L. (2003). *Pathophysiology: Clinical concepts of disease processes*. St. Louis, MO: Mosby.

Roldan, C., & Abrams, J. (2002). *Evaluation of the patient with heart disease: Integrating the physical exam and echocardiography*. Philadelphia: Lippincott, Williams & Wilkins.

PART V

Bullock, B., & Henze, R. (2000). *Focus on pathophysiology*. Philadelphia: Lippincott, Williams & Wilkins.

Janssen, J., & McDermott, M. (2007). Update on benign thyroid disorders in women. *The Female Patient*, Vol. 32 pgs. 49–56.

Lu, R., & Burman, K. (2006). Interpretation of thyroid function tests. *Women's Health in Primary Care*, September-October 2006, pgs. 30–40.

Porth, C. (2005). *Pathophysiology: Concepts of altered health states* (7th ed.). Philadelphia: Lippincott, Williams & Wilkins.

Price, S., & Wilson, L. (2003). *Pathophysiology: Clinical concepts of disease processes*. St. Louis, MO: Mosby.

Stan, M., & Fatourechi, V. (2007). Thyroid nodules and goiters: current standards of care. *Consultant*, 47, January 2007, pgs. 49–56.

Youngkin, E., & Davis, M. (2004). *Women's health: A primary care clinical guide* (3rd ed.). Upper Saddle River, NJ: Pearson Prentice Hall.

PART VI

Dambro, M. R. (Ed.). (2001). *Griffith's 5-minute clinical consultant.* Philadelphia: Lippincott, Williams & Wilkins.

Groer, M. W. (2001). *Advanced pathophysiology: Application to clinical practice.* Philadelphia: Lippincott, Williams & Wilkins.

Hansen, M. (1998). *Pathophysiology: Foundations of disease and clinical interventions.* Philadelphia: W. B. Saunders.

Huether, S. E., & McCance, K. L. (2004). *Understanding pathophysiology* (3rd ed.). St. Louis, MO: Mosby.

Langford, R. W., & Thompson, J. D. (2000). *Mosby's handbook of diseases* (2nd ed.). St. Louis, MO: C. V. Mosby Co.

LeMone, P., & Burke, K. M. (2004). *Medical surgical nursing: Critical thinking in client care* (3rd ed.). Upper Saddle River, NJ: Prentice Hall Health.

McPhee, S., Papadakis, M., & Tierney, L. Jr. (Eds). (2007). *Current medical diagnosis and treatment* (46th ed.). New York: McGraw-Hill.

Pagana, K. D., & Pagana, T. J. (2006). *Mosby's diagnostic and laboratory tests* (3rd ed). St. Louis, MO: Mosby.

Porth, C. M. (2005). *Pathophysiology: Concepts of altered health* (7th ed.). Philadelphia: Lippincott, Williams & Wilkins.

Zollo, A. J. (2004). *Medical secrets* (4th ed.). Philadelphia: Hanley & Belfus.

PART VII

Bullock, B., & Henze, R. (2000). *Focus on pathophysiology.* Philadelphia: Lippincott, Williams & Wilkins.

Dubin, D. (2000). *Rapid interpretation of EKGs* (6th ed.). Tampa, FL: Cover Publishing.

Grundy, S., Cleeman, J., Daniels, S., Donato, K., Ecket, R., Franklin, B., Gordon, D., Krauss, R., Savage, P., Smith, S., Spertus, J., & Costa, F. (2005). Diagnosis and management of the metabolic syndrome. An American Heart Association/National Heart, Lung, and Blood Institute scientific statement. *Circulation.* Sept. 12, 2005, circ.ahajournals.org.

Huether, S., & McCance, K. (2004). *Understanding pathophysiology* (3rd ed.). St. Louis, MO: Mosby.

Porth, C. (2005). *Pathophysiology: Concepts of altered health states* (7th ed.). Philadelphia: Lippincott, Williams & Wilkins.

Price, S., & Wilson, L. (2003). *Pathophysiology: Clinical concepts of disease processes.* St. Louis, MO: Mosby.

Roldan, C., & Abrams, J. (2002). *Evaluation of the patient with heart disease: Integrating the physical exam and echocardiography.* Philadelphia: Lippincott, Williams & Wilkins.

Seventh Report of the Joint National Committee on Prevention, Detection, Evaluation and Treatment of High Blood Pressure (JNC 7). U.S. Department of Health and Human Services, NIH Publication No. 03-5231, May 2003.

PART VIII

Bullock, B., & Henze, R. (2000). *Focus on pathophysiology.* Philadelphia: Lippincott, Williams & Wilkins.

Huether, S., & McCance, K. (2004). *Understanding pathophysiology* (3rd ed.). St. Louis, MO: Mosby.

Landzberg, B. (2006). Celiac disease: Could you be missing the diagnosis? *Consultant,* Nov. 2006, Vol 46 No. 11, pgs. 1458-1466.

Porth, C. (2005). *Pathophysiology: Concepts of altered health states* (7th ed.). Philadelphia: Lippincott, Williams & Wilkins.

PART IX

Dambro, M. R. (Ed). (2001). *Griffith's 5-minute clinical consultant.* Philadelphia: Lippincott, Williams & Wilkins.

Groer, M. W. (2001). *Advanced pathophysiology: Application to clinical practice.* Philadelphia: Lippincott, Williams & Wilkins.

Hansen, M. (1998). *Pathophysiology: Foundations of disease and clinical interventions.* Philadelphia: W. B. Saunders.

Huether, S. E., & McCance, K. L. (2004). *Understanding pathophysiology* (3rd ed.). St. Louis, MO: C. V. Mosby Co.

Langford, R. W., & Thompson, J. D. (2000). *Mosby's handbook of diseases* (2nd ed.). St. Louis, MO: C. V. Mosby Co.

LeMone, P. & Burke, K. M. (2004). *Medical surgical nursing: Critical thinking in client care* (3rd ed.). Upper Saddle River, NJ: Prentice Hall Health.

McPhee, S., Papadakis, M., & Tierney, L. Jr. (Eds). (2007). *Current medical diagnosis and treatment* (46th ed.). New York: McGraw-Hill.

Pagana, K. D., & Pagana, T. J. (2006). *Mosby's diagnostic and laboratory tests* (3rd ed.). St. Louis, MO: Mosby.

Porth, C. M. (2005). *Pathophysiology: Concepts of altered health* (7th ed.). Philadelphia: Lippincott, Williams & Wilkins.

Zollo, A. J. (2004). *Medical secrets* (4th ed.). Philadelphia: Hanley & Belfus.

PART X

Bullock, B., & Henze, R. (2000). *Focus on pathophysiology.* Philadelphia: Lippincott, Williams & Wilkins.

Edmunds, M., & Mayhew, M. (2004). *Pharmacology for the primary care provider.* St. Louis, MO: Mosby.

Ettinger, B. (2006). What's new in osteoporosis management. *The Female Patient, 31*, Vol 31, pgs. 26-27.

Huether, S., & McCance, K. (2004). *Understanding pathophysiology* (3rd ed.). St. Louis, MO: Mosby.

Porth, C. (2005). *Pathophysiology: Concepts of altered health states* (7th ed.). Philadelphia: Lippincott, Williams & Wilkins.

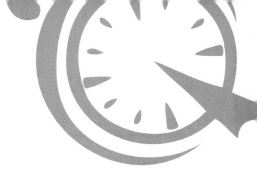

Index

Note: Page numbers followed by *f* and *t* indicate figures and tables, respectively.

A

AAT. *See* α₁-antitrypsin
abdominal distention, with intestinal obstruction, 402, 404
abscess(es), crypt, 389
accessory muscles of respiration, 208–209
  in emphysema, 234
acetaminophen, for low back pain, 555
acetylcholine, 114, 145
5-acetylsalicylic acid, for ulcerative colitis, 389–390
achlorhydria, 99
acid, 27
acid–base balance, 25–31
  laboratory evaluation of, 206*f*
acid–base imbalance, 17, 28–31. *See also* acidosis; alkalosis
  in chronic renal failure, 508*t*
  management of, 29
acidosis, 17, 28. *See also* acid–base imbalance; metabolic acidosis; renal tubular acidosis; respiratory acidosis
  causes of, 28–29
  and oxygen-hemoglobin bond, 210
  signs and symptoms of, 26*f*

acne, 185
acquired active immunity, 59
acquired immunodeficiency syndrome, 67–73
  associated disorders, 70, 73*f*
  diagnosis of, 71–72
  diagnostic criteria for, 70, 73*f*
  encephalitis in, 128
  epidemiology of, 69
  management of, 72–73
  pathophysiology of, 68*f*, 69–71
  prevention of, 68*f*
  stages of, 68*f*
  treatment of, 68*f*
  and tuberculosis, 253
action potential(s), cardiac, 276
active transport, 6
acute respiratory distress syndrome, 221
  causes of
    pulmonary, 225*t*
    systemic, 225*t*
  epidemiology of, 223
  manifestations of, 225–226
  pathophysiology of, 222*f*, 224–226
  phases of, 222*f*, 224–225
  prevention of, 223
  risk factors for, 223
  sequelae, 223
  treatment of, 222*f*, 226
acute tubular necrosis, 502*f*, 503

Addison's disease, 185
  and chronic gastritis, 367
  management of, 186
  pathophysiology of, 186
adenocarcinoma
  colorectal, 419, 424*f*
  esophageal, 421
  of lung, 240–241
  pancreatic, 451–452
adenoma(s), colorectal, 422, 423
adenosine triphosphate, 205
  formation of, 283
adenovirus, meningitis caused by, 126
ADH. *See* antidiuretic hormone
adhesions, 402*f*
  and intestinal obstruction, 402, 403
adipose tissue, 283
adrenal cortex, 182
  hormones from, 162*f*
adrenal glands, 181–187
  age-related changes in, 184*f*, 185
  anatomy of, 182
  dysfunction of, 185–187
  hormones secreted by, 163, 182
  physiology of, 182–185
adrenaline. *See* epinephrine
adrenal insufficiency, 186
  and hyperphosphatemia, 23
adrenal medulla, 114, 182
  disorders of, 187

3